The Nasal Valve

Editors

ROBIN W. LINDSAY
SHEKHAR K. GADKAREE

OTOLARYNGOLOGIC CLINICS OF NORTH AMERICA

www.oto.theclinics.com

Consulting Editor
SUJANA S. CHANDRASEKHAR

April 2025 • Volume 58 • Number 2

ELSEVIER

1600 John F. Kennedy Boulevard • Suite 1800 • Philadelphia, Pennsylvania, 19103-2899

http://www.oto.theclinics.com

OTOLARYNGOLOGIC CLINICS OF NORTH AMERICA Volume 58, Number 2
April 2025 ISSN 0030-6665, ISBN-13: 978-0-443-34407-7

Editor: Stacy Eastman
Developmental Editor: Malvika Shah

Otolaryngologic Clinics of North America (ISSN 0030-6665) is published bimonthly by Elsevier, Inc., 360 Park Avenue South, New York, NY 10010-1710. Months of issue are February, April, June, August, October, and December. Business and Editorial Offices: 1600 John F. Kennedy Blvd., Suite 1800, Philadelphia, PA 19103-2899. Customer Service Office: 6277 Sea Harbor Drive, Orlando, FL 32887-4800. Periodicals postage paid at New York, NY and additional mailing offices. Subscription prices are $492.00 per year (US individuals), $100.00 per year (US & Canadian student/resident), $641.00 per year (Canadian individuals), $699.00 per year (international individuals), $270.00 per year (international student/resident). For institutional access pricing please contact Customer Service via the contact information below. Foreign air speed delivery is included in all *Clinics*' subscription prices. All prices are subject to change without notice. Orders, claims, and journal inquiries: Please visit our Support Hub page https://service.elsevier.com for assistance.

Reprints. For copies of 100 or more of articles in this publication, please contact the Commercial Reprints Department, Elsevier Inc., 360 Park Avenue South, New York, NY 10010-1710. Tel.: 212-633-3874; Fax: 212-633-3820; E-mail: reprints@elsevier.com.

Otolaryngologic Clinics of North America is also published in Spanish by McGraw-Hill Interamericana Editores S.A., P.O. Box 5-237, 06500 Mexico D.F., Mexico.

Otolaryngologic Clinics of North America is covered in *MEDLINE/PubMed (Index Medicus), Current Contents/Clinical Medicine, Excerpta Medica, BIOSIS, Science Citation Index,* and *ISI/BIOMED.*

Contributors

CONSULTING EDITOR

SUJANA S. CHANDRASEKHAR, MD, FACS, FAAO-HNS
Consulting Editor, Otolaryngologic Clinics of North America, President, American
Otological Society, Past President, American Academy of Otolaryngology-Head and Neck
Surgery, Partner, ENT & Allergy Associates, LLP, Clinical Professor, Department of
Otolaryngology-Head and Neck Surgery, Zucker School of Medicine at Hofstra-Northwell,
Clinical Associate Professor, Department of Otolaryngology-Head and Neck Surgery,
Icahn School of Medicine at Mount Sinai. New York, New York, USA

EDITORS

ROBIN W. LINDSAY, MD
Associate Professor of Otolaryngology, Harvard Medical School, Facial Plastic and
Reconstructive Surgeon, Otolaryngology, Massachusetts Eye and Ear Infirmary, Boston,
Massachusetts, USA

SHEKHAR K. GADKAREE, MD
Assistant Professor of Otolaryngology–Head and Neck Surgery, University of Miami Miller
School of Medicine, Miami, Florida, USA

AUTHORS

ERIC BARBARITE, MD
Assistant Professor, Department of Otolaryngology–Head and Neck Surgery, Washington
University in St. Louis, Saint Louis, Missouri, USA

CARLEY BOYCE, MD
Resident, Department of Otolaryngology–Head and Neck Surgery, Louisiana State
University Health Sciences Center, New Orleans, Louisiana, USA

CIERSTEN A. BURKS, MD
Instructor, Department of Otolaryngology–Head and Neck Surgery, Harvard Medical
School, Facial Plastic and Reconstructive Surgery, Massachusetts Eye and Ear, Boston,
Massachusetts, USA

SYDNEY C. BUTTS, MD, FACS
Associate Professor and Interim Chair, Chief, Facial Plastic and Reconstructive Surgery,
SUNY Downstate Health Sciences University, Brooklyn, New York, USA

HAILEY CHEN
Student Research Associate, Department of Otolaryngology–Head and Neck Surgery,
University of California Irvine, Orange, California, USA

J. MADISON CLARK, MD, FACS
W. Paul Biggers Distinguished Professor, Chief, Division of Facial Plastic and
Reconstructive Surgery, University of North Carolina, Chapel Hill, North Carolina, USA

ADEEB DERAKHSHAN, MD
Assistant Professor, Division of Facial Plastic and Reconstructive Surgery, Department of Otolaryngology–Head and Neck Surgery, Loma Linda University Health, Loma Linda, California, USA

LANE B. DONALDSON, MD
Resident Physician, Department of Otolaryngology–Head and Neck Surgery, Henry Ford Hospital, Detroit, Michigan, USA

JAMES ENG, MD
Division of Facial Plastics and Reconstructive Surgery, University of South Florida, Tampa, Florida, USA

SHAYAN FAKURNEJAD, MD
Resident Physician, Department of Otolaryngology–Head and Neck Surgery, University of California, San Francisco, San Francisco, California, USA

MAX FENG, MD
Resident Physician, Department of Otolaryngology–Head and Neck Surgery, Loma Linda University Health, Loma Linda, California, USA

JENNIFER FULLER, MD
Assistant Professor, Division of Facial Plastic and Reconstructive Surgery, Department of Otolaryngology–Head and Neck Surgery, Loma Linda University Health, Loma Linda, California, USA

SHEKHAR K. GADKAREE, MD
Assistant Professor, Department of Otolaryngology–Head and Neck Surgery, University of Miami Miller School of Medicine, Miami, Florida, USA

ISABELLE GENGLER, MD
Resident, Facial Plastic and Reconstructive Surgery, Department of Otolaryngology–Head and Neck Surgery, University of Cincinnati College of Medicine, Cincinnati, Ohio, USA

LAURA HETZLER, MD
Professor and Vice Chair, Department of Otolaryngology–Head and Neck Surgery, Louisiana State University Health Sciences Center, New Orleans, Louisiana, USA; Our Lady of the Lake Regional Medical Center, Baton Rouge, Louisiana, USA

TSUNG-YEN HSIEH, MD
Assistant Professor, Facial Plastic and Reconstructive Surgery, Department of Otolaryngology–Head and Neck Surgery, University of Cincinnati College of Medicine, Cincinnati, Ohio, USA

LAMONT R. JONES, MD, MBA
Staff Physician, Division of Facial Plastic and Reconstructive Surgery, Department of Otolaryngology–Head and Neck Surgery, Henry Ford Hospital, Detroit, Michigan, USA; Co-Director Cleft and Craniofacial Clinic, Associate Chief Medical Officer Henry Ford Medical Group, Clinical Professor, Department of Surgery, Michigan State University, East Lansing, Michigan, USA; Clinical Professor, Wayne State University School of Medicine, Detroit, Michigan, USA

HAILEY JUSZCZAK, MD
Resident, Department of Otolaryngology, SUNY Downstate Health Sciences University, Brooklyn, New York, USA

PHILIP DANIEL KNOTT, MD
Professor and Director, Division of Facial Plastic and Reconstructive Surgery, Department of Otolaryngology–Head and Neck Surgery, University of California, San Francisco, San Francisco, California, USA

JACLYN LEE, MD
Resident Physician, Department of Otolaryngology–Head and Neck Surgery, Vanderbilt University Medical Center, Nashville, Tennessee, USA

JESSYKA G. LIGHTHALL, MD, FACS
Associate Professor, Department of Otolaryngology–Head and Neck Surgery, Penn State Health Milton S. Hershey Medical Center, Division Chief, Facial Plastic and Reconstructive Surgery, Associate Professor, Department of Otolaryngology–Head and Neck Surgery, Penn State College of Medicine, Director, Facial Nerve Clinic, Medical Director, Esteem Penn State Health Cosmetic Associates, Hershey, Pennsylvania, USA

DEREK H. LIU, MD
Resident Physician, Department of Otolaryngology–Head and Neck Surgery, University of California Irvine, Orange, California, USA

SOFIA LYFORD-PIKE, MD
Associate Professor, Facial Plastic and Reconstructive Surgery, Department of Otolaryngology–Head and Neck Surgery, University of Minnesota, Minneapolis, Minnesota, USA

WILLIAM MASON, MD
Resident Physician, Department of Otolaryngology–Head and Neck Surgery, Henry Ford Hospital, Detroit, Michigan, USA

SURESH MOHAN, MD
Assistant Professor, Facial Plastic and Reconstructive Surgery, Division of Otolaryngology, Yale School of Medicine, New Haven, Connecticut, USA

SAM P. MOST, MD
Professor and Chief, Division of Facial Plastic and Reconstructive Surgery, Department of Otolaryngology–Head and Neck Surgery, Stanford University School of Medicine, Stanford, California, USA

UCHE NWAGU, MD
Resident Physician, Department of Otolaryngology–Head and Neck Surgery, Thomas Jefferson University, Philadelphia, Pennsylvania, USA

ALYSSA K. OVAITT, MD
Assistant Professor, Department of Otolaryngology–Head and Neck Surgery, Louisiana State University Health Sciences Center, New Orleans, Louisiana, USA

ANIRUDDHA C. PARIKH, MD
Fellow, Department of Otolaryngology–Head and Neck Surgery, Penn State Health Milton S. Hershey Medical Center, Hershey, Pennsylvania, USA

PRIYESH N. PATEL, MD
Assistant Professor, Facial Plastic and Reconstructive Surgery, Department of Otolaryngology–Head and Neck Surgery, Vanderbilt University Medical Center, Nashville, Tennessee, USA

TIFFANY T. PHAM, MD, MS
Fellow Physician, Department of Otolaryngology–Head and Neck Surgery, University of Miami Miller School of Medicine, Miami, Florida, USA

TYLER M. RIST, MD
Facial Plastic and Reconstructive Surgery Fellow, Department of Otolaryngology, University of North Carolina, Chapel Hill, North Carolina, USA

JON ROBITSCHEK, MD
Associate Professor, Division of Facial Plastics and Reconstructive Surgery, University of South Florida, Tampa, Florida, USA

MONICA K. ROSSI-MEYER, MD
Clinical Instructor, Division of Facial Plastic and Reconstructive Surgery, Department of Otolaryngology–Head and Neck Surgery, Stanford University School of Medicine, Stanford, California, USA; Assistant Professor, Facial Plastic and Reconstructive Surgery, Department of Otolaryngology–Head and Neck Surgery, Vanderbilt University Medical Center, Nashville, Tennessee, USA

RAHUL SETH, MD
Volunteer Associate Professor, Golden State Plastic Surgery, Division of Facial Plastic and Reconstructive Surgery, Department of Otolaryngology–Head and Neck Surgery, University of California, San Francisco, San Francisco, California, USA

MUNISH SHANDILYA, MS(ENT), FRCS Ed(OTO), FRCS(ORL-HNS)
Rhinoplasty Surgeon, The Nose Clinic, Dublin, Ireland

SCOTT J. STEPHAN, MD
Associate Professor, Carol and John S. Odess Chair, Facial Plastic and Reconstructive Surgery, Department of Otolaryngology–Head and Neck Surgery, Vanderbilt University Medical Center, Nashville, Tennessee, USA

DANIEL SUAREZ, MD
Resident, Department of Otolaryngology, SUNY Downstate Health Sciences University, Brooklyn, New York, USA

TRAVIS T. TOLLEFSON, MD, MPH, FACS
Professor and Director, Facial Plastic and Reconstructive Surgery, Department of Otolaryngology–Head and Neck Surgery, University of California Davis Medical Center, University of California Davis, Sacramento, California, USA

ANDREW A. WINKLER, MD
Associate Professor, Department of Otolaryngology–Head and Neck Surgery, University of Colorado School of Medicine, Aurora, Colorado, USA

BRIAN J-F. WONG, MD, PhD
Professor and Fellowship Director, Facial Plastic Surgery Department of Otolaryngology–Head and Neck Surgery, University of California Irvine, Beckman Laser Institute, Department of Biomedical Engineering, Samueli School of Engineering, University of California Irvine, Irvine, California, USA;

RUI XAVIER, MD, PhD
Otolaryngologist, Department of Otorhinolaryngology, Hospital Luz Arrabida, Porto, Portugal

VIVIAN XU, MD
Resident Physician, Department of Otolaryngology–Head and Neck Surgery, Thomas Jefferson University, Philadelphia, Pennsylvania, USA

SHIAYIN F. YANG, MD
Associate Professor, Facial Plastic and Reconstructive Surgery, Department of Otolaryngology–Head and Neck Surgery, Vanderbilt University Medical Center, Nashville, Tennessee, USA

Contents

The nasal valves are not simple, 2-dimensional cross-sections but rather a complex, 3-dimensional, collapsible, and heterogeneous structure. Historically, the internal nasal valve (INV) is defined by the septum medially, the caudal margin of the upper lateral cartilage laterally, and the inferior turbinate inferiorly. Typically located 1.3 cm deep into the nasal cavity, the INV angle delineated by the upper lateral cartilage and septum typically measures 10° to 15° in the Caucasian population. As computational methods reveal new insights into nasal valve function, a new conceptual framework is needed to guide rhinoplasty surgical decision-making.

Although no gold-standard test exists for measuring the success of surgery in functional rhinoplasty, the patient's own subjective experience of their nasal airway obstruction and its impact on quality of life is paramount in outcomes assessment. Patient-reported outcome measures (PROMs) are questionnaires designed to evaluate both disease-specific nasal functional and esthetic domains and global health-related quality of life domains. Ideal PROMs are derived from patient input, psychometrically validated, reliable, and responsive. Assessment at both preoperative and postoperative visits allows for quantitative analysis of surgical outcomes and helps promote communication between the patient and surgeon.

The diagnosis of nasal valve compromise (NVC) is clinical. However, objective evaluation of the nasal airway can support the clinical diagnosis of NVC and quantify the derangement produced by NVC in nasal airflow and in nasal airway resistance. Computational fluid dynamics analysis can quantify disturbances of the normal nasal airway conditions and, furthermore, localize these disturbances to the nasal valve. Objective evaluation of the nasal airway is useful to assess the results of surgery addressing the nasal valve, being able to quantify the improvement in

Successful treatment of nasal airway obstruction depends on accurate diagnosis of the underlying etiology. Lateral wall insufficiency (LWI) is a common cause of obstructed nasal breathing and should be recognized and treated accordingly by the rhinoplasty surgeon. LWI refers to dynamic collapse of the lateral nasal sidewalls at the internal (zone 1) and external (zone 2) nasal valves. This article serves as an overview of the important aspects in evaluation and management of LWI.

▶ Video content accompanies this article at http://www.oto.theclinics. com.

Persistent nasal airway obstruction from inadequately addressed nasal valve compromise is common. Many techniques exist to perform nasal valve repair. Historically, spreader grafts are the most commonly used, despite a relative lack of evidence demonstrating its superiority over other methods. The butterfly graft is an alternative method of nasal valve repair and detailed surgical description from over 20 years of innovation follows in this section. There is growing evidence to suggest that the butterfly graft may be superior to spreader grafts with similar acceptability of the esthetic outcomes.

▶ Video content accompanies this article at http://www.oto.theclinics. com.

The internal nasal valve, the narrowest portion of the nasal airway, is prone to collapse and is often targeted for improvement in nasal reconstruction and rhinoplasty. Endonasal techniques can reduce surrounding trauma and reduce operative times compared to traditional open methods. Options include the use of spreader, butterfly and alar batten grafts, suspension and flaring sutures, and Z-plasty for scarring. These techniques offer structural support and improved airflow with less risk of external changes, but also the challenges of limited visibility and the need for precise graft placement.

The number of non-Caucasian patients with nasal valve compromise seeking functional rhinoplasty is projected to increase in tandem with an increasingly diverse population in the United States. Gaining a deeper appreciation for the variances in nasal morphology amongst different ethnicities will help rhinoplasty surgeons perform accurate preoperative evaluations, optimize functional and esthetic outcomes, and maintain ethnic congruence with surgery.

Gender-affirming facial surgery is increasing in prevalence, and rhinoplasty plays an integral role in its success. The nose displays considerable gender dimorphism, and maneuvers performed during gender-affirming rhinoplasty may differ considerably from those performed during cis-gender surgery. During feminization rhinoplasty in particular, cosmetic goals often rely on reductive techniques such as osteotomies, dorsal reduction, sidewall narrowing, tip narrowing, and alar base narrowing. These maneuvers collectively have important ramifications when considering the functional aspects of the nose. Herein, we outline the status of feminization rhinoplasty, and the interplay of cosmetic and functional considerations of the field.

The saddle nose deformity is associated with dorsal collapse and can have both function and cosmetic problems. The saddle nose can cause nasal obstruction by narrowing the nasal cavities, eliciting dynamic internal and external nasal valve narrowing, and abnormally widening the internal and external nasal valves altering airflow dynamics, sinonasal passageways, and olfaction. The saddle nose is challenging to treat due to skin contracture, lack of donor tissue, and difficulties in esthetic integration. A focus on balancing the functional and esthetic concerns during treatment is paramount.

Nasal airway obstruction is a frequent complaint in an otolaryngology clinic and is often multifactorial. Anatomic contributors may include a nasal septal deviation, inferior turbinate hypertrophy, and nasal valve compromise. Septoplasty and inferior turbinate reduction are one of the most common procedures performed by an otolaryngologist. A variety of techniques have been described to strengthen the lateral crura; however, the lateral crural strut graft should be considered in the revision rhinoplasty patient as studies have suggested it is more powerful than other methods without requiring other techniques to strengthen the lateral crura.

Cleft lip and palate, the most common congenital orofacial anomalies, result in complex nasal deformities due to deficient bony maxilla, dentoalveolar arch, teeth, and soft tissues. This article explores nasal deformities in patients with cleft lip and palate, surgical techniques and considerations in cleft rhinoplasty, particularly focusing on nasal valves in both unilateral and bilateral cases. Unilateral cleft lip deformities include asymmetry of the nasal tip, flattened nostril, and displaced caudal septum, while bilateral cleft lip deformities present a wider and flatter nose with complex nasal features.

Ciersten A. Burks and Sofia Lyford-Pike

Facial paralysis significantly impacts the form and function of patients. Assessment of the face in zones is important to ensure no functional area of the face is neglected. Nasal valve compromise in patients with facial paralysis, for example, is often overlooked yet should be addressed to correct nasal obstruction. In flaccid facial paralysis, inferomedial displacement of the alar base and lateral nasal sidewall insufficiency contribute to nasal valve compromise. For surgical candidates, static suspension of the nasal valve in a superolateral vector is an ideal technique to address the etiology of nasal obstruction in patients with facial paralysis.

Daniel Suarez, Hailey Juszczak, and Sydney C. Butts

Airway obstruction is a possible sequela following reconstruction of the nose after Mohs excision of skin cancers. While the principles and goals of tissue replacement after Mohs micrographic surgery are well-established, less attention has been paid to the evaluation of the nasal airway after reconstruction. Reconstructive planning begins with understanding the risk factors associated with the development of nasal valve compromise. Several approaches to prevent and correct nasal valve narrowing will be reviewed as part of a unified reconstructive plan for patients after skin cancer excision in high risk areas.

OTOLARYNGOLOGIC CLINICS OF NORTH AMERICA

SERIES OF RELATED INTEREST

Facial Plastic Surgery Clinics
Available at: **https://www.facialplastic.theclinics.com/**

THE CLINICS ARE AVAILABLE ONLINE!
Access your subscription at:
www.theclinics.com

Foreword

Sniffing Out an Important Anatomical Problem

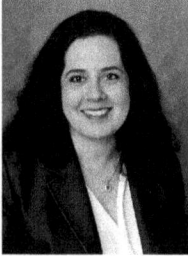

SUJANA S. CHANDRASEKHAR, MD, FAAO-HNS, FAOS, FACS
Consulting Editor

Dr Robin Lindsay, one of the two Guest Editors of this issue of *Otolaryngologic Clinics of North America* on The Nasal Valve, and I were walking along the beach in Florida some months ago, during a break at a national meeting, when our conversation turned to interesting topics that had enough breadth, depth, and interest to merit an entire issue of *Otolaryngologic Clinics of North America*. Perhaps seeing me trying to keep up with her pace and breathing in as hard as I could, she alit on the problem of the nasal valve. Initially, I couldn't grasp how such a small anatomical area, the narrowest portion of the nose, could hold that much interest. I quickly learned how mistaken an ear surgeon can be. From the first description by Mink in 1903 as the narrow opening formed between the caudal portion of the superior lateral cartilage and the nasal septum, comprising a 10° to 15° angle, and thus as the region of maximum nasal resistance, to the systematic understanding of today, this small and important area has been appropriately subdivided and understood anatomically, physiologically, and with patient-reported outcomes measures.

Dr Lindsay and co-Guest Editor Dr Shekhar Gadkaree have compiled a deep dive issue that will be appreciated by rhinoplasty surgeons and comprehensive otolaryngologists alike. The 17 articles in this issue give us a thorough understanding of the anatomy, physiology, and methods of objective and subjective assessment of the nasal valve. The particular challenges of ethnically diverse nasal shapes and of gender affirmation care are explored fully. Care is to be taken in cases of revision surgery, in patients with cleft lip and palate or facial palsy, and after tissue-sparing Moh surgery for cancer in the area.

Otolaryngol Clin N Am 58 (2025) xv–xvi
https://doi.org/10.1016/j.otc.2024.09.005
0030-6665/25/© 2024 Published by Elsevier Inc.

oto.theclinics.com

It is easy to ignore the nasal valves when they are working well. After reading this issue of *Otolaryngologic Clinics of North America*, you will know with certainty that when they do not, one intervention certainly does not fit all.

Sujana S. Chandrasekhar, MD, FAAO-HNS, FAOS, FACS
Consulting Editor
Otolaryngologic Clinics of North America
President, American Otological Society
Past President, American Academy of Otolaryngology-Head and Neck Surgery
Partner, ENT & Allergy Associates
LLP Clinical Professor
Department of Otolaryngology-Head and Neck Surgery
Zucker School of Medicine at Hofstra-Northwell
Clinical Associate Professor
Department of Otolaryngology–Head and Neck Surgery
Icahn School of Medicine at Mount Sinai
18 East 48th Street, 2nd Floor
New York, NY 10017, USA

E-mail address:
SSC@NYOTOLOGY.COM

Preface

The Evolution of Nasal Valve Treatment

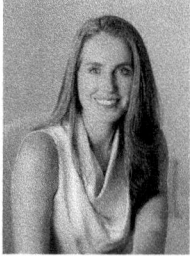

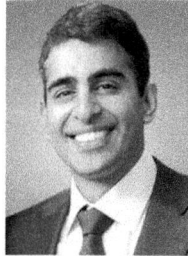

Robin W. Lindsay, MD   Shekhar K. Gadkaree, MD
Editors

The term nasal valve (NV) is not new, but our ability to understand the impact of the NV anatomy on nasal airflow and the impact of airflow on patient quality of life has dramatically increased over the past several decades with the development and utilization of patient-reported outcomes measures (PROMs), objective measures, new surgical techniques, and refinement of the anatomic description of the NV.

Mink first coined the term NV in 1903,[1] describing what we now refer to as the internal NV. Butterfly grafts, described by Hage in 1964,[2] and spreader grafts described by Sheen in 1984[3] were some of the early surgical techniques used to treat nasal obstruction caused by the NV. Many early studies followed patient outcomes, but a validated disease-specific metric to measure patient outcomes did not exist until the development of the Nasal Obstruction Symptom Evaluation score (NOSE) in 2004 by Stewart and colleagues.[4] In 2015, the FACE-q score was developed by Klassen and colleagues in 2015,[5] which allowed for evaluation of patient-perceived nasal aesthetics. This was followed by the SCHNOS, developed by Most in 2018[6] to evaluate both nasal form and function. Utilization of PROMS in hundreds of studies has allowed our field to demonstrate the disease-specific quality-of-life improvement after surgical correction of the NV and that corrections can be made without a negative impact on nasal aesthetics. PROMs have now become the gold standard in the care of patients with nasal obstruction, and their use will continue to improve the quality of care that we provide to our patients as we continue to develop and refine our surgical techniques.

As with all surgical procedures, accurate diagnosis is vital to providing the correct surgical treatment. This could not be truer for the surgical management of NV compromise. In 2010, Rhee led a consensus panel on the diagnosis and management of NV compromise to organize and disseminate information about the NV. The consensus

Otolaryngol Clin N Am 58 (2025) xvii–xviii
https://doi.org/10.1016/j.otc.2024.09.004
0030-6665/25/© 2024 Published by Elsevier Inc.

statement defined the anatomy of the internal and external NV, stated that the NV was a distinct clinical cause of nasal obstruction apart from the septum and the turbinates, discussed important clinical exam findings, and expressed the need for more standardized outcome studies.

The lack of use of standard terminology and the use of interchangeable terms as the treatment of NV compromise has evolved have complicated the evaluation of different surgical treatments. We put forth that the term NV compromise be standardized and used as the umbrella term for the nasal obstruction caused by an anatomic defect of the NV anatomy, including internal NV narrowing, external NV narrowing, and NV collapse/lateral wall insufficiency. The etiology of each cause of NV compromise can stem from several different anatomic defects, each with specific surgical treatments designed to treat the specific anatomic cause of the NV compromise. An individual patient may have one or all three causes of NV compromise and thus requires an individualized treatment plan.

DISCLOSURES

S.K. Gadkaree, and R.W. Lindsay, no financial disclosures.

Robin W. Lindsay, MD
Otolaryngology, Harvard Medical School
Massachusetts Eye and Ear Infirmary
Boston, MA, USA

Shekhar K. Gadkaree, MD
Otolaryngology–Head and Neck Surgery
University of Miami Miller School of Medicine
Miami, FL, USA

E-mail addresses:
Robin_Lindsay@meei.harvard.edu (R.W. Lindsay)
sgadkaree@miami.edu (S.K. Gadkaree)

REFERENCES

1. Mink PJ. Le nez comme voie respiratorie. Belgium: Presse Otolaryngol; 1903. p. 481–96.
2. Hage J. Collapsed alae strengthened by conchal cartilage (the butterfly cartilage graft). Br J Plast Surg 1965;18:92–6.
3. Sheen JH. Spreader graft: a method of reconstructing the roof of the middle nasal vault following rhinoplasty. Plast Reconstr Surg 1984;73(2):230–9.
4. Stewart MG, Witsell DL, Smith TL, et al. Development and validation of the Nasal Obstruction Symptom Evaluation (NOSE) scale. Otolaryngol Head Neck Surg 2004;130(2):157–63.
5. Klassen AF, Cano SJ, Schwitzer JA, et al. FACE-Q scales for health-related quality of life, early life impact, satisfaction with outcomes, and decision to have treatment: development and validation. Plast Reconstr Surg 2015;135(2):375–86.
6. Moubayed SP, Ioannidis JPA, Saltychev M, Most SP. The 10-Item Standardized Cosmesis and Health Nasal Outcomes Survey (SCHNOS) for Functional and Cosmetic Rhinoplasty. JAMA Facial Plast Surg 2018;20(1):37–42.

Anatomy and Physiology of the Nasal Valves

Derek H. Liu, MD[a], Hailey Chen[a], Brian J-F. Wong, MD, PhD[a,b,c,d],*

KEYWORDS

- Internal nasal valve • External nasal valve • Lateral wall insufficiency
- Dynamic valve collapse • Nasal obstruction

KEY POINTS

- The external nasal valve is defined by the cross-section of the ala, whereas the internal nasal valve is defined by the septum, caudal margin of the upper lateral cartilage, and the inferior turbinate.
- Nasal valve function is defined by complex, 3-dimensional structures composed of cartilage, muscle, connective tissue, and skin which provide both static and dynamic support.
- Normal nasal airflow has been described with widely accepted concepts, including a critical internal nasal valve angle, the Bernoulli principle, and Poiseuille's equation, which may be insufficient to capture the 3-dimensional, patient-specific nature of nasal obstruction.
- Computational fluid dynamics has emerged as a potential noninvasive technique for assessing nasal valve physiology while accounting for the complexities of the nasal airway geometry.

THE NASAL VALVE

Mink first described the nasal valve in 1903 as a region of narrowing in the nasal vestibule. He defined the nasal valve as a region bounded medially by the septum and laterally by the limen nasi, where the caudal border of the upper lateral cartilage (ULC) overlaps the lateral crus of the lower lateral cartilage (LLC).[1–3] Since then, there has been variation in the use of the term "nasal valve." Most commonly, authors refer to 2 separate regions within the nasal vault as the external nasal valve (ENV) and internal nasal valve (INV) (**Fig. 1**).

The ENV is operationally defined simply as the 2-dimensional (2D) cross-section of the ala. The borders are composed of the lateral crura of the LLCs, the columella and medial crura medially, and the nasal floor inferiorly.[1] Some have defined the external

---

[a] Department of Otolaryngology, Head and Neck Surgery, University of California Irvine, 101 The City Drive South, ZOT 5386, Orange, CA 92868, USA; [b] Beckman Laser Institute, University of California Irvine, Irvine, CA, USA; [c] Department of Biomedical Engineering, Samueli School of Engineering, University of California Irvine, Irvine, CA, USA; [d] Facial Plastic Surgery
* Corresponding author. 101 The City Drive South, ZOT 5386, Orange, CA 92868.
E-mail address: bjwong@uci.edu

Otolaryngol Clin N Am 58 (2025) 189–203
https://doi.org/10.1016/j.otc.2024.09.001
0030-6665/25/© 2024 Elsevier Inc. All rights reserved, including those for text and data mining, AI training, and similar technologies.

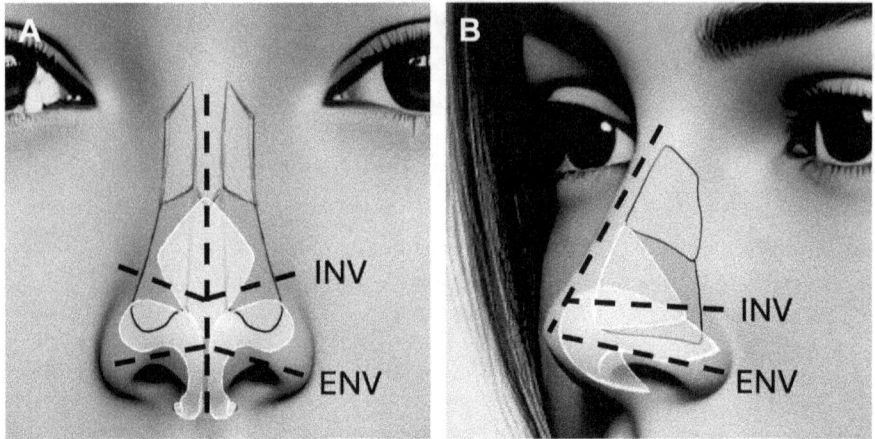

Fig. 1. External and internal nasal valves, (*A*) frontal and (*B*) oblique views. The ENV is located at the ala, while the INV is at the level of the caudal border of the ULC. ENV, external nasal valve; INV, internal nasal valve.

valve as a 3-dimensional (3D) volume, bordered caudally by the nostril anteroinferiorly and the internal nasal valve posteriorly.[4,5]

Most definitions of the INV demarcate this region as the plane through the nasal vault with the smallest cross-sectional area (CSA). Historically, the INV is defined by the septum medially, the caudal margin of the ULC laterally, and the inferior turbinate inferiorly. Typically located 1.3 cm deep into the nasal cavity, the INV angle delineated by the ULC and septum typically measures 10° to 15° in the Caucasian population. In practice, precise identification of the valve is difficult both clinically and even using diagnostic imaging (eg, CT). Valve angle measurement using the naked eye is, at best, a crude estimate.

ANATOMY
Muscles

The muscles of the nose can be organized as intrinsic, with origins and insertions contained within the nasal region, or extrinsic, which are outside this domain but act to alter nasal shape position (**Fig. 2**).[6] They can be classified by function, as listed below.[7] Some have also included the zygomaticus minor and orbicularis oris as relevant to nasal dynamics.[8]

1. Elevators: procerus, levator labii superioris alaequae nasi, and anomalous nasi
2. Depressors: alar nasalis (dilator naris posterior) and depressor septi nasi
3. Compressors: transverse nasalis and compressor narium minor
4. Dilators: dilator naris anterior

Electromyographic studies highlighted the role of specific nasal muscles in nasal valve function.[9,10] The nasalis forms the muscular component of the nasal superficial musculoaponeurotic system (SMAS).[11] The transverse portion, known as the pars transversalis, attaches to the nasal skin and indirectly stabilizes the nasal valve and sidewall. The alar portion, known as the par alaris and alternatively referred to as the dilator naris posterior, originates from the maxilla and attaches to the accessory cartilage medially, providing lateral stability of the ala.[12,13] The dilator naris anterior,

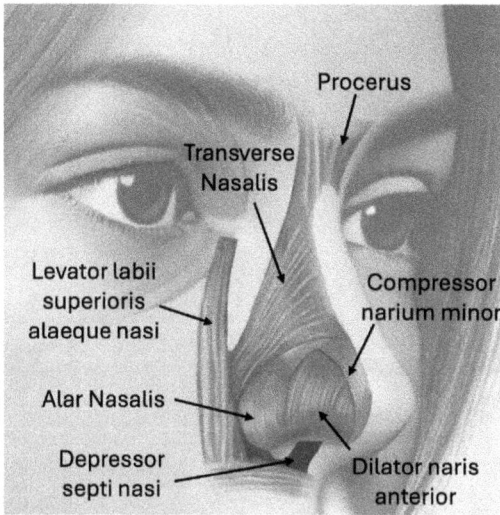

Fig. 2. Muscles of the nose.

also referred to the apices nasi, originates from the lateral crus to attach to the alar groove. Previous studies disagreed regarding the presence of an independent dilator naris muscle, with some recent studies referring to a dilator naris vestibularis which occupies and surrounds nearly the entire nasal ala.[14–18]

The importance of nasal muscles function is best illustrated in patients with facial nerve injury, who often experience nasal obstruction. While a significant contributor to nasal valve collapse is the weight of the unsupported cheek tissues, the nasal muscles both actively flare the nostrils and provide static support against gravity.[13,19] For example, temporary paralysis of nasal muscles with lidocaine results in reductions in alar stiffness along with flow restriction measured by rhinomanometry. This suggests that resting muscle tone is critical in supporting nasal airway patency.[20] Loss of muscular activity results in ENV narrowing and collapse, and surgical interventions for facial paralysis patients such as suture suspension or fascia lata slings are associated with improved Nasal Obstruction and Septoplasty Effectiveness (NOSE) survery scores.[21]

Lower Lateral Cartilages

The paired LLCs are divided into 3 segments: the medial, intermediate, and lateral crura. The LLCs define the structure and shape of both the nasal tip and the ENV. The shape of the LLC is complex and defies taxonomy. Functionally, the LLC is a dome-shaped structure that maintains the nasal aperture and functions to resist forces of deformation generated during inspiration. One specific LLC morphology, alar malposition, warrants further discussion. Malpositioned lateral crura, now referred to more specifically as cephalic malposition, were a concept first defined by Sheen and Sheen.[22] The axis of the lateral crus may be defined as a line which begins at the dome medially and roughly bisects the length of the lateral crura (**Fig. 3A–D**). This axis should be oriented toward the lateral canthus of the ipsilateral eye. Cephalically malpositioned lateral crura have an axis which points toward the ipsilateral medial canthus.[23] In other words, cephalic lateral crura are more perpendicular to the alar rim, rather than parallel.

Cephalic malposition is associated with tip bulbosity and the compound tip deformity, external valve weakness, and collapse.[24] Constantian estimated that 50% of

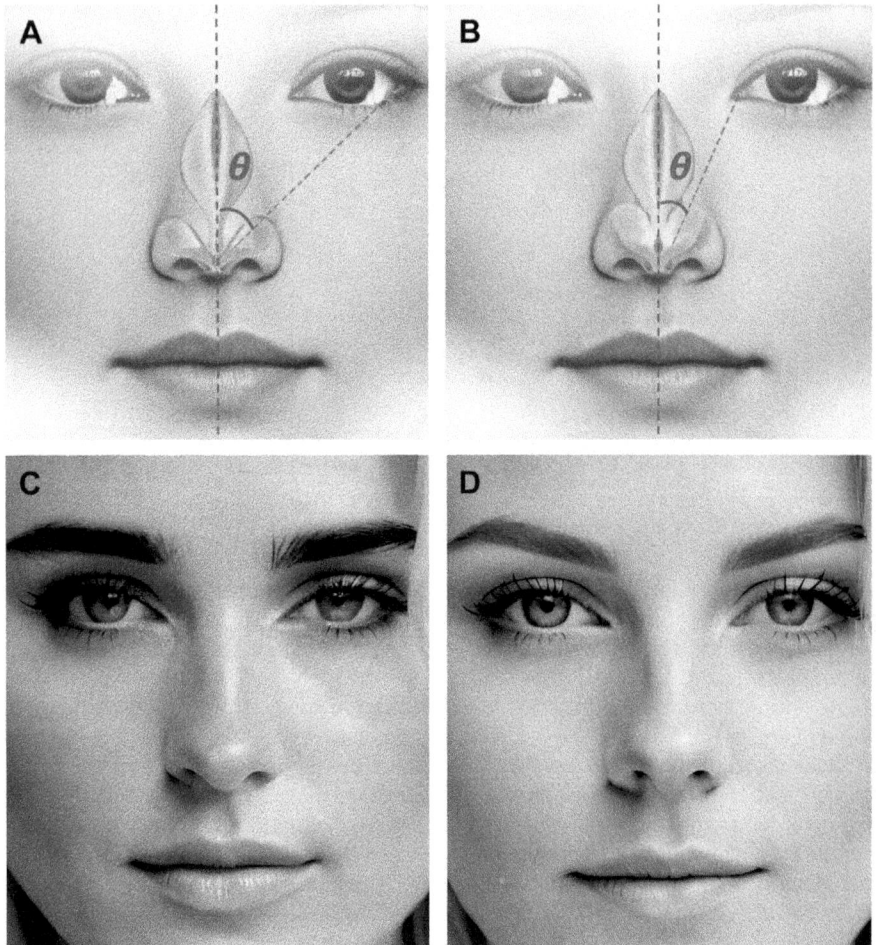

Fig. 3. Orientations of the lower lateral crus longitudinal axis (*A*) toward the lateral canthus (*B*) cephalically malpositioned toward the medial canthus (*C*) nasal tip with appropriately positioned lower lateral crura (*D*) malposition resulting in a broad nasal tip.

patients with external valve obstruction had cephalic lateral crura.[25–27] Different treatment strategies have been proposed, including repositioning of the lateral crura.[28] Using this technique, Toriumi advocated that the axis of the lateral crus and the mid-sagittal plane should ideally form an angle greater than 30°.[24,29] Lateral crural tensioning (LCT) can also accomplish this objective of improving the airway. First described by Davis, this technique combines a lateral crural steal with a caudal septal extension graft to increase tension and stabilize the sidewall.[30] Combining this tensioning with articulated alar rim grafts to support the alar margin, LCT may achieve similar improvements in airway but requires less cartilage and is potentially less likely to crowd the airway when compared with lateral crural strut grafts (LCSG).[31–35]

Upper Lateral Cartilages

The ULCs are paired, triangular cartilages which articulate with the septum medially, the pyriform aperture cephalically, and the LLCs caudally.[36] Stability is provided to the ULC via muco-periosteal, muco-perichondrial, and fibrous articulations to adjacent structures. At the dorsal aspect of the cephalic margin, the ULC joins the cartilaginous and bony septum and the nasal bones to form the keystone area. The cephalic portion of the ULC attaches to the undersurface of the nasal bones, overlapping by 6 to 8 mm.[37] The ULC is additionally attached to the pyriform aperture by the pyriform ligament, which contributes to the static support of the cartilaginous midvault.[38,39] Caudally, the ULC attaches to the LLC at the scroll area, which provides key structural support to the INV.[40,41]

Scroll Complex

The LLC cephalic edge turns down to form a hook, while the ULC caudal edge turns up to form a ledge. The 2 interdigitate, creating the characteristic scroll-like shape, and giving this region its name of "scroll" area or region.[42] There are numerous variations of this arrangement, and a keen understanding of the anatomic variations is essential for any intercartilaginous approaches to the nasal dorsum. Within this region complex, fibrous attachments are collectively referred to as the scroll ligament.[43] This complex includes a longitudinal scroll ligament which spans the junction between the ULC and LLC and is transected during intercartilaginous incisions. In addition, a vertical scroll ligament has been suggested, which connects the longitudinal scroll ligament to the overlying deep SMAS layer.[44]

The scroll complex is widely accepted as one of 3 major tip support mechanisms but also plays a significant role in nasal valve function. The scroll ligament provides support to the external valve by supporting and raising the caudal edge of the lateral crus of the LLC. Given its location at the lateral wall of the INV, the overlapping cartilages provide key structural stiffness. Additionally, the vertical scroll attachments to the overlying skin-soft tissue envelope provide further support to the INV.[45] Some authors advocate a subperichondrial dissection during rhinoplasty in order to elevate and preserve the overlying scroll ligaments.[46] Two prospective studies of open rhinoplasty patients found that scroll reconstruction was associated with improved nasal patency.[47,48]

Nasal Septum

The nasal septum is a vertical midline structure which separates the left and right nasal cavities, and is a composite structure of bone, cartilage, and mucosa. The quadrangular cartilage forms the anterior cartilaginous portion. Posteriorly, the perpendicular plate of ethmoid superiorly, the vomer inferiorly, and the nasal crest of the maxilla and palatine bones form the osseous portion. The vomer divides the choanae posteriorly, which separates the nasal cavity from the nasopharynx. The membranous septum, located anteriorly between the nasal columella and the caudal quadrangular cartilage, is formed by the union of septum mucous membranes and acts as a flexible buffer which may protect the cartilaginous septum[49]

Several classification systemsof septal deformities have been proposed. Multiple authors described deviations based on common patterns including a straight septal tilt, a C-shaped deformity, or an S-shaped deformity. For example, Guyuron described 6 classes of septal deviations, which includes the C- and S-shaped deformities each in the vertical and horizontal planes, the straight septal tilt, and a localized spur. Notable alternative classification systems include Rao and Mladina's description of 7 patterns of deviations, Baumann and Baumann's 6 types, and Buyukertan's division of the septum into 10 areas of interest.[50–54] Septal deviations may cause obstruction at various levels, and small deviations specifically in the region of the nasal valve cause significant narrowing of the INV angle.[55,56] Caudal deviations may also cause obstruction at the level of the ENV.

Inferior Turbinates

The 3 pairs of nasal turbinates arise from the lateral nasal sidewall, consisting of thin scrolls of bone covered in erectile tissue and mucoperiosteum. Whereas the superior and middle turbinates arise from the ethmoid bone, the inferior turbinates are separate bony structures. Covered in pseudostratified ciliated columnar epithelium, the bulk of the inferior turbinate is made of the lamina propria, which houses a rich network of venous sinusoids. This erectile tissue regulates the volume of the inferior turbinates in response to autonomic stimulation.[57] Inferior turbinate hypertrophy may be caused by enlargement of the bone, the mucosa, or both. Soft tissue hypertrophy is common and is typically seen in chronic rhinitis.[58]

PHYSIOLOGY
Airway Resistance

Airway resistance, the opposition to airflow, is defined by Ohm's law as the pressure gradient divided by the flow rate.

$$R = \frac{\Delta P}{Q}$$

With inspiration, a negative pressure gradient is generated between the nasopharynx and the nares, which causes air to flow through the nose with an inverse relationship to resistance. Thus, as resistance increases, flow decreases.

Nasal resistance may be measured by rhinomanometry, which uses a flow measuring device and 2 pressure sensors to measure pressure gradient. Active rhinomanometry uses physiologic airflow from the patient's own respiratory cycle, whereas passive rhinomanometry introduces extrinsic air typically via an air pump. Posterior rhinomanometry places a pressure sensor in the oral oropharynx, whereas anterior manometry places the sensor in the contralateral nasal cavity. Active anterior techniques are most common; active is more physiologic and anterior avoids the difficulty of the gag reflex.[59,60]

The significance of anatomic variations in determining the resistance of the nasal airway can be illustrated using Poiseuille's law, which describes the drop in pressure of laminar flow of an incompressible fluid in a long cylindrical pipe.

$$R = \frac{8\eta L}{\pi r^4}$$

Importantly, resistance varies inversely with the fourth power of the radius. A slight narrowing of the airway may cause an exponential increase in resistance. Given that the INV is the narrowest point of the nasal airway, any further reduction in CSA can greatly increase resistance, and significant attention has been focused on improving the patency of the INV.

Nasal Cycle

The nasal cycle refers to the spontaneous congestion and decongestion of the nasal mucosa, where the decongestion of one side is accompanied by the congestion of the contralateral side. Congestion of one side causes narrowing of the nasal airway, including at the INV and may contribute to nasal obstruction. First described by Kayser in 1895, the nasal cycle is driven by asymmetric blood flow to the erectile tissue in the nasal septum and inferior turbinate. The mechanisms which regulate blood flow are not clear, but significant attention has been focused on the autonomic nervous system. Sympathetic branches of the superior cervical ganglion give rise to the deep petrosal nerve, which joins parasympathetic preganglionic fibers from the greater superficial petrosal nerve to form the Vidian nerve. At the pterygopalatine ganglion, the parasympathetic fibers synapse with postganglionic neurons. Both sympathetic and parasympathetic fibers then travel along with nasal branches of the maxillary nerve (V2) through the sphenopalatine foramen to innervate the nasal mucosa.

These Vidian nerve fibers are targeted in patients with refractory rhinitis who continue to have rhinorrhea despite medical therapy. Historically, this involved resection of the neurovascular bundle at the level of the sphenopalatine foramen. While effective, Vidian neurectomy was also associated with cheek and palate numbness, dry eyes, and potentially unfavorable changes to the blood supply to the posterior nasal cavity. Instead, selective techniques which target postganglionic nerve branches have been proposed to reduce morbidity.[61,62] Various methods have been described, including surgical ablation, cryotherapy, and laser ablation. Radiofrequency ablation has received increasing interest, particularly since the Food and Drug Administration approval of the RhinAer radiofrequency system in 2020.[63,64]

Dynamic Collapse

Dynamic obstruction is lateral nasal sidewall collapse during inspiration. The Bernoulli principle explains that total airflow at any point along the nasal airway must be equal, and thus in narrower regions, velocity increases. Due to the conservation of energy, as velocity increases, a negative internal pressure is generated. Given that the INV is considered the narrowest point in the nasal airway, airflow reaches a maximum velocity at this point, leading to negative pressure which can lead to a transmural difference that overcomes the rigidity of the nasal sidewall and causes collapse. This collapse causes additional narrowing of the airway, which further increases resistance and decreases airflow.

Acoustic Rhinometry

Acoustic rhinometry is a noninvasive technique used to evaluate the geometry of the nasal cavity. A probe is sealed against a patient's nostril, a sound impulse is generated, and reflected sound waves are recorded. Changes in the CSA of the airway are assumed to correlate with changes in acoustic impedance. The time delay until the reflected sound is detected is used to calculate the distance traveled by the sound impulse along the airway. These data are used to generate CSA as a function of distance, and nasal cavity volume can be calculated as the integral of this curve.[65,66] Using acoustic rhinometry, previous studies have identified minimal cross-sectional areas (mCSAs) corresponding to 3 anatomic sources of obstruction, specifically the INV, the anterior half of the inferior and/or head of the middle turbinate, and the middle-posterior portion of the middle turbinate.[67,68] Unfortunately, acoustic rhinometry is not used routinely, due to significant experimental error, overestimation of the posterior nose due to sound leakage into the sinuses, and weak correlations between mCSA and nasal resistance.[69]

RETHINKING THE NASAL VALVE

The previous section represents the currently accepted concepts related to nasal airflow. Unfortunately, these principles rely on numerous assumptions which are invalid when considering normal human physiologic conditions. The nasal airway involves complex and dynamic interactions between airflow and a heterogeneous, collapsible structure.

Geometry

The idea of a critical INV angle of 10° to 15° is widely accepted, but most rhinoplasty surgeons would not approach nasal airway obstruction with a singular focus.[70] For one, the INV is not always a simple angle defined by 2 straight lines, but instead may be classified into several shapes and is sometimes occupied by the septal body.[71] Further, estimating the INV angle can vary significantly depending on the plane of measurement. For example, standard coronal CT images may significantly underestimate or overestimate the nasal valve angle compared with reformatted images which reflect the true orientation of the INV.[72] Even with the improved accuracy of reformatted images, measurements of the INV demonstrated no correlation to preoperative-modified Cottle maneuver scores, suggesting the limited clinical utility of the INV angle.[73]

Even when considering the 2D CSA of the INV rather than a simple angle, there is a poor correlation between mCSA and subjective scores of nasal patency.[74] The rate of persistent subjective symptoms after rhinoplasty remains high despite adequate increases in mCSA, affecting up to 53% of patients postoperatively.[75] Recent computational studies have suggested that the correlation between mCSA and resistance only becomes relevant below a critical area threshold which is only present in severely constricted nasal cavities. Therefore, in most patients, nasal resistance is significantly dependent on the geometry of regions throughout the nasal cavity other than the INV alone.[69,75]

The geometry of the nose is complex. Both Poiseuille's law and the Bernoulli principle describe flow through cylindrical pipes, but the shape of the nasal airway hardly resembles a cylinder and varies profoundly from one individual to another. Studies of nasal airflow unsurprisingly demonstrate significant inter-individual differences.[76] Computational fluid dynamics (CFD) has emerged as a technique to account for each patient's individual anatomy. A patient's CT scan is used to generate a 3D model of their individual nasal airway, which is then used to simulate nasal airflow. An example using an average nasal airflow created using statistical-shape modeling is shown in **Fig. 4**A–D, demonstrating the ability to calculate various parameters including airflow velocity, static pressure, and wall shear stress.[77] While their clinical applicability remains limited, these computational models have yielded significant new insights into nasal airflow physiology. For example, previous CFD studies have demonstrated that heat flux is a better correlate to subjective scores of obstruction.[78,79] Others have highlighted that the major flow path is through the middle meatus in some and through the inferior meatus in others, which may contribute to differences in perception of nasal airway patency.[80]

Reynolds Number

The Reynolds number is a nondimensional ratio of inertial forces to viscous forces within a fluid. At low Reynolds numbers, viscous forces dominate, leading to laminar flow in which fluid moves smoothly in layers without mixing perpendicular to the direction of flow. In contrast, at high Reynolds numbers, inertial forces dominate and produce a chaotic flow characterized by irregularity, eddies, and vortices. When describing flow through a long pipe, laminar flow typically occurs at Reynolds numbers less than 2300, turbulent flow at Reynolds numbers greater than 4000. Transitional flow, which is defined by central turbulent flow and peripheral laminar flow, occurs at intermediate Reynolds numbers between 2300 and 4000.

Nasal airflow is often accepted as laminar during "quiet" inspiration, however, this remains highly controversial. Estimates of the Reynolds number of nasal airflow range from 600 to 2000, however, the threshold at which flow becomes turbulent is

A   Velocity Contours   B   Velocity Vectors

C   Pressure   D   Wall Shear Stress

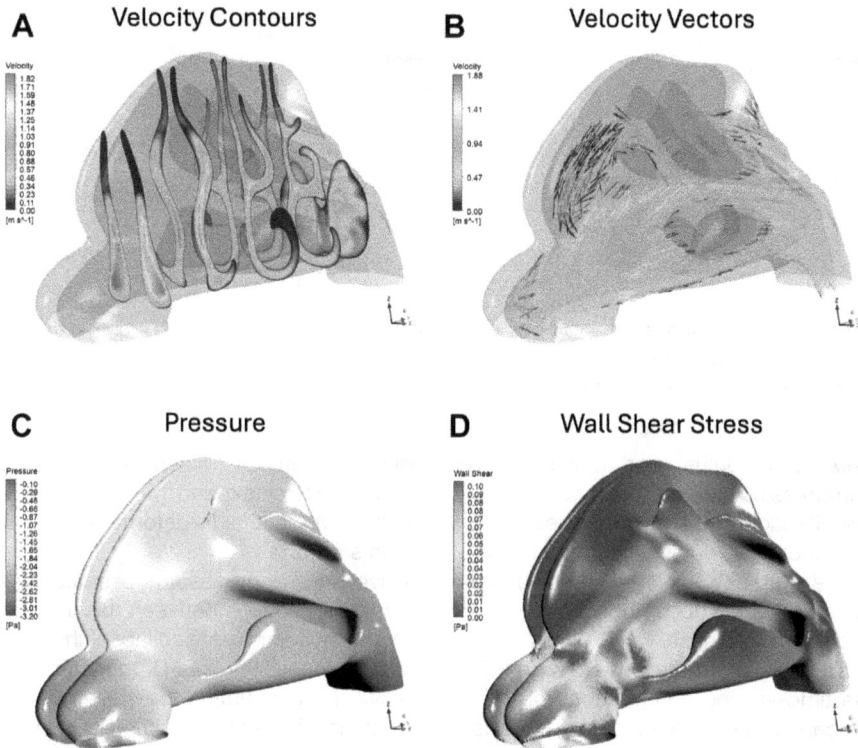

Fig. 4. CFD model of steady-state inspiration in an average nasal airway geometry. Multiple parameters can be calculated and visualized including (A) velocity contours at evenly spaced coronal planes, (B) velocity vectors along a para-sagittal plane demonstrating an anterior dorsal vortex, (C) static pressure distribution, and (D) wall shear stress.

dependent on the flow geometry.[80,81] Complex geometries may cause disruption in flow such that turbulence occurs at much lower Reynolds numbers within a range of 100 to 1000, with one study estimating a critical Reynolds of the nasal airway as low as 450.[82] Estimates of Reynolds number in the nasal airway often exceed this lower threshold, which implies transitional or turbulent flow even during quiet inspiration (**Fig. 5**). Turbulent flow is hypothesized to enhance heat and moisture transfer at the mucosa but also results in increased shear stress at the cavity walls and may lead to increased airway resistance.[70,83] Rather than describing the entire nasal cavity with a single Reynolds number, models which represent the valve and main nasal cavity as independent regions demonstrated higher accuracy, again highlighting the nuances of the complex nasal airway geometry.[84]

Fluid Structure Interaction

An accurate description of nasal airflow must account for the material properties of the nasal valve, which is a dynamic and collapsible structure.[85] The mechanical behavior of a material can be described by describing its change in response to an applied force, or load. These loads may be linear, including tensile or compressive loads which cause elongation or contraction respectively. The degree of deformation, referred to as strain, can be measured as a function of the force applied, referred to as stress. When a stress–strain curve is linear, the slope is known as the elastic modulus, or

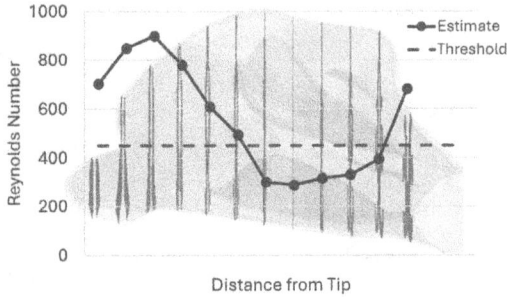

Fig. 5. Computational estimates of Reynolds number at evenly distributed cross-sections of the nasal airway. Anteriorly in the nasal valve region, these estimates exceed a lower threshold of 450 (*dashed line*).

Young's modulus, and describes the material's stiffness. When elongation or compression occurs, the material must also constrict or expand perpendicular to the direction of the applied stress. The tendency of a material to deform in direction perpendicular to a load is known as the Poisson's ratio.[86]

The currently accepted models of nasal valve physiology assume a static, rigid structure which does not account for the dynamic interactions between nasal airflow and the mobile nasal valve. Given the importance of dynamic valve collapse, there is a need for fluid-structure interaction (FSI) models, an extension of CFD, to incorporate the time-varying deformations of the nasal valve. By accounting for these material properties, one FSI model of the nasal valve during inspiratory sniffing conditions demonstrated good agreement with in vivo estimates of nasal valve collapse. Interestingly, they found that a dynamic model predicted a minimal increase in resistance of the nasal airway when compared with a model of the nasal airway as a static structure. In other words, during forceful inspiration, the increase in resistance caused by narrowing of the nasal valve and Poiseuille's law may be clinically insignificant.[87] Additional FSI models are warranted to investigate the contribution of dynamic valve collapse to nasal airway resistance, particularly during restful breathing.

Understanding the mechanisms of dynamic valve collapse is critical to surgical decision-making. Zoumalan and colleagues proposed a technique for real-time intraoperative assessment of the nasal valve, utilizing a suction at the nasal sill to generate a negative pressure. This produced airflow out of the nose in a direction analogous to expiration, while paradoxically causing depression of the nasal valve.[87] In a commentary, Rhee highlighted the obvious that physiologic expiration causes dilation of the nasal valve rather than collapse.[88] If the Bernoulli principle were accurately applied, then the INV should collapse as air flows into a narrowed segment, which should occur regardless of the direction of airflow during inspiration versus expiration. Alternatively, a simpler explanation may be that pressure inside the nasal airway is negative during inspiration and positive during expiration. With increasingly forceful nasal inspiration, negative pressure increases and overcomes the structural rigidity of the nasal sidewall, which is more similar to the Starling resistor commonly used to describe pharyngeal collapse in obstructive sleep apnea. The Bernoulli principle may still be relevant, but its relative significance is unclear. As Rhee noted, approaching surgery to increase the diameter of a "narrowed straw" is fundamentally different from approaching surgery to increase the rigidity of the lateral nasal wall.[88] Understanding the relevant importance of structural elasticity versus the Bernoulli principle is key to choosing the best surgical approach.

SUMMARY

The nasal valves are not simple, 2D cross-sections, but rather a complex, 3D, collapsible, and heterogenous structure. Nasal valve physiology has been often described with an emphasis on a critical INV angle, with the Bernoulli principle and Poiseuille's equation used to explain its singular significance in nasal obstruction. The geometry of the nasal airway is 3D and complex, however, and cannot be fully explained by our current understanding. As computational methods reveal new insights into nasal valve function, a new conceptual framework is needed to guide rhinoplasty surgical decision-making.

CLINICS CARE POINTS

- In addition to the cartilages and nasal bones, the skin and soft tissue envelope of the nose also plays a critical role in both form and function.

- Nasal valve dysfunction may be caused by septal deviations, turbinate hypertophy, and the shape and stiffness of the upper lateral cartilages. Identifying the correct sources of obstruction is key to a succesful surgical plan.

- Nasal obstruction is often more than simply a narrowed two-dimensional angle of the internal nasal valve. The nasal airway should be evaluated comprehensively with an appreciation for each patient's unique anatomy and geometry.

DISCLOSURE

The authors have nothing to close.

REFERENCES

1. Wexler DB, Davidson TM. The nasal valve: a review of the anatomy, imaging, and physiology. Am J Rhinol 2004;18:143–50.
2. Mink PJ. Physiologie Der Oberen Luftwege. Leipzig, Germany: F.C.W. Vogel; 1920.
3. Barrett DM, Casanueva FJ, Cook TA. Management of the nasal valve. Facial Plast Surg Clin North Am 2016;24(3):219–34.
4. Sinkler MA, Wehrle CJ, Elphingstone JW, et al. Surgical management of the internal nasal valve: a review of surgical approaches. Aesthetic Plast Surg 2021;45(3):1127–36.
5. Hamilton GS. The external nasal valve. Facial Plast Surg Clin North Am 2017;25(2):179–94.
6. Howard BK, Rohrich RJ. Understanding the nasal airway: principles and practice. Plast Reconstr Surg 2002;109(3):1128–46 [quiz: 1145–6].
7. GRIESMAN B. Muscles and cartilages of the nose from the standpoint of a typical rhinoplasty. Arch Otolaryngol Head Neck Surg 1944;39(4):334–41.
8. Hoeyberghs JL, Desta K, Matthews RN. The lost muscles of the nose. Aesthetic Plast Surg 1996;20(2):165–9.
9. Aksoy F, Veyseller B, Yildirim YS, et al. Role of nasal muscles in nasal valve collapse. Otolaryngol Head Neck Surg 2010;142(3):365–9.
10. Bruintjes TD, van Olphen AF, Hillen B, et al. Electromyography of the human nasal muscles. Eur Arch Oto-Rhino-Laryngol 1996;253(8):464–9.

11. Letourneau A, Daniel RK. The superficial musculoaponeurotic system of the nose. Plast Reconstr Surg 1988;82(1):48–57.
12. Bruintjes TD, Van Olphen AF, Hillen B, et al. A functional anatomic study of the relationship of the nasal cartilages and muscles to the nasal valve area. Laryngoscope 1998;108(7):1025–32.
13. Pou JD, Patel KG, Oyer SL. Treating nasal valve collapse in facial paralysis: what I do differently. Facial Plast Surg Clin North Am 2021;29(3):439–45.
14. Rohrich RJ, Malafa MM, Ahmad J, et al. Managing alar flare in rhinoplasty. Plast Reconstr Surg 2017;140(5):910–9.
15. Goffinet L, Barbier D, Lascombes P, et al. Nostrilplasty by manipulating the dilator naris muscles: a pilot study. Plast Reconstr Surg 2017;139(5):1208e–10e.
16. Hur MS, Hu KS, Youn KH, et al. New anatomical profile of the nasal musculature: dilator naris vestibularis, dilator naris anterior, and alar part of the nasalis. Clin Anat 2011;24(2):162–7.
17. Bruintjes TD, van Olphen AF, Hillen B. Review of the functional anatomy of the cartilages and muscles of the nose. Rhinology 1996;34(2):66–74. Available at: http://www.ncbi.nlm.nih.gov/pubmed/8876065.
18. Sakarya EU, Kar M, Bafaqeeh SA. Surgical anatomy of the external and internal nose. In: Cingi C, Muluk NB, editors. All around the nose. Cham, Germany: Springer International Publishing; 2020. p. 39–47. https://doi.org/10.1007/978-3-030-21217-9_4.
19. Soler ZM, Rosenthal E, Wax MK. Immediate nasal valve reconstruction after facial nerve resection. Arch Facial Plast Surg 2008;10(5):312–5.
20. Kienstra MA, Gassner HG, Sherris DA, et al. Effects of the nasal muscles on the nasal airway. Am J Rhinol 2005;19(4):375–81.
21. Lindsay RW, Bhama P, Hohman M, et al. Prospective evaluation of quality-of-life improvement after correction of the alar base in the flaccidly paralyzed face. JAMA Facial Plast Surg 2015;17(2):108–12.
22. Sheen JH, Sheen AP. Aesthetic rhinoplasty. St Louis, MO: CV Mosby; 1987.
23. Xavier R, Azeredo-Lopes S, Menger DJ, et al. Cephalic malposition of the lateral crura and parenthesis deformity: a cadaver study in caucasians. Aesthetic Plast Surg 2020;44(6):2244–52.
24. Toriumi DM, Asher SA. Lateral crural repositioning for treatment of cephalic malposition. Facial Plast Surg Clin North Am. 2015;23(1):55–71.
25. Constantian MB, Clardy RB. The relative importance of septal and nasal valvular surgery in correcting airway obstruction in primary and secondary rhinoplasty. Plast Reconstr Surg 1996;98(1):38–54 [discussion: 55–8].
26. Constantian MB. The two essential elements for planning tip surgery in primary and secondary rhinoplasty: observations based on review of 100 consecutive patients. Plast Reconstr Surg 2004;114(6):1571–81 [discussion: 1582–5].
27. Constantian MB. Functional effects of alar cartilage malposition. Ann Plast Surg 1993;30(6):487–99.
28. Gunter JP, Friedman RM. Lateral crural strut graft: technique and clinical applications in rhinoplasty. Plast Reconstr Surg 1997;99(4):943–52 [discussion: 953–5].
29. Bared A, Rashan A, Caughlin BP, et al. Lower lateral cartilage repositioning objective analysis using 3-dimensional imaging. JAMA Facial Plast Surg 2014;16(4):261–7.
30. Davis RE. Lateral crural tensioning for refinement of the wide and underprojected nasal tip: rethinking the lateral crural steal. Facial Plast Surg Clin North Am 2015;23(1):23–53.

31. Best CAE, Wong BJF. Nasal valve management: the case to move away from grafts to tensioning. Curr Otorhinolaryngol Rep 2023;11(3):260–5.
32. Kondo M, Orgain C, Alvarado R, et al. The effects of lateral crural tensioning with an articulated alar rim graft versus lateral crural strut graft on nasal function. Facial Plast Surg Aesthet Med 2020;22(4):281–5.
33. Goodrich JL, Wong BJF. Optimizing the soft tissue triangle, alar margin furrow, and alar ridge aesthetics: analysis and use of the articulate alar rim graft. Facial Plast Surg 2016;32(6):646–55.
34. Foulad A, Volgger V, Wong B. Lateral crural tensioning for refinement of the nasal tip and increasing alar stability: a case series. Facial Plast Surg 2017;33(3): 316–23.
35. Hismi A, Burks CA, Locascio JJ, et al. Comparative effectiveness of cartilage grafts in functional rhinoplasty for nasal sidewall collapse. Facial Plast Surg Aesthet Med 2022;24(3):240–6.
36. Toriumi DM. Management of the middle nasal vault in rhinoplasty. Operative Techniques in Plast Reconstr Surg 1995;2(1):16–30.
37. Rohrich RJ, Adams WP, Ahmad J, et al. Dallas rhinoplasty nasal surgery by the masters. New York, NY: Thieme Medical Pub; 2014.
38. Rohrich RJ, Hoxworth RE, Thornton JF, et al. The pyriform ligament. Plast Reconstr Surg 2008;121(1):277–81.
39. Craig JR, Bied A, Landas S, et al. Anatomy of the upper lateral cartilage along the lateral pyriform aperture. Plast Reconstr Surg 2015;135:406–11.
40. Janeke JB, Wright WK. Studies on the support of the nasal tip. Arch Otolaryngol 1971;93(5):458–64.
41. Saban YC, Amodeo A, Hammou JC, et al, An anatomical study of the nasal superficial musculoaponeurotic system surgical applications in rhinoplasty. Vol 10, Available at: www.liebertpub.com, (Accessed 18 May 2024), 2008.
42. Cunningham B, McKinney P. The alar scroll: an important anatomical structure in lobule surgery. Operat Tech Plast Reconstr Surg 2000;7(4):187–93.
43. Daniel RK, Palhazi P. The nasal ligaments and tip support in rhinoplasty: an anatomical study. Aesthet Surg J 2018;38(4):357–68.
44. Saban Y, Andretto Amodeo C, Hammou JC, et al. An anatomical study of the nasal superficial musculoaponeurotic system: surgical applications in rhinoplasty. Arch Facial Plast Surg 2008;10(2):109–15.
45. Bitik O, Uzun H, Konaş E. Scroll reconstruction: fine tuning of the interface between middle and lower thirds in rhinoplasty. Aesthet Surg J 2019;39(5):481–94.
46. Çakir B, Öreroğlu AR, Doğan T, et al. A complete subperichondrial dissection technique for rhinoplasty with management of the nasal ligaments. Aesthet Surg J 2012; 32(5):564–74.
47. Barone M, Salzillo R, De Bernardis R, et al. Reconstruction of scroll and pitanguy's ligaments in open rhinoplasty: a controlled randomized study. Aesthetic Plast Surg 2023. https://doi.org/10.1007/s00266-023-03725-0.
48. Ozturk A, Eroglu S, Timur B, et al. Functional role of scroll reconstruction in open rhinoplasty. Aesthetic Plast Surg 2021. https://doi.org/10.1007/s00266.
49. Stovin JS. The importance of the membranous nasal septum. AMA Arch Otolaryngol 1958;67(5):540.
50. Mladina R, Čujić E, Šubarić M, et al. Nasal septal deformities in ear, nose, and throat patients. An international study. American Journal of Otolaryngology - Head and Neck Medicine and Surgery 2008;29(2):75–82.

51. Lin JK, Wheatley FC, Handwerker J, et al. Analyzing nasal septal deviations to develop a new classification system: a computed tomography study using MATLAB and OsiriX. JAMA Facial Plast Surg 2014;16(3):183–7.
52. Buyukertan M, Keklikoglu N, Kokten G. A morphometric consideration of nasal septal deviations by people with paranasal complaints; a computed tomography study. Rhinology 2003;41(1):21–4. Available at: http://www.ncbi.nlm.nih.gov/pubmed/12677736.
53. Baumann I, Baumann H. A new classification of septal deviations. Rhinology 2007;45(3):220–3. Available at: http://www.ncbi.nlm.nih.gov/pubmed/17956023.
54. Guyuron B, Uzzo CD, Scull H. A practical classification of septonasal deviation and an effective guide to septal surgery. Plast Reconstr Surg 1999;104(7):2202–9 [discussion: 2210–2].
55. Fettman N, Sanford T, Sindwani R. Surgical management of the deviated septum: techniques in septoplasty. Otolaryngol Clin North Am 2009;42(2):241–52.
56. Clark DW, Signore AG Del, Raithatha R, et al, Nasal airway obstruction: prevalence and anatomic contributors. Vol 97, Available at: www.entjournal.com173, (Accessed 28 April 2024).
57. Berger G, Balum-Azim M, Ophir D. The normal inferior turbinate: histomorphometric analysis and clinical implications. Laryngoscope 2003;113(7):1192–8.
58. Hsu DW, Suh JD. Anatomy and physiology of nasal obstruction. Otolaryngol Clin North Am 2018;51(5):853–65.
59. Naito K, Horibe S, Tanabe Y, et al. Objective assessment of nasal obstruction. Fujita medical journal 2023;9(2):53–64.
60. Clement PAR, Gordts F. Standardisation committee on objective assessment of the nasal airway I and E. Consensus report on acoustic rhinometry and rhinomanometry. Rhinology 2005;43(3):169–79.
61. Kikawada T. Endoscopic posterior nasal neurectomy: an alternative to vidian neurectomy. Operat Tech Otolaryngol Head Neck Surg 2007;18(4):297–301.
62. Takahara D, Takeno S, Hamamoto T, et al. Management of intractable nasal hyperreactivity by selective resection of posterior nasal nerve branches. Int J Otolaryngol 2017;2017:1–5.
63. Yu AJ, Tam B, Wrobel B, et al. Radiofrequency neurolysis of the posterior nasal nerve: a systematic review and meta-analysis. Laryngoscope 2024;134(2):507–16.
64. Stolovitzky JP, Ow RA, Silvers SL, et al. Effect of radiofrequency neurolysis on the symptoms of chronic rhinitis: a randomized controlled trial. OTO Open 2021;5(3). https://doi.org/10.1177/2473974X211041124.
65. Roithmann R, Cole P, Chapnik J, et al. Acoustic rhinometry in the evaluation of nasal obstruction. Laryngoscope 1995;105(3):275–81.
66. Hilberg O, Jackson AC, Swift DL, et al. Acoustic rhinometry: evaluation of nasal cavity geometry by acoustic reflection. J Appl Physiol (1985) 1989;66(1):295–303.
67. Mamikoglu B, Houser SM, Corey JP. An interpretation method for objective assessment of nasal congestion with acoustic rhinometry. Laryngoscope 2002;112(5):926–9.
68. Corey JP. Acoustic rhinometry: should we be using it? Curr Opin Otolaryngol Head Neck Surg 2006;14(1):29–34.
69. Garcia GJM, Hariri BM, Patel RG, et al. The relationship between nasal resistance to airflow and the airspace minimal cross-sectional area. J Biomech 2016;49(9):1670–8.

70. Tripathi PB, Elghobashi S, Wong BJF. The myth of the internal nasal valve. JAMA Facial Plast Surg 2017;19(4):253–4.
71. Miman MC, Deliktaş H, Özturan O, et al. Internal nasal valve: revisited with objective facts. Otolaryngol Head Neck Surg 2006;134(1):41–7.
72. Poetker DM, Rhee JS, Mocan BO, et al. Computed tomography technique for evaluation of the nasal valve. Arch Facial Plast Surg 2004;6(4):240–3.
73. Bloom JD, Sridharan S, Hagiwara M, et al. Reformatted computed tomography to assess the internal nasal valve and association with physical examination. Arch Facial Plast Surg 2012;14:331–5. Available at: www.liebertpub.com.
74. André RF, Vuyk HD, Ahmed A, et al. Correlation between subjective and objective evaluation of the nasal airway. A systematic review of the highest level of evidence. Clin Otolaryngol 2009;34(6):518–25.
75. Campbell DA, Moghaddam MG, Rhee JS, et al. Narrowed posterior nasal airway limits efficacy of anterior septoplasty. Facial Plast Surg Aesthet Med 2021;23(1):13–20.
76. Segal RA, Kepler GM, Kimbell JS. Effects of differences in nasal anatomy on airflow distribution: a comparison of four individuals at rest. Ann Biomed Eng 2008;36(11):1870–82.
77. Brüning J, Hildebrandt T, Heppt W, et al. Characterization of the airflow within an average geometry of the healthy human nasal cavity. Sci Rep 2020;10(1). https://doi.org/10.1038/s41598-020-60755-3.
78. Kimbell JS, Frank DO, Laud P, et al. Changes in nasal airflow and heat transfer correlate with symptom improvement after surgery for nasal obstruction. J Biomech 2013;46(15):2634–43.
79. Sullivan CD, Garcia GJM, Frank-Ito DO, et al. Perception of better nasal patency correlates with increased mucosal cooling after surgery for nasal obstruction. Otolaryngol Head Neck Surg 2014;150(1):139–47.
80. Zhao K, Jiang J. What is normal nasal airflow? A computational study of 22 healthy adults. Int Forum Allergy Rhinol 2014;4(6):435–46.
81. Johnsen SG. Computational rhinology: unraveling discrepancies between in silico and in vivo nasal airflow assessments for enhanced clinical decision support. Bioengineering 2024;11(3). https://doi.org/10.3390/bioengineering11030239.
82. O'neill G, Tolley NS. Modelling nasal airflow coefficients: an insight into the nature of airflow. Rhinology 2021;59(1):66–74.
83. Chen XB, Lee HP, Chong VFH, et al. Assessment of septal deviation effects on nasal air flow: a computational fluid dynamics model. Laryngoscope 2009;119(9):1730–6.
84. O'neill G, Tolley NS. The complexities of nasal airflow: theory and practice. J Appl Physiol 2019;127:1215–23.
85. Shi B, Huang H. Computational technology for nasal cartilage-related clinical research and application. Int J Oral Sci 2020;12(1). https://doi.org/10.1038/s41368-020-00089-y.
86. Callister Jr WD, Rethwisch DG. Materials science and engineering: an introduction. 10th edition. Wiley; 2018.
87. Zoumalan RA, Larrabee WF, Murakami CS. Intraoperative suction-assisted evaluation of the nasal valve in rhinoplasty. Arch Facial Plast Surg 2012;14(1):34–8.
88. Rhee JS, Kimbell JS. The nasal valve dilemma: the narrow straw vs the weak wall. Arch Facial Plast Surg 2012;14(1):9–10.

Patient-Reported Outcome Measures in Nasal Valve Repair and Nasal Obstruction

Max Feng, MD[a], Adeeb Derakhshan, MD[b], Jennifer Fuller, MD[b],*

KEYWORDS

- Functional rhinoplasty • Nasal valve • Nasal obstruction
- Patient-reported outcome measures • Quality of life

KEY POINTS

- Patient-reported outcome measures (PROMs) are important for assessing outcomes in functional rhinoplasty and facilitating communication between the patient and surgeon.
- Ideal PROMs should be patient-derived, psychometrically validated, reliable, and responsive.
- PROMs can gauge disease-specific nasal functional and esthetic outcomes, as well as global health-related quality of life outcomes.
- Functional, esthetic, and global health-related quality of life outcomes should be evaluated, because functional rhinoplasty is shown to impact all 3 domains.

INTRODUCTION

Assessing outcomes in functional rhinoplasty is difficult due to the multifactorial nature of nasal obstruction. There are multiple elements involved, including the patient's subjective perception of their nasal airflow, the clinician's objective assessment of the nasal airway, the anatomic area and volume of the nasal cavity, and the degree of dynamic airflow passing through the nasal cavity during breathing.[1] Multiple modalities exist for assessing nasal obstruction, such as rhinometry, clinician-graded outcomes, patient-reported outcomes, and imaging. However, there is currently no gold-standard outcome assessment in functional rhinoplasty. Ultimately, a patient's own perception of nasal obstruction and its impact on quality of life (QoL) is central in measuring the success of surgery. Thus, patient-reported outcome measures

[a] Department of Otolaryngology–Head & Neck Surgery, Loma Linda University Health, 11234 Anderson Street, Room 2586A, Loma Linda, CA 92354, USA; [b] Division of Facial Plastic and Reconstructive Surgery, Department of Otolaryngology–Head & Neck Surgery, Loma Linda University Health, 11234 Anderson Street, Room 2586A, Loma Linda, CA 92354, USA
* Corresponding author. 11234 Anderson Street, Room 2586A, Loma Linda, CA 92354.
E-mail address: JEFuller@llu.edu

Otolaryngol Clin N Am 58 (2025) 205–214
https://doi.org/10.1016/j.otc.2024.08.005
0030-6665/25/© 2024 Elsevier Inc. All rights reserved, including those for text and data mining, AI training, and similar technologies.

oto.theclinics.com

(PROMs) are increasingly used in rhinoplasty to evaluate surgical outcomes. In the clinical consensus statement on nasal valve compromise, there is a strong consensus that PROMs are valid indicators of a successful intervention.[2] The rhinoplasty clinical practice guidelines recommend incorporating PROMs in rhinoplasty surgery to allow patients to express satisfaction and communicate with the clinician.[3]

Disease-specific instruments aim to gauge the impact of nasal obstruction on patient QoL. These instruments can be divided into functional and/or esthetic assessments. Global health-related QoL PROMs can help determine the impact of nasal obstruction on a patient's general health. An ideal PROM would allow for comparison of techniques, quantify positive effects, identify patients most likely to benefit from nasal valve surgery, and provide a follow-up standard and benchmark for future studies.[4] Furthermore, the PROM should be psychometrically validated. The ideal PROM questionnaire is succinct in the number of items being assessed, effective in capturing the degree to which nasal obstruction impacts QoL, written in plain language, and administered in an accessible format.[5] There is currently no clear consensus on a gold-standard PROM. In this section, validated, reliable, and responsive PROMs that are used in functional and/or esthetic rhinoplasty are highlighted (**Tables 1** and **2**).

DISCUSSION
Functional-Only Patient-Reported Outcome Measures

Nasal Obstruction Symptom Evaluation scale
The Nasal Obstruction Symptom Evaluation (NOSE) scale is the first validated disease-specific QoL instrument designed for assessing nasal obstruction. The tool was initially developed for use in patients undergoing septoplasty but has since become among the most widely used PROMs in functional rhinoplasty. The questionnaire is valid, reliable, and responsive in measuring QoL disturbances of nasal obstruction.[6] The questionnaire is also brief and easy to complete, with minimal patient response burden.

The NOSE evaluates the impact of nasal obstruction on patient QoL over the past 4 weeks. The questionnaire contains 5 questions based on a 5-point Likert scale, with a score of 0 representing no problem and 4 representing severe problem. Scoring is reported on a scale of 0 to 100 by adding the individual scores and multiplying the raw score by 5. NOSE scores have been used to classify nasal obstruction as mild (5–25), moderate (30–50), severe (55–75), and extreme (80–100). A cutoff score of 30 has been used to differentiate between patients with and without significant nasal airway

Table 1	
Validated patient-reported outcome measure instruments in functional rhinoplasty	
Outcome Type	**Instrument**
Functional only	NOSE
	SNOT-22
Esthetic only	FACE-Q rhinoplasty module
Functional and esthetic	SCHNOS
	SNOT-23
Global health-related quality of life	EQ5D

Abbreviations: EQ5D, EuroQol 5-Dimension Questionnaire; NOSE, Nasal Obstruction Symptom Evaluation Scale; SCHNOS, Standardized Cosmesis and Health Nasal Outcomes Survey; SNOT, Sino-Nasal Outcomes Test.

Table 2
Patient-reported outcome measure characteristics

Instrument	Domain(s) Assessed	Items	Scale	Score Range	Recall Period	Mean Baseline Score	Mean Follow-up Score	Mean Change	Severity Classes	MCID
NOSE	Nasal obstruction symptoms	5	5-Point Likert, 0–4	0–100 (Higher score = better outcome)	Past 4 wk	65 ± 22	23 ± 20	42	Mild (5–25), moderate (30–50), severe (55–75), extreme (80–100)	19.4
Nasal obstruction VAS	Overall nasal obstruction	1	Continuous	Variable (higher score = worse outcome)	Current	6.7 ± 2.3 on 0–10 scale	2.1 ± 2.2 on 0–10 scale	4.6 on 0–10 scale	N/A	3.0 on 0–10 scale
SNOT-22	Symptoms related to rhinosinusitis and its impact on quality of life	22	6-Point Likert, 0–5	0–110 (Higher score = worse outcome)	Past 2 wk	39.95 ± 2.47	21.22 ± 2.24	18.7	N/A	N/A
SNOT-23	Same as SNOT-22, with the addition of nasal shape question	23	6-point Likert, 0–5	0–115 (Higher score = worse outcome)	Past 2 wk	51.6 ± 26.2	25.7 ± 22.0	25.9	N/A	N/A
FACE-Q Rhinoplasty Module	Satisfaction with appearance of nose and nostrils, adverse effects after surgery	10 (Satisfaction with nose), 5 (satisfaction with nostrils), 4 (adverse effects)	4-Point Likert, 1–4	Rasch transformation to 0–100 (higher score = better outcome)	Past week	39.2 ± 16.6 (nose), 50.1 ± 28.9 (nostrils)	74.0 ± 23.3 (nose), 80.0 ± 24.9 (nostrils)	34.8 (nose), 29.9 (nostrils)	N/A	11.1 (nose), 14.0 (nostrils)

(continued on next page)

Table 2
(continued)

Instrument	Domain(s) Assessed	Items	Scale	Score Range	Recall Period	Mean Baseline Score	Mean Follow-up Score	Mean Change	Severity Classes	MCID
SCHNOS	Nasal obstruction symptoms, patient perception of nasal cosmesis and its impact on mood/self-esteem	4 (Obstructive), 6 (cosmesis)	6-Point Likert, 0–5	0–100 Obstructive and cosmesis (higher score = worse outcome)	Past 4 wk	72.9 ± 17.8 (SCHNOS-O), 30.1 ± 28.2 (SCHNOS-C)	31.4 ± 28.1 (SCHNOS-O), 8.7 ± 15.3 (SCHNOS-C)	41.5 (SCHNOS-O), 21.4 (SCHNOS-C)	Mild (<40), moderate (45–70), severe (75–100) (SCHNOS-O); mild (<33.3), moderate (33.3–66.6), severe (>66.6) (SCHNOS-C)	28.3 (SCHNOS-O), 18.0 (SCHNOS-C)
EQ5D	Mobility, self-care, usual activities, pain/discomfort, anxiety/depression	5	3-Point Likert, 0–2	Conversion to HUV of 0–1.0 (higher score = better outcome)	Current	0.87	0.93 (12 mo)	0.06	N/A	N/A
EQ5D VAS	Overall health	1	Continuous	0–100 (Higher score = better outcome)	Current	75.7	82.0	6.3	N/A	9.5

Abbreviations: EQ5D, EuroQol 5-Dimension Questionnaire; HUV, health utility value; MCID, minimum clinically important difference; N/A, not applicable or no data; NOSE, Nasal Obstruction Symptom Evaluation scale; SCHNOS-C, Standard Cosmesis and Health Nasal Outcomes Survey-cosmesis domain; SCHNOS-O, SCHNOS obstruction domain; SNOT, Sino-Nasal Outcomes Test; VAS, visual analog scale.

obstruction (NAO) with a sensitivity of 93.7% and specificity of 90.3%.[7] Although NOSE scores have not shown a significant correlation with objective measures, particularly as diagnostic tools, a 2019 study did show a significant correlation between improvement in NOSE scores and improvement in peak nasal inspiratory flow following functional rhinoplasty.[8]

NOSE scores have also been extensively used to assess functional rhinoplasty outcomes. A meta-analysis of pooled NOSE data found a mean preoperative score of 67.4, with a range of 34.8 to 86.5. Postrhinoplasty NOSE scores improved by 49.8 points (95% confidence interval [CI], 45.2–54.3) at 3- to 6-month follow-up, by 43.4 points (95% CI, 35.8–51.0) at 6- to 12-month follow-up, and by 48.7 points (95% CI, 39.0–58.4) at 12-month follow-up.[9] A systematic review of 20 NOSE articles reported a weighted average of 65 ± 22 preoperatively, decreasing to 23 ± 20 postoperatively, with a mean decrease of 42 points.[10] The mean clinically important difference (MCID) has been reported as 19.4 points.[11]

Visual analog scale

The nasal obstruction visual analog scale (VAS) is a self-assessment of nasal airflow based on a continuous scale. The patient's subjective degree of nasal obstruction is typically graded from 0 (no obstruction) to 5 (complete obstruction).[12] However, variations in the numerical range exist, and this range can be increased to encompass more values, such as from 0 to 100.[1] The VAS can also be used to compare the degree of left- and right-sided nasal obstruction, NAO in different positions such as supine and sitting, and NAO before and after topical decongestants.[1,13] Lam and colleagues[1] found that the nasal obstruction VAS was significantly associated with both upright and supine minimum cross-sectional area (MCA), which indicated that a 0.1-cm^2 decrease in MCA corresponded to an ∼3% increase in subjective nasal obstruction. However, the VAS was not associated with volume or flow.[1] Mean preoperative and postoperative VAS scores were 6.7 ± 2.3 and 2.1 ± 2.2 (on a 0–10 scale), respectively. The MCID was calculated to be 3.0 on a 0- to 10-point scale.[10]

The benefit of the VAS is that it consists of a single question and can be easily completed by patients. Unlike the NOSE, which asks patients to rate the severity of their nasal obstruction in the past month, the VAS only asks at a single point in time. Owing to the single measure, the VAS does not adequately measure internal consistency and does not provide meaningful QoL information. VAS can also have significant intrarater and interrater variability. The high variability in scaling makes comparisons across studies difficult.[1,12,13]

Sino-Nasal Outcomes Test-22

The Sino-Nasal Outcomes Test-22 (SNOT-22) is an extensively studied disease-specific QoL PROM used to assess outcomes of intervention for sinonasal disease. Although primarily used to measure outcomes in inflammatory nasal disease, the tool contains a single question that addresses nasal obstruction and has been used to evaluate outcomes in functional rhinoplasty.[14–17] The test consists of 22 questions measuring various aspects of the severity and frequency of sinonasal disease symptoms using a 6-point Likert scale, with 0 being "no problem" and 5 being "problem as bad as it can be." A final total score of 0 to 110 is calculated using the sum of the individual question scores, with a higher total score indicating greater disease severity.[18]

The mean preoperative SNOT-22 in 76 patients undergoing functional rhinoplasty was 39.95 ± 2.47. The mean postoperative score was 21.22 ± 2.24. Specifically, the score pertaining to nasal blockage decreased from 3.45 to 1.58.[17]

Esthetic-Only Patient-Reported Outcomes Measures

FACE-Q rhinoplasty

The FACE-Q was developed by Klassen and colleagues[19] for measuring outcomes in surgical and nonsurgical facial esthetic procedures. The patient-derived questionnaire contains multiple modules and includes more than 40 independently functioning scales and checklists, encompassing facial appearance, QoL, and adverse effects.[19] The FACE-Q rhinoplasty module specifically measures patient-perceived changes in nasal appearance and postoperative adverse effects after rhinoplasty in the past week. The questionnaire consists of a 10-question "satisfaction with nose" scale and a 5-question "satisfaction with nostrils" scale measured on a 4-point Likert scale, in which 1 is "very dissatisfied" and 4 is "very satisfied." The raw score is then converted into equivalent linear interval data from 0 to 100 generated by a Rasch transformation. Higher scores indicate better outcomes.[20] This tool has been psychometrically validated and is easy to read and understand.[20–22] A separate postoperative checklist measures adverse effects over the past 2 days. This checklist contains 4 questions measured on a 4-point Likert scale, in which 1 is "not at all" and 4 is "extremely." The questions include how much a patient has been bothered by skin thickness or swelling, tenderness, difficulty breathing through the nose, and unnatural-appearing bumps or hollows on the nose.[20]

The mean preoperative and postoperative scores were 39.2 (±16.6) and 74.0 (±23.3) for the satisfaction with nose scale and 50.1 (±28.9) and 80.0 (±24.9) for the satisfaction with nostrils scale, respectively, following rhinoplasty.[20] The normal range was found to be 47 to 100 for the satisfaction with nose scale and 64 to 100 for the satisfaction with nostrils scale. Values less than these thresholds were considered abnormal and indicative of unhappy patients.[23] In a study of patients undergoing functional rhinoplasty with spreader grafts, the satisfaction with nose score increased by 21.6 (±23.8) and the satisfaction with nostrils score increased by 24.8 (±27.7). The MCID was calculated as 11.1 for satisfaction of nose and 14.0 for satisfaction of nostrils.[24] Further work remains for developing severity classification ranges.

Functional and Esthetic Patient-Reported Outcome Measures

Standardized Cosmesis and Health Nasal Outcomes Survey

The Standardized Cosmesis and Health Nasal Outcomes Survey (SCHNOS) was developed with patient input to evaluate functional and cosmetic outcomes in rhinoplasty. The questionnaire consists of 10 questions divided into a 4-item nasal obstruction domain (SCHNOS-O) and a 6-item nasal cosmesis domain (SCHNOS-C). The questionnaire evaluates the severity of nasal obstruction symptoms and patient perception of nasal cosmesis and its impact on mood and self-esteem over the past 1 month. The questions are ranked on a 6-point Likert scale, in which 0 is "no problem" and 5 is "extreme problem." Each domain is separately scored and based off a maximum score of 100. To calculate the scores, the sum of the obstructive component is divided by 20 and multiplied by 100, whereas the sum of the cosmesis component is divided by 30 and multiplied by 100.[25]

An SCHNOS-O score of 40 was found to differentiate between patients with and without nasal obstruction (sensitivity 85.7, specificity 82.4), making it a good screening tool.[26] Patients with nasal obstruction can be categorized into mild (<40), moderate (45–70), and severe (75–100) based on the obstructive score. An SCHNOS-C score of 30 differentiated patients with and without esthetic concerns (sensitivity 92.1, specificity 62.4), and the esthetic concerns can be categorized into mild (<33.3), moderate (33.3–66.6) and severe (>66.6) based on the cosmesis score.[26] The SCHNOS question

5, "decreased mood and self-esteem due to my nose," has been shown to be highly predictive of revisions and body dysmorphic disorder (BDD) in patients who undergo cosmetic rhinoplasty, suggesting that the question can serve as a screening tool for BDD.[27,28]

A study of 90 patients undergoing functional rhinoplasty found mean SCHNOS-O and SCHNOS-C preoperative scores of 72.9 (±17.8) and 30.1 (±28.2), respectively. These scores decreased to 31.4 (±28.1) and 8.7 (±15.3) within 2 months after surgery with a sustained improvement at 12-month follow-up in both domains.[25] The MCID was determined to be 28.3 for SCHNO-O and 18.0 for SCHNOS-C.[29]

SCHNOS-O and NOSE scores have a very strong correlation (Spearman r = 0.943), suggesting that the SCHNOS-O and NOSE scores are fairly equivalent in evaluating obstructive outcomes.[30] Furthermore, the NOSE and SCHNOS-O have been cocalibrated into a common scale, allowing for comparison between the 2 scores.[31]

Sino-Nasal Outcomes Test-23

Takhar and colleagues[32] developed a modification of the SNOT-22 by adding an additional question regarding "concern with shape of the nose," dubbed the Sino-Nasal Outcomes Test-23 (SNOT-23). The total score range was increased to 0 to 115 with the additional question. In a study of 69 patients undergoing functional rhinoplasty, the mean preoperative and postoperative SNOT-23 scores were 51.6 (±26.2) and 25.7 (±22.0), respectively. The average score was 10.4 (±10.4) in the group without NAO. SNOT-23 scores demonstrated high correlation with the VAS (Spearman R^2 = 0.74) and NOSE (Spearman R^2 = 0.82) scores. There was no correlation with nasal inspiratory peak flow. The tool is validated and reliable.[32]

Global Health-Related Quality of Life Patient-Reported Outcome Measures

EuroQol 5-Dimension questionnaire

Although disease-specific PROMs allow for the assessment of nasal obstruction and nasal cosmesis outcomes in rhinoplasty, the overall impact of nasal surgery on somatic, social, and psychological domains are not captured. Broader QoL instruments are necessary for understanding the effect of nasal obstruction and nasal airway surgery on a patient's overall health status, including physical and mental health.[33]

The EuroQol 5-Dimension (EQ5D) questionnaire is widely used in health outcomes research to measure the cost-effectiveness of health care interventions.[34] The instrument consists of 5 questions measuring 5 domains at the time the survey is taken: mobility, self-care, usual activities, pain/discomfort, and anxiety/depression. Each domain is rated as "no problems," "moderate problems," or "severe problems." This instrument has a low user burden and can be completed in approximately 2 minutes. EQ5D includes a VAS in which participants score their overall health on a continuous scale from 0 to 100.[35]

In a study from Yamasaki and colleagues[36] of 567 patient undergoing rhinoplasty with or without inferior turbinate reduction for functional or dual functional and cosmetic purposes, the mean preoperative EQ5D VAS was 75.7 for the rhinoplasty alone group (95% CI, 74.6–76.8; n = 292) and 74.6 for the rhinoplasty and turbinate group (95% CI, 73.1–76.2; n = 137). This improved to 82.0 (95% CI, 81.1–82.8; n = 259) for the rhinoplasty alone group and 82.1 (95% CI, 80.9–83.4; n = 126) for the rhinoplasty and turbinate group. There was a weak negative correlation between change in NOSE score and change in EQ5D VAS (r = −0.38).[36] Similarly, Fuller and colleagues[37] reported a moderate negative correlation (r = −0.37) between NOSE and EQ5D VAS scores. The MCID of EQ5D VAS was calculated at 9.5. Patients reporting problems with pain/discomfort and usual activity had higher preoperative NOSE scores than those without. The percentage of patients reporting problems in usual activity and pain/discomfort decreased by more than half at long-term follow-up.[37]

EQ5D results can be converted into health utility values (HUVs) using population-based data of the adult US population, allowing for the translation of HUVs into cost utility analysis and quality-adjusted life year data.[38] An HUV of 1.00 denotes a perfect state of health. In a study from Gadkaree and colleagues[38] of 463 patients undergoing functional rhinoplasty, the mean preoperative HUV was 0.87, which improved to 0.91 at 2 months and 0.93 at 12 months. Mean preoperative VAS was 73.8, which increased to 81.2 at 2 months and 81.3 at 12 months. There was a weak positive correlation between change in EQ5D VAS and HUV scores ($r = 0.22$).[38]

SUMMARY

PROMs are essential for quantifying the impact of functional rhinoplasty on nasal obstruction and facilitating communication between patient and surgeon. Although the primary goal of functional rhinoplasty is to address nasal obstruction, nasal cosmesis is invariably impacted, necessitating the need for instruments that also measure nasal esthetic outcomes. Furthermore, the impact of nasal valve surgery on somatic, social, and psychological domains should also be captured with global health-related QoL assessments.

CLINICS CARE POINTS

- PROMs are essential for understanding the impact of nasal valve surgery on patient-perceived nasal obstruction, nasal esthetics, and general QoL.
- PROMs include functional only, esthetic only, combined esthetic and functional, and general QoL assessments.
- The NOSE scale andSNOT-22 are validated instruments for assessing functional outcomes.
- The FACE-Q rhinoplasty module is a validated instrument for assessing esthetic outcomes.
- The SCHNOS and SNOT-23 are validated instruments for assessing both functional and esthetic outcomes.
- EQ5D is a validated instrument for assessing global health-related QoL outcomes.

DISCLOSURES

The authors have nothing to disclose.

REFERENCES

1. Lam DJ, James KT, Weaver EM. Comparison of anatomic, physiological, and subjective measures of the nasal airway. Am J Rhinol 2006;20(5):463–70.
2. Rhee JS, Weaver EM, Park SS, et al. Clinical consensus statement: diagnosis and management of nasal valve compromise. Otolaryngol Neck Surg 2010;143(1):48–59.
3. Ishii LE, Tollefson TT, Basura GJ, et al. Clinical practice guideline: improving nasal form and function after rhinoplasty executive summary. Otolaryngol Neck Surg 2017;156(2):205–19.
4. Barone M, Cogliandro A, Di Stefano N, et al. A systematic review of patient-reported outcome measures after rhinoplasty. Eur Arch Oto-Rhino-Laryngol 2017;274(4):1807–11.

5. Warinner C, Loyo M, Gu J, et al. Patient-reported outcomes measures in rhino-plasty: need for use and implementation. Facial Plast Surg FPS 2023;39(5): 517–26.

6. Stewart MG, Witsell DL, Smith TL, et al. Development and validation of the nasal obstruction symptom evaluation (NOSE) scale1. Otolaryngol Neck Surg 2004; 130(2):157–63.

7. Lipan MJ, Most SP. Development of a severity classification system for subjective nasal obstruction. JAMA Facial Plast Surg 2013;15(5):358–61.

8. Fuller JC, Gadkaree SK, Levesque PA, et al. Peak nasal inspiratory flow is a useful measure of nasal airflow in functional septorhinoplasty. Laryngoscope 2019; 129(3):594–601.

9. Floyd EM, Ho S, Patel P, et al. Systematic review and meta-analysis of studies evaluating functional rhinoplasty outcomes with the NOSE score. Otolaryngol Neck Surg 2017;156(5):809–15.

10. Rhee JS, Sullivan CD, Frank DO, et al. A systematic review of patient-reported nasal obstruction scores: defining normative and symptomatic ranges in surgical patients. JAMA Facial Plast Surg 2014;16(3):219–25 [quiz: 232].

11. Stewart MG, Smith TL, Weaver EM, et al. Outcomes after nasal septoplasty: re-sults from the nasal obstruction septoplasty effectiveness (NOSE) study. Otolar-yngol Neck Surg 2004;130(3):283–90.

12. Armengot M, Campos A, Zapater E, et al. Upper lateral cartilage transposition in the surgical management of nasal valve incompetence. Rhinology 2003;41(2): 107–12.

13. Sipilä J, Suonpää J, Silvoniemi P, et al. Correlations between subjective sensation of nasal patency and rhinomanometry in both unilateral and total nasal assess-ment. ORL J Otorhinolaryngol Relat Spec 1995;57(5):260–3.

14. Palesy T, Pratt E, Mrad N, et al. Airflow and patient-perceived improvement following rhinoplastic correction of external nasal valve dysfunction. JAMA Facial Plast Surg 2015;17(2):131–6.

15. Strazdins E, Nie YF, Ramli R, et al. Association between mental health status and patient satisfaction with the functional outcomes of rhinoplasty. JAMA Facial Plast Surg 2018;20(4):284–91.

16. Taş BM, Erden B. Evaluation of the effect of conventional rhinoplasty with autos-preader flap and let-down technique on nasal functions. Facial Plast Surg FPS 2021;37(3):302–5.

17. Poirrier AL, Ahluwalia S, Goodson A, et al. Is the sino-nasal outcome Test-22 a suitable evaluation for septorhinoplasty? Laryngoscope 2013;123(1):76–81.

18. Hopkins C, Gillett S, Slack R, et al. Psychometric validity of the 22-item sinonasal outcome test. Clin Otolaryngol 2009;34(5):447–54.

19. Klassen AF, Cano SJ, Scott A, et al. Measuring patient-reported outcomes in facial aesthetic patients: development of the FACE-Q. Facial Plast Surg FPS 2010;26(4):303–9.

20. Klassen AF, Cano SJ, East CA, et al. Development and psychometric evaluation of the FACE-Q scales for patients undergoing rhinoplasty. JAMA Facial Plast Surg 2016;18(1):27–35.

21. Klassen AF, Cano SJ, Schwitzer JA, et al. FACE-Q scales for health-related quality of life, early life impact, satisfaction with outcomes, and decision to have treat-ment: development and validation. Plast Reconstr Surg 2015;135(2):375–86.

22. Pusic AL, Klassen AF, Scott AM, et al. Development and psychometric evaluation of the FACE-Q satisfaction with appearance scale: a new patient-reported

outcome instrument for facial aesthetics patients. Clin Plast Surg 2013;40(2):
249–60.

23. Radulesco T, Mancini J, Penicaud M, et al. Assessing normal values for the
FACE-Q rhinoplasty module: an observational study. Clin Otolaryngol 2018;
43(4):1025–30.

24. Fuller JC, Levesque PA, Lindsay RW. Analysis of patient-perceived nasal appearance evaluations following functional septorhinoplasty with spreader graft placement. JAMA Facial Plast Surg 2019;21(4):305–11.

25. Kandathil CK, Saltychev M, Patel PN, et al. Natural history of the standardized
cosmesis and health nasal outcomes survey after rhinoplasty. Laryngoscope
2021;131(1). https://doi.org/10.1002/lary.28831.

26. Patel PN, Wadhwa H, Okland T, et al. Comparison of the distribution of standardized cosmesis and health nasal outcomes survey scores between symptomatic
and asymptomatic patients. Facial Plast Surg Aesthetic Med 2022;24(4):305–9.

27. Wei EX, Kimura KS, Abdelhamid AS, et al. Prevalence and characteristics associated with positive body dysmorphic disorder screening among patients presenting for cosmetic facial plastic surgery. Facial Plast Surg Aesthetic Med
2024;26(3):262–9.

28. Okland TS, Patel P, Liu GS, et al. Using nasal self-esteem to predict revision in
cosmetic rhinoplasty. Aesthetic Surg J 2021;41(6):652–6.

29. Kandathil CK, Saltychev M, Abdelwahab M, et al. Minimal clinically important difference of the standardized cosmesis and health nasal outcomes survey.
Aesthetic Surg J 2019;39(8):837–40.

30. Moubayed SP, Ioannidis JPA, Saltychev M, et al. The 10-item standardized cosmesis and health nasal outcomes survey (SCHNOS) for functional and cosmetic
rhinoplasty. JAMA Facial Plast Surg 2018;20(1):37–42.

31. van Zijl FV, Declau F, Rizopoulos D, et al. The rhinoplasty rosetta stone: using rasch
analysis to create and validate crosswalks between the NOSE and SCHNOS functional subscale. Plast Reconstr Surg 2024. https://doi.org/10.1097/PRS.000000
0000011438.

32. Takhar A, Stephens J, Randhawa PS, et al. Validation of the sino-nasal outcome
test-23 in septorhinoplasty surgery. Rhinology 2014;52(4):301–4.

33. Xavier R, Azeredo-Lopes S, Menger DJ, et al. Generic health-related quality-of-
life changes after rhinoplasty: a prospective study with long-term results. Facial
Plast Surg 2023;39(02):164–72.

34. Essink-Bot ML, Stouthard ME, Bonsel GJ. Generalizability of valuations on health
states collected with the EuroQolc-questionnaire. Health Econ 1993;2(3):237–46.

35. Devlin N, Parkin D, Janssen B. An introduction to EQ-5D instruments and their applications. In: Methods for analysing and reporting EQ-5D data. Cham,
Switzerland: Springer International Publishing; 2020. p. 1–22.

36. Yamasaki A, Levesque PA, Bleier BS, et al. Improvement in nasal obstruction and
quality of life after septorhinoplasty and turbinate surgery. Laryngoscope 2019;
129(7):1554–60.

37. Fuller JC, Levesque PA, Lindsay RW. Assessment of the EuroQol 5-dimension
questionnaire for detection of clinically significant global health-related quality-
of-life improvement following functional septorhinoplasty. JAMA Facial Plast
Surg 2017;19(2):95–100.

38. Gadkaree SK, Fuller JC, Justicz NS, et al. Health utility values as an outcome
measure in patients undergoing functional septorhinoplasty. JAMA Facial Plast
Surg 2019;21(5):381–6.

Objective Outcome Measures in Nasal Valve Repair and Nasal Obstruction

Rui Xavier, MD, PhD[a],*,
Munish Shandilya, MS(ENT), FRCS Ed(OTO), FRCS(ORL-HNS)[b]

KEYWORDS

- Nasal airway obstruction • Nasal valve compromise
- Objective evaluation of the nasal airway • Acoustic rhinometry • Rhinomanometry
- Peak nasal inspiratory flow • Computational fluid dynamics

KEY POINTS

- Diagnosis of nasal valve compromise (NVC) is clinical, but objective evaluation of the nasal airway may corroborate this diagnosis and quantify the extent of its impairment on nasal airflow.
- Computational fluid dynamics (CFD) analysis may demonstrate changes of the normal nasal airway conditions and localize these changes to the nasal valve.
- Surgery is the treatment of choice for nasal airway obstruction caused by NVC.
- Results of surgical treatment of NVC may be assessed by different methods of objective evaluation of the nasal airway, demonstrating changes in nasal valve dimensions and in nasal airflow or in nasal airway resistance.
- The demonstration of improvement of the various parameters of the nasal airway by objective methods of evaluation stands for the recognition of the efficacy of surgery for treating NVC and corroborates that surgery should be considered in patients with NVC.

INTRODUCTION

Nasal airway obstruction (NAO) can significantly impair quality-of-life, negatively affecting nearly all domains of health-related quality-of-life.[1–4] Nasal valve compromise (NVC) has been recognized as a distinct etiologic factor for NAO, being able to cause NAO *per se* or in combination with other etiologic factors.[5]

Surgery has been considered the treatment of choice for NVC by a Consensus Statement of the American Academy of Otolaryngology.[5] Before a decision to proceed

[a] Department of Otorhinolaryngology, Hospital Luz Arrabida, Porto, Portugal; [b] The Nose Clinic, Dublin, Ireland
* Corresponding author. Department of Otorhinolaryngology, Hospital Luz Arrabida, Praceta Henrique Moreira 150, Vila Nova de Gaia 4400-346, Portugal.
E-mail address: rjxavier65@gmail.com

Otolaryngol Clin N Am 58 (2025) 215–226
https://doi.org/10.1016/j.otc.2024.08.006
0030-6665/25/© 2024 Elsevier Inc. All rights are reserved, including those for text and data mining, AI training, and similar technologies.

to surgery is taken it is crucial that NVC is properly identified and that its impairment on nasal breathing is assessed. Also importantly, results of surgery of NVC should be evaluated, so that the surgical options leading to more significant and more consistent improvements of NAO may be offered to and discussed with each patient with NVC.

PRE-OPERATIVE ASSESSMENT OF PATIENTS WITH NASAL VALVE COMPROMISE

The diagnosis of NVC is a clinical one. Complementary examinations may be used to exclude other causes of NAO and may, in selected cases, support the clinical diagnosis of NVC. Imaging studies of the nasal airway such as computed tomography (CT) or MRI can be used to measure the internal nasal valve (INV) angle and area (**Figs. 1** and **2**). These measurements should preferably be obtained from reformatted coronal oblique planes, perpendicular to the nasal dorsum in a sagittal plane (**Fig. 3**), as these planes more accurately reflect the path of the nasal airflow at the INV.[6–8] Measurements obtained from these imaging examinations may possibly demonstrate a narrow INV angle or a decreased INV area,[9,10] documenting static NVC at the INV. INV area—but not INV angle—may also be evaluated by acoustic rhinometry (AR), which is considered the most accurate method to measure the cross-sectional area of the INV.[6] However, normal values of INV angle and area taken from AR or from imaging studies do not exclude NVC at the INV, as these measurements may fail to demonstrate dynamic NVC.

NVC at the external nasal valve (ENV) is most frequently a dynamic dysfunction, therefore rarely apparent in imaging studies or in AR measurements. Furthermore, the position of the AR probe at the entrance of the nasal airway may prevent dynamic collapse of the ENV to be fully apparent, thus limiting the usefulness of AR to assess NVC at the ENV.

Measurements of nasal airway resistance or of nasal airflow by rhinomanometry (RMM) or by peak nasal inspiratory flow (PNIF) may be useful to evaluate the impairment of nasal breathing in each individual case, but this impairment is not specific of NVC. Furthermore, in cases of severe lateral wall insufficiency (LWI) it may be

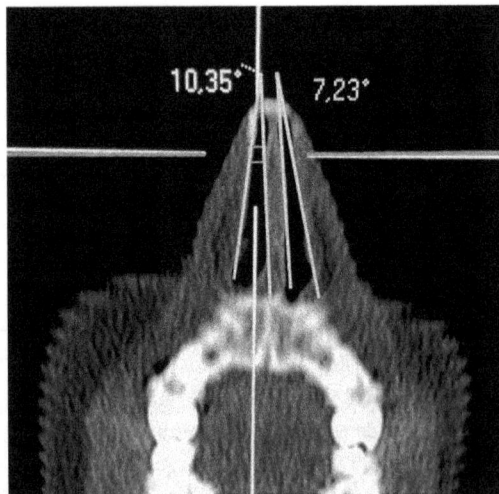

Fig. 1. The nasal valve angle was measured along the medial and lateral margins of the airway lumen averaging the contour irregularities.

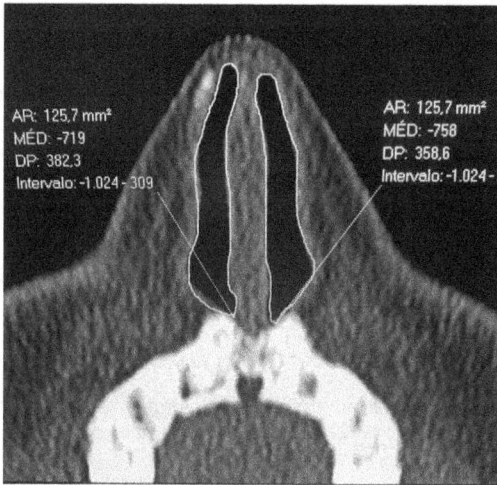

Fig. 2. The cross-section area of the nasal valve was measured along the margins of the airway lumen.

impossible to obtain measurements of nasal airflow with PNIF due to total collapse of the nasal airway.

The same lack of specificity for NVC applies to patient-reported assessment of nasal breathing. This assessment will quantify the impairment in nasal breathing experienced by the patient, but the score thus produced will not be specific of NVC.

Computational fluid dynamics (CFD) analysis of the nasal airway can identify changes of nasal airflow, of nasal airway pressure, of nasal cavity wall shear stress, of nasal mucosal heat transfer, of nasal airflow paths and of other physics' variables inside the nasal airway due to NVC. Not only CFD can determine the precise location

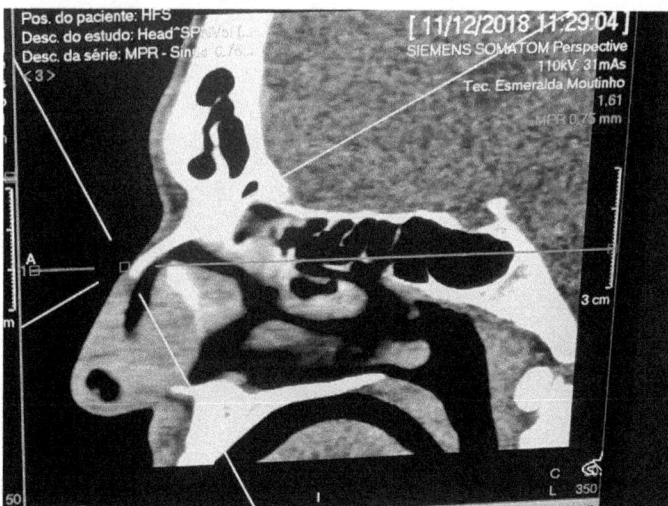

Fig. 3. The reformatted coronal oblique plane, perpendicular to the nasal dorsum in a sagittal plane.

of these changes inside the nasal airway, thereby identifying the anatomic area responsible for these derangements, but it can also predict variations of these physics' variables secondary to modifications of the nasal airway on virtual surgery (**Figs. 4** and **5**). This unique capacity of CFD also applies to surgical enlargement of the nasal valve.[11,12] Nevertheless, it may be more difficult to predict the effect on physics' variables inside the nasal airway of surgical reinforcement of the lateral nasal wall due to technical limitations to produce this reinforcement with virtual surgery. Even so, CFD analysis may be useful to the diagnostic assessment of NVC and to assist the clinical decision of selecting the surgical technique or combination of techniques that will likely better address the cause of NVC and improve nasal breathing in each individual case.

EVALUATION OF RESULTS OF SURGERY OF NASAL VALVE COMPROMISE

Surgery is the treatment of choice for NVC.[5] Systematic reviews of studies addressing results of surgery for NVC have found that surgery targeted to the specific cause or causes of NVC improves NAO.[13–17]

The results of surgical treatment of NVC may be evaluated by several different ways: measuring changes of nasal airflow, of nasal airway resistance, of nasal valve dimensions, of nasal breathing sensation and of the degree of LWI. Additionally, CFD analysis of the nasal airway may be conducted after surgery for NVC.

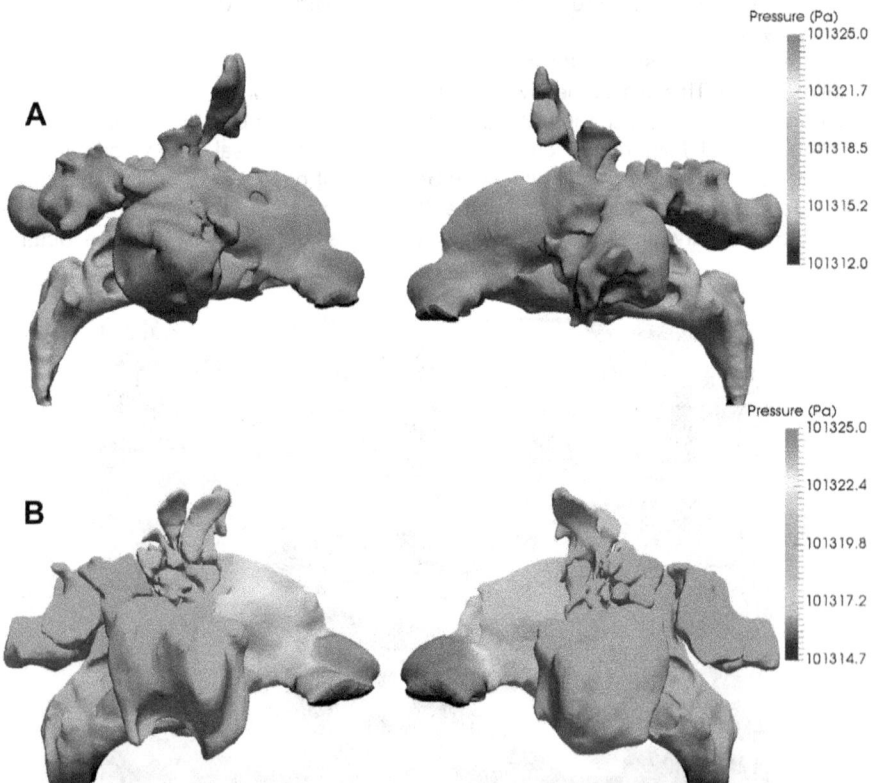

Fig. 4. CFD analysis of airway pressure of a nasal airway with septal perforation. (*A*) Before virtual closure and (*B*) after virtual closure of the perforation (inhaled air pressure101325 Pa, nasopharynx pressure 101,312 Pa).

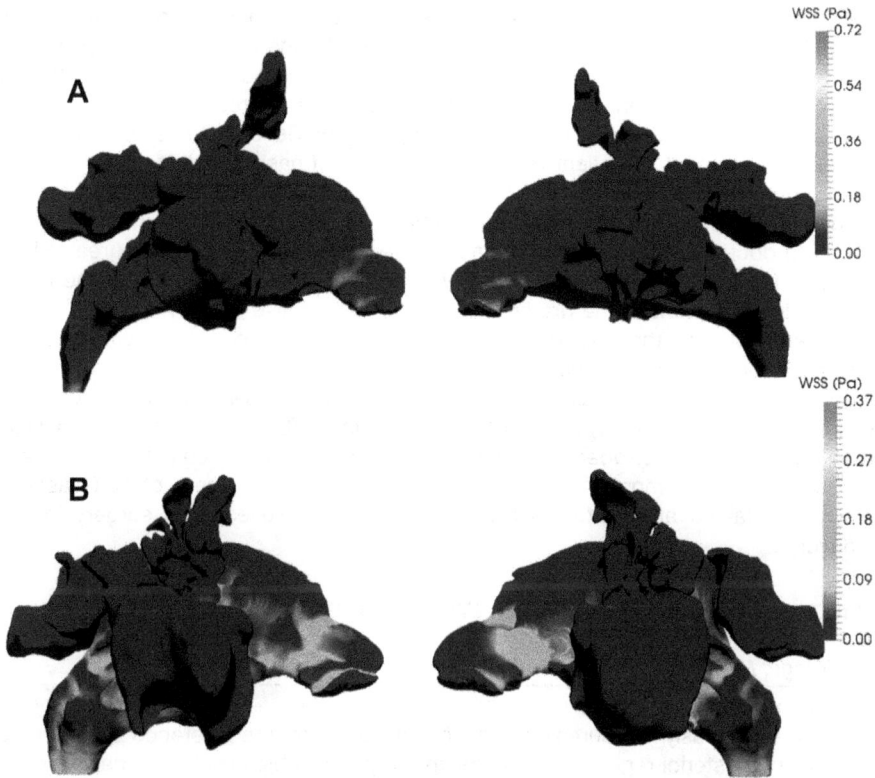

Fig. 5. CFD analysis of wall shear stress of a nasal airway with septal perforation. (*A*) Before virtual closure and (*B*) after virtual closure of the perforation (inhaled air pressure 101325 Pa, nasopharynx pressure 101,312 Pa, airflow rate 6.37 L/min before virtual surgery and 14.26 L/min after virtual surgery).

Methods used for the evaluation of results of nasal valve surgery may be classified as.

- Physiologic methods
- Anatomic methods
- Patient-reported evaluation of nasal breathing
- Physician-derived evaluation of NVC
- CFD analysis of the nasal airway

Physiologic methods measure nasal airflow or nasal airway resistance. These methods include measurements made by RMM and by PNIF. Several studies using physiologic methods have demonstrated an improvement of nasal airflow and a decrease of nasal airway resistance after surgery addressing NVC.[18–20]

Anatomic methods include measurements of the nasal valve dimensions produced by AR or obtained from imaging studies of the nasal airway such as CT or MRI. Anatomic methods have demonstrated enlargement of INV area or widening of INV angle after surgery to address NVC.[19,21] However, anatomic methods may fail to demonstrate changes introduced by surgery aiming to reinforce lateral wall resistance as to improve LWI and hence a lack of demonstration of increased dimensions of the nasal valve does not imply an unfavourable result of surgery.

Patient-reported evaluation of nasal breathing uses validated disease-specific scales to assess the degree of NAO as appreciated by the patient. This assessment of nasal breathing has the advantage of quantifying the degree of subjective sensation of nasal breathing experienced by the patient and the degree of interference with routine daily activities caused by breathing impairment. Several studies have demonstrated improvement of patient-reported evaluation of nasal breathing after surgery aiming to correct NVC.[4,13,14,19,21–28]

Physician-derived evaluation of NVC relies on the assessment made by the attending doctor of modifications in nasal valve dimensions or in the degree of LWI achieved by surgery. Several studies have demonstrated enlargement of the nasal valve or improvement of the grade of LWI after nasal valve surgery.[11,20,29,30] It has been demonstrated that this physician-derived evaluation correlates with patient-reported scoring of nasal breathing.[4,20,30]

CFD analysis of the nasal airway may demonstrate changes in several physics' variables inside the nasal airway after surgery addressing NVC. However, for this analysis to be conducted a post-operative imaging study is required, which is rarely clinically justified. Therefore, most studies using CFD to evaluate surgery of NVC assess changes obtained after virtual surgery or changes achieved after surgery in the cadaver.

OBJECTIVE OUTCOME METHODS FOR EVALUATION OF RESULTS OF SURGERY OF NASAL VALVE COMPROMISE
Physiologic Methods

Rhinomanometry
RMM simultaneously measures nasal airflow and the pressure difference between the anterior and posterior regions of the nose, thereby being able to calculate nasal airway resistance. These measurements of nasal airway resistance and of nasal airflow allow an objective evaluation of nasal breathing in each individual case. Therefore, comparing pre and post-operative measurements obtained by RMM may evaluate and quantify changes of nasal airflow and of nasal airway resistance achieved by surgery addressing NVC.

RMM has demonstrated an increase of nasal airflow after surgery of the nasal valve. This increase has been quantified as a 2x increase after surgery of the INV, as a 2.6x increase after surgery of the ENV, as a 3.8x increase after surgery of both INV and ENV and as a 4.9x increase after surgery of both nasal valves plus septoplasty.[18] RMM has also demonstrated that an enlargement of INV angle leads to a decrease of nasal airway resistance[31] as would be expected from Poiseulle's Law. The decrease of nasal airway resistance after using different surgical techniques to address NVC has also been measured with RMM. Nasal airway resistance was decreased in patients with NVC by both spreader grafts and autospreader flaps, with no significative difference in the decrease obtained between these 2 surgical techniques.[32] A systematic review of studies addressing results of functional rhinoplasty has found that RMM measurements were improved by surgery addressing NVC.[16]

Peak nasal inspiratory flow
Peak nasal inspiratory flow allows a readily available measurement of the peak inspiratory flow, using an inverted peak flow meter connected to a size appropriated facial mask. Despite its simplicity, the reproducibility of the results obtained by PNIF measurements has been demonstrated.[33,34] Despite the significant variation in PNIF values obtained from different asymptomatic individuals, PNIF measurements obtained from the same patient at diverse occasions effectively assess changes in nasal

airflow. An immediate increase in the value of PNIF after applying nasal dilators in patients with NVC has been demonstrated.[35] In the same line, PNIF measurements taken from the same patient before and after surgery addressing NVC may be used to evaluate changes in nasal airflow achieved by surgery.

The value of PNIF increases after surgery of the nasal valve with both spreader grafts and autospreader flaps, but bilateral spreader grafts produce a significantly higher increase than autospreader flaps or a combination of autospreader flaps plus a unilateral spreader graft.[36] A significant association between INV area and the value of PNIF has been demonstrated.[37] A linear correlation between the increase in the INV area and the increase in PNIF value has been demonstrated, with this correlation being maintained even after adjusting the value of INV area with the value of the corresponding INV angle.[37]

An improvement of the value of PNIF after surgery addressing the ENV has also been demonstrated. Suspension suture of the lateral crura improved PNIF measurement.[38] The same was demonstrated after lateral crural strut grafts and after lateral crural turn-in flaps for treatment of NVC at the ENV.[19]

ANATOMIC METHODS
Acoustic Rhinometry

Acoustic rhinometry has been considered the best method for measuring the dimensions of the anterior part of the nasal airway and, specifically, of the cross-sectional area of the INV.[6] Equally, AR measurements have been considered superior to measurements taken from CT imaging of the nasal airway for assessing results of surgery addressing the INV.[39] AR is also superior to RMM as an objective method to evaluate results of surgery of the INV, with higher sensitivity and higher specificity.[40]

NVC at the INV is usually a static obstruction and, as so, most surgical techniques addressing INV aim to enlarge the INV. Enlargement of the INV area after nasal valve surgery has been demonstrated by studies using AR.[41,42] The specific effect of different surgical techniques on INV area has been studied by AR measurements. An enlargement of INV cross-sectional area has been demonstrated when spreader grafts are used,[42] when a combination of spreader grafts and flaring suture is used,[29,43] but not when spreader flaps are the surgical option.[44] The individual contribution to the increase in INV cross-sectional area produced by spreader grafts and by flaring suture has also been quantified by AR: an increase in INV cross-sectional area of 9.1% when only a flaring suture is used and an increase of 18.7% when a flaring suture is used in combination with spreader grafts.[29]

Imaging Methods

Measurements of nasal valve dimensions may also be made on CT and MRI imaging studies of the nasal airway. The capacity for measuring the INV angle is a distinct advantage of imaging studies over AR. However, after surgery of the nasal valve there is rarely clinical indication for imaging studies of the nasal airway, hence the sparsity of studies comparing pre and post-operative dimensions of the nasal valve using imaging studies. Measurements obtained from imaging studies have been used to assess INV dimensions preoperatively, but their reliability to assess results of surgery of the nasal valve has been questioned.[9,39] However, this disbelieve refers to studies evaluating measurements of the INV obtained from standard axial planes instead of the reformatted coronal oblique planes, perpendicular to the nasal dorsum in a sagittal plane (see **Fig. 3**). These planes should be chosen as they more accurately reflect the path of the nasal airflow at the INV.[6–8] An increase in INV area after surgery using spreader grafts and spreader flaps has been documented on imaging studies of the nasal airway.[45] Equally, an increase in the cross-sectional area of the nasal airway after surgery of the ENV has been documented by measurements made on CT scan.[46]

Computational Fluid Dynamics

CFD analysis of the nasal airway requires an imaging study, as CT or MRI of the nasal airway, to create the virtual 3D model of the nasal airway into which CFD analysis runs. As mentioned above, this limits the use for post-operative CFD analysis, as imaging studies are rarely indicated after surgery of the nasal valve. As so, most studies using CFD analysis to evaluate the functional effect of surgical techniques addressing NVC have been conducted in cadaver specimens. Nevertheless, in the rare occasion in which a postoperative imaging study is clinically indicated, such as failure of symptomatic improvement after surgery of NVC, CFD analysis can provide crucial information of the conditions inside the nasal airway.

Similarly to other objective physiologic evaluation methods, the results produced by CFD analysis reflect not only the modifications of nasal valve dimensions achieved by surgery but also the possible surgical reinforcement of the lateral nasal wall for correction of LWI. In contrast with other objective physiologic studies, though, CFD analysis is performed under close to reality airway conditions, not requiring, for example, higher than normal nasal airflow rates. More than any other objective evaluation of the nasal airway, results of CFD analysis correlate with patient-reported assessment of nasal breathing. Changes in peak mucosal cooling inside the nasal airway, for example, are known to be related to modifications of the subjective sensation of nasal breathing. After surgery of the INV, changes in peak nasal airway mucosal cooling have been demonstrated by CFD, despite no measurable modification of nasal airflow or of nasal airway resistance.[47]

CFD analysis has been used to assess surgery of the INV in the cadaver, finding that spreader grafts improve nasal airflow but may worsen nasal airway resistance.[11] The same study also addressed the role of the flaring suture and found the location of the suture to be determinant to its functional outcome, with a more significant functional improvement when a medially placed or a modified flaring suture is used.[11]

CFD analysis has demonstrated a decrease in nasal airway resistance after butterfly grafts and after spreader grafts, with the decrease being more significant when a butterfly graft was used.[12] A different study using mucosal heat transfer has found spreader grafts to be functionally as efficient as a butterfly graft.[48]

Evaluation of Nasal Valve Compromise Surgery in Clinical Practice

The evaluation of results of nasal valve surgery made by these different methods allows different perspectives of the changes produced on the nasal airway by nasal valve repair. Anatomic methods essentially assess modifications of the dimensions of the nasal valve after surgery. As such, these methods are most suitable to evaluate surgery targeted to an enlargement of the nasal valve, particularly at the INV, the location where these methods can prove most useful. Conversely, physiologic methods assess improvements of nasal airflow and decreases of nasal airway resistance achieved by surgery of INV or ENV and after surgery aiming to enlarge the nasal valve or to reinforce the lateral nasal wall. Therefore, physiologic methods may be used to evaluate the efficacy of all surgical techniques designed to address NVC.

However, and with the exception of CFD analysis, objective evaluation of the nasal airway does not always correlate with patient-reported assessment of nasal breathing. In clinical practice, patient-reported evaluation has thus emerged as the most frequently used method for NAO assessment, including NAO caused by NVC. In line with this, many studies have evaluated the results of nasal valve surgery by using predominantly or exclusively patient-reported assessment of nasal breathing.[15–17,28]

Nevertheless, objective evaluation of changes in nasal airway dimensions, resistance or in nasal airflow achieved by different surgical techniques will provide valuable information to estimate the efficacy of each surgical technique to effectively fulfill its purposes. This information will prove useful to assist on the clinical decision of choosing the most adequate surgical technique in each individual clinical scenario of NVC.

In clinical practice, knowledge of the changes achieved by surgery in nasal airflow or in nasal airway resistance or dimensions in combination with patient-reported evaluation of nasal breathing can enlighten the circumstance of clinical unsuccess of surgical treatment of NVC. This piece of objective information, well interpreted, will assist the surgeon on understanding the reasons for this surgical failure and on deciding the most appropriate way to provide symptomatic improvement of NVC.

A combination of objective and patient-reported evaluations may also prove useful in the preoperative assessment of patients with NAO due to NVC, by helping to decide which patients will most likely improve from an enlargement of the nasal valve or from a reinforcement of the mechanical resistance of the lateral nasal wall.

On a different angle, the demonstration of improvement of the various parameters of the nasal airway by objective methods of evaluation stands for the recognition of the efficacy of surgery for treating NVC and corroborates that surgery should certainly be offered to most patients with NVC.

SUMMARY

The diagnosis of NVC is clinical. However, objective evaluation of the nasal airway may corroborate this diagnosis and quantify the extent of its impairment on nasal airflow. Anatomic methods measure the dimensions of the nasal valve while physiologic methods quantify the impairment on nasal airflow and on nasal airway resistance produced by NVC. Furthermore, CFD analysis may demonstrate changes of the normal nasal airway conditions and localize these changes to the nasal valve. Objective data can be useful to quantify the impairment caused by NVC and to assist on the clinical decision of choosing the most adequate surgical technique in each clinical case of NVC.

Surgery is the treatment of choice for NVC. Results of surgery may be assessed by objective evaluation of the nasal airway. Anatomic methods may be used to quantify modifications of the dimensions of the nasal valve after surgery. These methods are most suitable to evaluate surgery targeted to an enlargement of the nasal valve, particularly at the INV. Physiologic methods may be used to quantify changes in nasal airflow and in nasal airway resistance achieved by any surgical technique addressing NVC.

Objective evaluation in combination with patient-reported evaluation of nasal breathing can enlighten the scenario of clinical unsuccess of surgical treatment of NVC. The demonstration of improvement of the various parameters of the nasal airway by objective methods of evaluation stands for the recognition of the efficacy of surgery for treating NVC and corroborates that surgery should be considered in patients with NVC.

CLINICS CARE POINTS

- Anatomic methods measure the dimensions of the nasal valve and may be used to quantify modifications of these dimensions after surgery. These methods are most suitable to evaluate surgery targeted to an enlargement of the nasal valve, particularly at the INV.

- Physiologic methods quantify the impairment on nasal airflow and on nasal airway resistance produced by NVC and may be used to quantify changes in these parameters achieved by surgery. Physiologic methods may be used to evaluate the efficacy of all forms of surgery of NVC.

- Objective data can be useful to quantify the impairment caused by NVC and to assist on the clinical decision of choosing the most adequate surgical technique in each clinical case of NVC.

- A combination of objective and patient-reported evaluations may prove useful in the preoperative assessment of patients with NAO due to NVC, by helping to decide which patients will most likely improve from an enlargement of the nasal valve or from a reinforcement of the mechanical resistance of the lateral nasal wall.

- Objective evaluation in combination with patient-reported evaluation of nasal breathing can enlighten the scenario of clinical unsuccess of surgical treatment of NVC.

DISCLOSURE

The authors have nothing to disclose.

REFERENCES

1. Fuller J, Levesque P, Lindsay R. Assessment of the EuroQol 5-dimension questionnaire for detection of clinically significant global health-related quality-of-life improvement following functional septorhinoplasty. JAMA Facial Plast Surg 2017;19:95–100.
2. Stewart M, Ferguson B, Fromer L. Epidemiology and burden of nasal congestion. Int J Gen Med 2010;3:37–45.
3. Rhee J, Book D, Burzynski M, et al. Quality of life assessment in nasal airway obstruction. Laryngoscope 2003;113:1118–22.
4. Rhee J, Poetker D, Smith L, et al. Nasal valve surgery improves disease-specific quality of life. Laryngoscope 2005;115:437–40.
5. Rhee J, Weaver E, Park S, et al. Clinical consensus statement: diagnosis and management of nasal valve compromise. Otolaryngol Head Neck Surg 2010; 143:48–59.
6. Cakmak O, Coskun M, Celik H, et al. Value of acoustic rhinometry for measuring nasal valve area. Laryngoscope 2003;113:295–302.
7. Poetker D, Rhee J, Mocan B, et al. Computed tomography technique for evaluation of the nasal valve. Arch Facial Plast Surg 2004;6:240–3.
8. Bakker N, Lohuis P, Menger D, et al. Objective computerized determination of the minimum cross-sectional area of the nasal passage on computed tomography. Laryngoscope 2005;115:1809–12.
9. Moche J, Cohen J, Pearlman S. Axial computed tomography evaluation of the internal nasal valve correlates with clinical valve narrowing and patient complaint. Int Forum Allergy Rhinol 2013;3:592–7.
10. Wu J, Wang X, Chen Y, et al. Radiographic study of the nasal valve in different CT evaluation method in Asian patients with unilateral cleft lip nose. Aesthetic Plast Surg 2024;48:2412–22.
11. Shadfar S, Shockley W, Fleischman G, et al. Characterization of postoperative changes in nasal airflow using a cadaveric computational fluid dynamics model: supporting the internal nasal valve. JAMA Facial Plast Surg 2014;16:319–27.
12. Brandon B, Stepp W, Basu S, et al. Nasal airflow changes with bioabsorbable implant, butterfly, and spreader grafts. Laryngoscope 2020;130:E817–23.

13. Rhee J, Arganbright J, McMullin B, et al. Evidence supporting functional rhinoplasty or nasal valve repair: a 25-year systematic review. Otolaryngol Head Neck Surg 2008;139:10–20.
14. Spielmann P, White P, Hussain S. Surgical techniques for the treatment of nasal valve collapse: a systematic review. Laryngoscope 2009;119:1281–90.
15. Kandathil C, Spataro E, Laimi K, et al. Repair of the lateral nasal wall in nasal airway obstruction: a systematic review and meta-analysis. JAMA Facial Plast Surg 2018;20:307–13.
16. Zhao R, Chen K, Tang Y. Effects of functional rhinoplasty on nasal obstruction: a meta-analysis. Aesthetic Plast Surg 2022;46:873–85.
17. Floyd E, Ho S, Patel P, et al. Systematic review and meta-analysis of studies evaluating functional rhinoplasty outcomes with the NOSE score. Otolaryngol Head Neck Surg 2017;156:809–15.
18. Constantian M, Clardy R. The relative importance of septal and nasal valvular surgery in correcting airway obstruction in primary and secondary rhinoplasty. Plast Reconstr Surg 1996;98:38–54.
19. Barham H, Knisely A, Christensen J, et al. Costal cartilage lateral crural strut graft vs cephalic crural turn-in for correction of external valve dysfunction. JAMA Facial Plast Surg 2015;17:340–5.
20. Abdelwahab M, Patel P, Kandathil C, et al. Effect of lateral crural procedures on nasal wall stability and tip aesthetics in rhinoplasty. Laryngoscope 2021;131:E1830–7.
21. Most S. Analysis of outcomes after functional rhinoplasty using a disease-specific quality-of-life instrument. Arch Facial Plast Surg 2006;8:306–9.
22. Toriumi D, Cristel R. Lateral crural repositioning: implications on nasal function. Facial Plast Surg 2023;39:547–55.
23. Recker C, Hamilton G. Evaluation of the patient with nasal obstruction. Facial Plast Surg 2016;32:3–8.
24. Silva E. The relation between the lower lateral cartilages and the function of the external nasal valve. Aesthetic Plast Surg 2019;43:175–83.
25. Calloway H, Heilbronn C, Gu J, et al. Functional outcomes, quantitative morphometry, and aesthetic analysis of articulated alar rim grafts in septorhinoplasty. JAMA Facial Plast Surg 2019;21:558–65.
26. Chambers K, Horstkotte K, Shanley K, et al. Evaluation of improvement in nasal obstruction following nasal valve correction in patients with a history of failed septoplasty. JAMA Facial Plast Surg 2015;17:347–50.
27. Yeung A, Hassouneh B, Kim DW. Outcome of nasal valve obstruction after functional and aesthetic-functional rhinoplasty. JAMA Facial Plast Surg 2016;18:128–34.
28. Schlosser R, Park S. Surgery for the dysfunctional nasal valve: cadaveric analysis and clinical outcomes. Arch Facial Plast Surg 1999;1:105–10.
29. Vaezeafshar R, Moubayed S, Most S. Repair of lateral wall insufficiency. JAMA Facial Plast Surg 2018;20:111–5.
30. Poirrier A, Ahluwalia S, Kwame I, et al. External nasal valve collapse: validation of novel outcome measurement tool. Rhinology 2014;52:127–32.
31. Miman M, Deliktas H, Ozturan O, et al. Internal nasal valve: revisited with objective facts. Otolaryngol Head Neck Surg 2006;134:41–7.
32. Zeid N, Mohamed A, ElSayed ElFouly M, et al. Objective comparison between spreader grafts and flaps for mid-nasal vault reconstruction: a randomized controlled trial. Plast Surg (Oakv) 2020;28(3):137–41.

33. Volstad I, Olafsson T, Steinsvik E, et al. Minimal unilateral peak nasal inspiratory flow correlates with patient reported nasal obstruction. Rhinology 2019;57: 436–43.

34. Ottaviano G, Pendolino A, Nardello E, et al. Peak nasal inspiratory flow measurement and visual analogue scale in a large adult population. Clin Otolaryngol 2019;44:541–8.

35. Lekakis G, Dekimpe E, Steelant B, et al. Managing nasal valve compromise patients with nasal dilators: objective vs. subjective parameters. Rhinology 2016;54: 348–54.

36. Xavier R, Azeredo-Lopes S, Menger D, et al. Comparative functional effect of alternative surgical techniques used in rhinoplasty. Ann Otol Rhinol Laryngol 2023;132:638–47.

37. Xavier R, Azeredo-Lopes S, Menger D, et al. Which nasal airway dimensions correlate with nasal airflow and with nasal breathing sensation? Facial Plast Surg Aesthet Med 2021. https://doi.org/10.1089/fpsam.2021.0148.

38. Manickavasagam J, Iqbal I, Wong S, et al. Alar suspension sutures in the management of nasal valve collapse. Ann Otol Rhinol Laryngol 2015;124:740–4.

39. AlEnazi A, Alshathri A, Alshathri A, et al. Assessment and diagnostic methods of internal nasal valve: systematic review and meta-analysis. JPRAS Open 2023;40: 158–69.

40. Ansari E, Rogister F, Lefebvre P, et al. Responsiveness of acoustic rhinometry to septorhinoplasty by comparison with rhinomanometry and subjective instruments. Clin Otolaryngol 2019;44:778–83.

41. Friedman M, Ibrahim H, Lee G, et al. A simplified technique for airway correction at the nasal valve area. Otolaryngol Head Neck Surg 2004;131:519–24.

42. Erickson B, Hurowitz R, Jeffery C, et al. Acoustic rhinometry and video endoscopic scoring to evaluate postoperative outcomes in endonasal spreader graft surgery with septoplasty and turbinoplasty for nasal valve collapse. J Otolaryngol Head Neck Surg 2016;12. 45:51.

43. Zoumalan R, Constantinides M. Subjective and objective improvement in breathing after rhinoplasty. Arch Facial Plast Surg 2012;14:423–8.

44. Saedi B, Amali A, Gharavis V, et al. Spreader flaps do not change early functional outcomes in reduction rhinoplasty: a randomized control trial. Am J Rhinol Allergy 2014;28:70–4.

45. Zeina A, El Zeheiry A, Bahaa El-Din A. True and average internal nasal valve area in septorhinoplasty: radiological and clinical outcomes. Ann Plast Surg 2020;84: 487–93.

46. Menger D, Swart K, Nolst Trenité G, et al. Surgery of the external nasal valve: the correlation between subjective and objective measurements. Clin Otolaryngol 2014;39:150–5.

47. Wu Z, Krebs J, Spector B, et al. Regional peak mucosal cooling predicts radiofrequency treatment outcomes of nasal valve obstruction. Laryngoscope 2021; 131:E1760–9.

48. Brandon B, Austin G, Fleischman G, et al. Comparison of airflow between spreader grafts and butterfly grafts using computational flow dynamics in a cadaveric model. JAMA Facial Plast Surg 2018;20:215–21.

Preoperative Assessment of the Nasal Valve

James Eng, MD, Jon Robitschek, MD*

KEYWORDS

- Internal nasal valve • External nasal valve • Cottle maneuver

KEY POINTS

- Nasal obstruction is a complex problem, attributable to physiologic and anatomic processes, particularly as it pertains to nasal valve compromise (NVC).
- NVC is broad it its anatomic scope to include columella width, caudal/dorsal septal deviation, inferior turbinate hypertrophy, and/or attenuation of the nasal sidewall/alar rim/upper lateral cartilage.
- The foundational pillar in the successful evaluation of the nasal valve relies on a comprehensive history and physical examination.

BACKGROUND

Nasal obstruction is often a multifactorial problem, attributable to physiologic and anatomic processes. Patients are commonly referred to otolaryngologists and facial plastic and reconstructive surgeons for evaluation of anatomic causes of nasal obstruction, particularly pertaining to nasal valve compromise (NVC). The nasal valve refers to the areas within the nose that contribute to greatest overall airway resistance, and has been described as having internal and external components. The internal nasal valve (INV) is formed by the septum, the head of the inferior turbinate, and the upper lateral cartilages.[1,2] The external nasal valve (ENV) refers to the area between the nasal sill and vestibule, the caudal septum and medial crura, and the nasal ala.[3] The caudal border of the upper lateral cartilages forms the superior lateral border of the ENV (**Fig. 1**A–C).

Nasal valve compromise may be static or dynamic in nature. This is an important distinction as the two are surgically managed differently. A static issue is attributed to baseline narrowing of the area of the valves, and has also been referred to as nasal valve insufficiency in the literature. Meanwhile, a dynamic process refers to inward collapse of the nasal airway during inspiration, resulting from weakness of the intrinsic cartilages and poor soft tissue support.[4,5] This occurs as a result of increased

Division of Facial Plastics and Reconstructive Surgery, University of South Florida, Tampa, FL, USA
* Corresponding author. 5802 North 30th Street, Tampa, FL 33610.
E-mail address: robitschekj@usf.edu

Otolaryngol Clin N Am 58 (2025) 227–235
https://doi.org/10.1016/j.otc.2024.07.011
0030-6665/25/Published by Elsevier Inc.

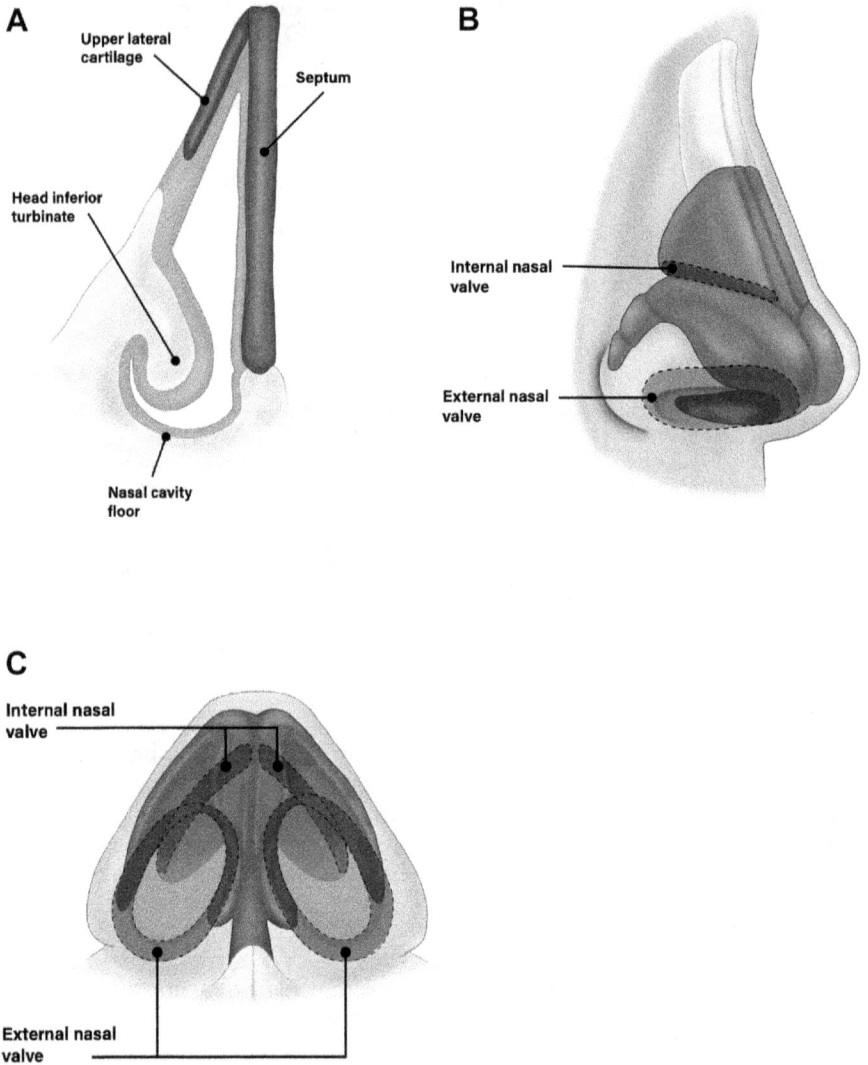

Fig. 1. Illustration depictions of (*A*) the components of the internal nasal valve, and the INV and ENV on (*B*) oblique view, and (*C*) basal view. (Image Courtesy: Haley Dragon, University of South Florida.)

transmural pressure with increased rates of airflow as described by Bernoulli principle.[1] For the purposes of this text, lateral wall insufficiency (LWI) will be used to delineate the dynamic component of nasal valve compromise.

Detailed assessment of the nasal valve is critical for appropriate preoperative planning. NVC may be implicated in up to 13% of adults suffering from chronic nasal obstruction, and is a common culprit in patients with persistent nasal obstruction following septoplasty surgery.[2] Evaluation of the nasal valve relies first and foremost on a comprehensive history and physical examination. Comparatively, other adjunctive measures such as rhinomanometry, acoustic manometry, and three-dimensional computed tomography (CT) have not proven universally useful in the diagnosis of NVC.

HISTORY AND PHYSICAL EXAMINATION

A comprehensive history should include onset of nasal obstruction, laterality, changes with positioning, and the extent to which these symptoms impact a patient's quality of life (QoL). Questions to consider when interviewing the patient might include

Are there any alleviating or exacerbating factors, and are the symptoms impacted by over-the-counter or prescription medications?
Is there a significant history of environmental or seasonal allergies?

It is also important to note any history of nasal trauma or any prior nasal surgeries. Other associated symptoms such as epistaxis, sinus pain or pressure, hyposmia or anosmia, and rhinorrhea would suggest other pathology besides NVC contributing to nasal obstruction.[2,6]

Subjective improvement in breathing with the use of nasal cones or other nasal dilators placed into the nasal vestibule may suggest ENV compromise.[3] Likewise, improvement with Breathe-Right Strips (CNS Incorporated, Minneapolis, Minnesota) could suggest LWI, INV, or ENV narrowing, depending on where along the nasal dorsum the strips are placed.[7] These devices have been shown to improve minimal cross-sectional area and nasal airflow resistance.[8] They are relatively noninvasive and inexpensive, provide potential therapeutic value to the patient, and can be used as diagnostic tools to the physician.[9,10]

According to a clinical consensus statement published by Rhee and colleagues in 2010, NVC may be attributable to a widened columella, a ptotic nasal tip, caudal or dorsal septal deviation, inferior turbinate hypertrophy, weakness of the nasal sidewall or alar rim, or collapse of the upper lateral cartilage. Additionally, there was agreement that audible or subjective improvement in nasal breathing during inspiration with stabilizing interventions (Cottle maneuver, manual intranasal lateralization of the lateral nasal sidewall) was also suggestive of NVC.[1]

External physical examination should evaluate the nose on frontal, lateral, and basal views, taking note of gross external deviations, and narrowing of the middle or lower third of the nose.[11] In particular, compromise of the internal nasal valve with associated structural loss of the nasal vault in the case of a saddle nose or inverted V deformity should be noted. Patients should be observed during both quiet and deep inspiration. Collapse of the alar rim or nasal sidewall seen with inspiration would suggest LWI.[12] Occasionally, a patient may demonstrate unilateral lateral wall collapse by occluding the contralateral nostril with his or finger. This should be discouraged, as the patient may be applying enough digital pressure to cause caudal septal and columellar deviation, creating a falsely severe degree of obstruction.[3]

Anterior rhinoscopy with a nasal speculum is a sufficient tool in identifying most internal factors contributing to obstruction, including but not limited to septal deviation or spurs, synechiae, turbinate hypertrophy, medial or lateral crura recurvature, cephalic malposition, and internal nasal valve narrowing. However, it should be noted that physical examination is not always specific, and observations of apparent abnormalities on physical examination are subject to examiner variability and may not prove to be consistently clinically significant.[13]

Palpation can provide insight into the strength of the nasal cartilages, and overall nasal tip support. Lifting the tip gently and assessing for improvement in breathing would suggest nasal tip ptosis as a potential contributor. In contrast to this, narrow nostrils appreciated on basal view can sometimes be attributed to an overprojected tip.[3]

The Cottle and modified Cottle maneuvers are commonly cited adjunctives to the physical examination designed to assess for NVC. The Cottle maneuver involves pulling the cheek and nasal sidewall laterally.[10,14] This maneuver is relatively nonspecific, and causes subjective improvement in breathing even in patients without NVC.[2] In the modified Cottle maneuver, an instrument such as a cotton tip applicator or an ear loop is used to lateralize the nasal soft tissues at the nasal valves.[9] The predictive outcomes using the modified Cottle maneuver have showed a statistically significant correlation with rhinoplasty postoperative outcomes for the ENV and INV.[15] It is important to keep in mind that the modified Cottle maneuver may still be falsely positive if excessive lateral force is applied by the examiner (**Fig. 2**A, B).

Nasal endoscopy is a powerful tool for the ENT surgeon, but has not been routinely implemented in the setting of nasal obstruction.[2] It may be useful in identifying other pathology that may not be otherwise appreciable on anterior rhinoscopy, such as obstructive concha bullosa, adenoid hypertrophy, choanal stenosis, and intranasal tumors. Lanfranchi and colleagues reported that 28 of their 95 patients presenting for rhinoplasty underwent additional surgery for findings seen on nasal endoscopy.[16] They argued that clinically relevant findings are discovered in a significant number of patients presenting with nasal obstruction symptoms, which otherwise would have been missed without a nasal endoscopy examination.

SUBJECTIVE MEASURES

Patient-reported outcome measures (PROMs) have been shown to be a more important instrument in the evaluation of nasal obstruction than any objective measure currently available. Many validated subjective tools have been developed to function as disease-specific health instruments in this patient population. Although these instruments cannot determine causes for nasal obstruction or site of obstruction, they are helpful in gauging the impact on a patient's QoL and the degree of improvement following a surgical intervention.

Visual analog scales (VAS) are one of the earliest and easiest tools applied to this patient population. Patients are asked to rate their degree of nasal symptoms on a

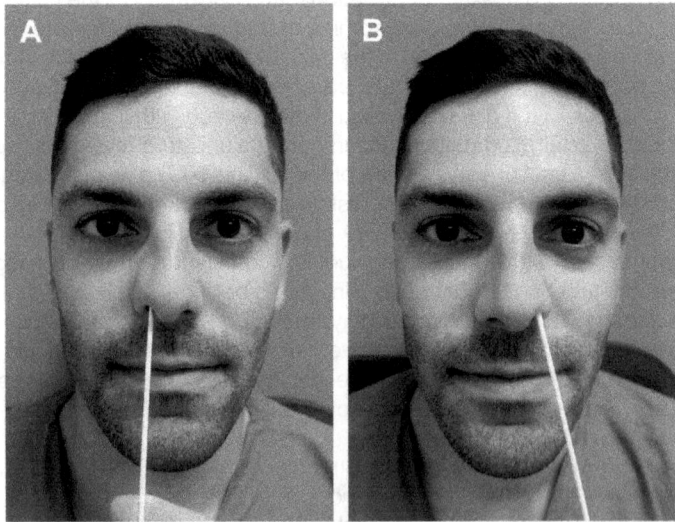

Fig. 2. Demonstration of the modified Cottle maneuver performed with the soft end of a cotton tip applicator. Having the patient inspire with the tip of the applicator stenting either the (A) middle vault or at the (B) nasal ala can delineate between INV or ENV compromise.

linear scale, from no obstruction to complete obstruction. Unlike other PROMs, the VAS can be used to assess each side of the nose separately, differentiating between unilateral or bilateral disease.[6] VAS can provide a quick picture of symptom severity, but exhibits high inter-rater and intrarater variability, and therefore has limited use as a standalone measure.[14,17]

A more specific instrument is the Nasal Obstruction Symptom Evaluation (NOSE) scale, which was introduced by Stewart and colleagues in 2003. Initially developed for patients undergoing septoplasty, this scale has 5 criteria: nasal congestion or stuffiness, nasal blockage or obstruction, trouble breathing through nose, trouble sleeping, and inability to get air through nose during exercise or exertion. A lower score correlates with a better QoL.[18] The NOSE scale has been used to show improvements in QoL for patients undergoing surgery specifically targeting NVC (**Fig. 3**).[19]

Another tool is the Sino-Nasal Outcome Test (SNOT-20), which was developed by Piccirillo and colleagues to assess multiple domains of symptom severity in patients with chronic rhinosinusitis. This has since been modified to the SNOT-22, with possible scores from 0 to 110, with a lower score correlating with higher QoL. These validated tools are able to measure clinical change in response to treatment.[20,21] SNOT-22 scores have been shown to correlate strongly with NOSE scale scores, implying that the SNOT may be used as a PROM even for patients suffering from nasal obstruction who do not have chronic rhinosinusitis.[22]

OBJECTIVE TESTS

Objective measures have not been shown to consistently correlate with subjective changes in nasal obstruction.[23,24] Additionally, objective tests often require specialized equipment, can be cost prohibitive, and may be operator dependent.[13] For these reasons, they have been used more frequently in research settings rather than clinical ones.

Peak nasal inspiratory flow measures maximal airflow during forced inspiration in liters per minute. This test depends on subject effort and may be affected by preexisting comorbidities such as pulmonary pathology. As airflow through the nose increases, the flow becomes turbulent, further limiting the ability to determine true peak flow.[25]

Rhinomanometry uses transnasal pressure differentials from the nares to the nasopharynx to measure airflow. The 3 methods of performing rhinomanometry are distinguished by the positioning of the pressure probe, and whether patients are breathing through the nose volitionally or if air is pumped through the nose with the machine, and are designated as active anterior, passive anterior, and active posterior. This tool assesses degrees of laminar or turbulent airflow, and creates pressure volume curve outputs. As each nostril is measured separately, rhinomanometry can compare resistance between the 2 sides of the nose, but cannot measure total nasal airway resistance. Rhinomanometry also cannot identify specific areas of obstruction within the nasal cavity. This technology is operator and equipment dependent, and lacks consistency in data reporting and pretest decongestion standardization.[10,26]

In acoustic rhinometry (AR), reflected sound waves recreate 2-dimensional portraits of nasal cavity geometry, which can then be used to measure volumes of cross-sectional areas. The output from AR is termed a rhinogram, a graph with characteristic notches that correspond with different areas of obstruction. The reliability of AR is operator technique and environment dependent, and although outcomes have correlated well with other objective measures, the same correlation has not been shown with PROMs and subjective nasal patency.[27,28]

Nasal Obstruction Symptom Evaluation (NOSE)
Instrument

Physician AAO-HNS#: __ __ __ __ __   Today's date: __ _/_ _/_ __ __ __

→ To the Patient: Please help us to better understand the impact of nasal obstruction on your quality of life by completing following survey. Thank You!

Over the past 1 month, how much of a problem were the following conditions for you?

Please circle the most correct response

	Not a problem	very mild problem	moderate problem	fairly bad problem	severe problem
1. Nasal congestion or stuffiness	0	1	2	3	4
2. Poor sense of smell	0	1	2	3	4
3. Snoring	0	1	2	3	4
4. Nasal blockage or obstruction	0	1	2	3	4
5. Trouble breathing through my nose	0	1	2	3	4
6. Trouble sleeping	0	1	2	3	4
7. Having to breathe through my mouth	0	1	2	3	4
8. Unable to get enough air through my nose during exercise or exertion	0	1	2	3	4
9. Feeling panic that I cannot get enough air through my nose	0	1	2	3	4
10. Embarrassment around friends and coworkers because I have trouble breathing through my nose	0	1	2	3	4
	Poor	Fair	Good	Very good	Excellent
11. In general, my health is	0	1	2	3	4

Please mark on this line how troublesome is your difficulty in breathing through your nose:

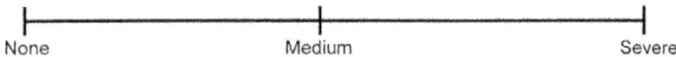

```
|------------------------|------------------------|
None                   Medium                  Severe
```

Fig. 3. The nasal obstruction symptom evaluation instrument. (Stewart MG, Witsell DL, Smith TL, Weaver EM, Yueh B, Hannley MT. Development and validation of the Nasal Obstruction Symptom Evaluation (NOSE) scale. Otolaryngol Head Neck Surg 2004;130:157-63. The NOSE Scale © 2003, the American Academy of Otolaryngology–Head and Neck Surgery Foundation.)

Nasal decongestant spray can be used with rhinomanometry and acoustic rhinometry to help elucidate whether the nasal obstruction is related to structural or mucosal causes.[26] For example, if there is no change in the volume at the minimal cross-sectional area identified on acoustic rhinometry before and after application of nasal decongestant spray, then a structural cause of obstruction would be favored.

IMAGING

Measurements of the narrowest portion of the nose at the INV angle can be made using CT. From a study by Poetker and colleagues published in 2004, coronal CT imaging data appeared to underpredict the INV angle. Meanwhile the nasal base view (NBV), perpendicular to the arc of nasal airflow through the nasal passageway known as the acoustic axis, demonstrated an INV angle more consistent with the classic teaching of 10° to 15°. Unfortunately, the determination of the acoustic axis is subjective, hence making the derived NBV and subsequent measurements inconsistent.[29]

CT results have been shown to correlate with acoustic rhinometry in postoperative patients.[30] However, there has not been a consistent relationship established between CT findings and patient subjective outcomes such as the NOSE. Additionally, there was poor correlation between the sidedness of nasal obstruction with the side of septal deviation.[31] The utility of CT in this population lies in ruling out other pathology such as sinusitis, large concha bullosa, nasal polyposis, or neoplasms, which may also be contributing to symptoms of nasal obstruction.

Computational fluid dynamics (CFD) software can be applied to CT or MRI data to predict airflow, heat transfer, and air humidification based off nasal cavity models. CFD variables of airflow resistance and heat flux have been shown to correlate with subjective nasal obstruction, and multiple studies already exist using CFD to evaluate the impact of surgical maneuvers in cadaveric specimens.[32,33] CFD modeling also has the potential to alter the shape of the nasal passageways to predict changes following surgery. Such technology is currently cost- and labor-prohibitive, and requires specialized software training, preventing its routine use in the clinical setting.[34] Models produced from these programs still hold significant promise in their potential to predict the impact of certain surgical maneuvers on nasal anatomy.

SUMMARY

The accurate diagnosis of NVC can be challenging. A comprehensive history and physical examination remain the gold standards in identifying ENV and INV pathology, or LWI as contributors to nasal obstruction. It is important to keep in mind that although physical examination is sensitive in identifying anatomic variations suggestive of NVC, in some instances, what is observed may still not necessarily be clinically relevant.[35] Subjective measures, specifically the NOSE scale, give helpful insight into the QoL implications from symptoms of nasal obstruction. PROMs are also useful in assessing for improvements in obstruction following surgery. Researchers have yet to identify an objective test that is readily accessible in the clinic setting, easily reproducible, and which strongly correlates with subjective nasal airflow. As a result objective measures are viewed as less important than subjective tests.[17] Finally, the routine use of radiographic imaging is not indicated in the evaluation of NVC. However, this may change as CFD continues to emerge as a promising means of evaluating patients with nasal obstruction and NVC.

CLINICS CARE POINTS

- History and physical examination are the key tools in establishing a diagnosis of NVC.
- Subjective measures demonstrate stronger correlation with NVC than any currently available objective test.
- Routine imaging is not needed in this patient population.

REFERENCES

1. Rhee JS, Weaver EM, Park SS, et al. Clinical consensus statement: diagnosis and management of nasal valve compromise. Otolaryngol Head Neck Surg 2010; 143(1):48–59.
2. Barrett DM, Casanueva FJ, Cook TA. Management of the nasal valve. Facial Plast Surg Clin North Am 2016;24(3):219–34.
3. Iii GSH. The external nasal valve. Facial Plast Surg Clin NA 2017;25(2): 179–94.
4. Spielmann PM, White PS, Hussain SSM. Surgical techniques for the treatment of nasal valve collapse: a systematic review. Laryngoscope 2009;119(7):1281–90.
5. Kandathil CK, Spataro EA, Laimi K, et al. Repair of the lateral nasal wall in nasal airway obstruction a systematic review and meta-analysis. JAMA Facial Plast Surg 2018;20(4):307–13.
6. Cannon DE, Rhee JS. Evidence-based practice. functional rhinoplasty. Otolaryngol Clin North Am 2012;45(5):1033–43.
7. Lin AY, Richards T. A predictive test and classification for valvular nasal obstruction using nasal strips. Plast Reconstr Surg 2010;126(1):143–5.
8. Peltonen LI, Vento SI, Simola M, et al. Effects of the nasal strip and dilator on nasal breathing - a study with healthy subjects. Rhinology 2004;42(3):122–5.
9. Gruber RP, Lin AY, Richards T. Nasal strips for evaluating and classifying valvular nasal obstruction. Aesthetic Plast Surg 2011;35(2):211–5.
10. Chandra RK, Patadia MO, Raviv J. Diagnosis of nasal airway obstruction. Otolaryngol Clin North Am 2009;42(2):207–25.
11. Chambers KJ, Horstkotte KA, Shanley K, et al. Evaluation of improvement in nasal obstruction following nasal valve correction in patients with a history of failed septoplasty. JAMA Facial Plast Surg 2015;17(5):347–50.
12. Constantian MB, Aiach G. The incompetent external nasal valve: pathophysiology and treatment in primary and secondary rhinoplasty. Plast Reconstr Surg 1994;93(5):919–33.
13. Rhee JS, Arganbright JM, McMullin BT, et al. Evidence supporting functional rhinoplasty or nasal valve repair: a 25-year systematic review. Otolaryngol Head Neck Surg 2008;139(1):10–20.
14. Keeler J, Most SP. Measuring nasal obstruction. Facial Plast Surg Clin North Am 2016;24(3):315–22.
15. Fung E, Hong P, Moore C, et al. The effectiveness of modified cottle maneuver in predicting outcomes in functional rhinoplasty. Plast Surg Int 2014; 2014:1–6.
16. Lanfranchi PV, Steiger J, Sparano A, et al. Diagnostic and surgical endoscopy in functional septorhinoplasty. Facial Plast Surg 2004;20(3):207–15.
17. Mohan S, Fuller JC, Ford SF, et al. Diagnostic and therapeutic management of nasal airway obstruction advances in diagnosis and treatment. JAMA Facial Plast Surg 2018;20(5):409–18.
18. Stewart MG, Witsell DL, Smith TL, et al. Development and validation of the Nasal Obstruction Symptom Evaluation (NOSE) scale. Otolaryngol Head Neck Surg 2004;130(2):157–63.
19. Most SP. Analysis of outcomes after functional rhinoplasty using a disease-specific quality-of-life instrument. Arch Facial Plast Surg 2006;8(5):306–9.
20. Piccirillo JF, Merritt MG, Richards ML. Psychometric and clinimetric validity of the 20-Item Sino-Nasal Outcome Test (SNOT-20). Otolaryngol Head Neck Surg 2002; 126(1):41–7.

21. Tait SD, Kallogjeri D, Chidambaram S, et al. Psychometric and clinimetric validity of the modified 25-item Sino-Nasal Outcome Test. Am J Rhinol Allergy 2019; 33(5):577–85.
22. Behnke J, Dundervill C, Bulbul M, et al. Using the Sino-Nasal Outcome Test (SNOT-22) to study outcome of treatment of nasal obstruction. Am J Otolaryngol - Head Neck Med Surg 2023;44(4):103879.
23. Gordon ASD, McCaffrey TV, Kern EB, et al. Rhinomanometry for preopoerative and postoperative assessment of nasal obstruction. Otolaryngol Head Neck Surg 1989;101(1):20–6.
24. Lam DJ, James KT, Weaver EM. Comparison of anatomic, physiological, and subjective measures of the nasal airway. Am J Rhinol 2006;20(5):463–70.
25. Bermüller C, Kirsche H, Rettinger G, et al. Diagnostic accuracy of peak nasal inspiratory flow and rhinomanometry in functional rhinosurgery. Laryngoscope 2008;118(4):605–10.
26. Nivatvongs W, Earnshaw J, Roberts D, et al. Re: Correlation between subjective and objective evaluation of the nasal airway. A systematic review of the highest level of evidence. Clin Otolaryngol 2011;36(2):181–2.
27. Lal D, Corey JP. Acoustic rhinometry and its uses in rhinology and diagnosis of nasal obstruction. Facial Plast Surg Clin North Am 2004;12(4):397–405.
28. Garcia GJM, Hariri BM, Patel RG, et al. The relationship between nasal resistance to airflow and the airspace minimal cross-sectional area. J Biomech 2016;49(9): 1670–8.
29. Poetker DM, Rhee JS, Mocan BO, et al. Computed tomography technique for evaluation of the nasal valve. Arch Facial Plast Surg 2004;6(4):240–3.
30. Prasun D, Jura N, Tomi H, et al. Nasal airway volumetric measurement using segmented HRCT images and acoustic rhinometry. Am J Rhinol 1999;13(2): 97–103.
31. Ardeshirpour F, McCarn KE, McKinney AM, et al. Computed tomography scan does not correlate with patient experience of nasal obstruction. Laryngoscope 2016;126(4):820–5.
32. Brandon BM, Austin GK, Fleischman G, et al. Comparison of airflow between spreader grafts and butterfly grafts using computational flow dynamics in a cadaveric model. JAMA Facial Plast Surg 2018;20(3):215–21.
33. Bu R, Oldenburg AL, Kimbell JS. Anatomic optical coherence tomography (aOCT) for evaluation of the internal nasal valve. Laryngoscope 2023;132(11): 2148–56.
34. Garcia GJM, Rhee JS, Senior BA, et al. Septal deviation and nasal resistance: an investigation using virtual surgery and computational fluid dynamics. Am J Rhinol Allergy 2010;24(1):46–53.
35. Spataro E, Most SP. Measuring nasal obstruction outcomes. Otolaryngol Clin North Am 2018;51(5):883–95.

Postoperative Pain and Perioperative Antibiotic Management in Functional Rhinoplasty

Jaclyn Lee, MD[a], Monica K. Rossi-Meyer, MD[b],
Shiayin F. Yang, MD[b], Scott J. Stephan, MD[b],
Priyesh N. Patel, MD[b],*

KEYWORDS

- Rhinoplasty • Pain management • Opioids • Antibiotic prophylaxis

KEY POINTS

- A multimodal pain regimen and preoperative counseling and expectations setting is recommended to reduce opioid use in postrhinoplasty pain control.
- Acetaminophen and nonsteroidal antiinflammatory drug combination regimens have demonstrated noninferiority to opioids for pain control and without increased risk of postoperative bleeding.
- A single intravenous dose of antibiotics before incision is equivalent to an additional postoperative oral course for most uncomplicated functional rhinoplasty. The American Academy of Otolaryngology recommends less than 24 hours of postoperative antibiotics if it is used.
- Certain patient and surgical characteristics may warrant consideration of additional oral antibiotics, including complex revision cases, allogenic or alloplastic grafts, implants, immunosuppression, or cardiac prosthesis.

INTRODUCTION

Rhinoplasty is one of the most frequently performed surgeries in the world, a highly popular cosmetic and functional procedure.[1] In functional rhinoplasty, the goal is to improve nasal obstruction and breathing by addressing any nasal valve insufficiency or septal deviation.[2] A successful functional rhinoplasty improves many quality-of-life metrics,

[a] Department of Otolaryngology–Head and Neck Surgery, Vanderbilt University Medical Center, 1215 21st Avenue South, Suite 7209, Medical Center East, South Tower, Nashville, TN 37232, USA; [b] Facial Plastic and Reconstructive Surgery, Department of Otolaryngology–Head and Neck Surgery, Vanderbilt University Medical Center, 1215 21st Avenue South, Suite 7209, Medical Center East, South Tower, Nashville, TN 37232, USA
* Corresponding author.
E-mail address: priyesh.patel.1@vumc.org

Otolaryngol Clin N Am 58 (2025) 237–245
https://doi.org/10.1016/j.otc.2024.07.028
0030-6665/25/© 2024 Elsevier Inc. All rights reserved, including those for text and data mining, AI training, and similar technologies.

oto.theclinics.com

including patient scores of Nasal Obstruction Symptom Evaluation,[3] Sino-Nasal Outcome Test-22,[4] and visual analog scale of obstruction scores.[5] The complexity of a successful rhinoplasty is related to the intricate anatomy and physiology of the nasal valve and internal nasal lining, each patient's unique anatomic concerns and areas of obstruction, and the aesthetic centerpiece of the nose on the face, showcasing details of even small microadjustments.[2,6]

There are several considerations regarding surgery of the nose and intranasal areas. First is the pain and sensitivity of this region, which is important when considering postoperative pain management strategies. Second is sterility, as the nasal passageways have classically been considered a less sterile area of the body. These surgical considerations influence considerations of perioperative antibiotic use and strategies for infection prevention. This review article aims to summarize the current breadth of data reported on these topics to provide an informed assessment of these two areas of clinical concern regarding functional rhinoplasty.

POSTOPERATIVE PAIN MANAGEMENT IN FUNCTIONAL RHINOPLASTY
Sensory Innervations to the Nose

The nose is intricately supplied by a network of multiple sensory nerves. Many contributions from various inputs create a complex network, making a single regional nerve block for rhinoplasty difficult to target.[7,8] The infratrochlear nerve, a secondary branch of V1 (ophthalmic division of trigeminal nerve), provides sensation to superior aspects of the external nose. Another V1 branch, the external nasal nerve, provides sensation to the nasal tip, internal nasal alae, and nasal dorsum.[7,8] The maxillary division of trigeminal nerve, V2, subsequently provides sensation to bilateral nasal dorsum and alae. Both V1 and V2 are also responsible for providing sensation to the internal nasal mucosa and nasal septum[7,9] (**Fig. 1**).

Post-Rhinoplasty Pain Control

Patient discomfort following rhinoplasty is generally related to the trauma of surgery, intraoperative nerve transections, and frequently, postoperative nasal packing and

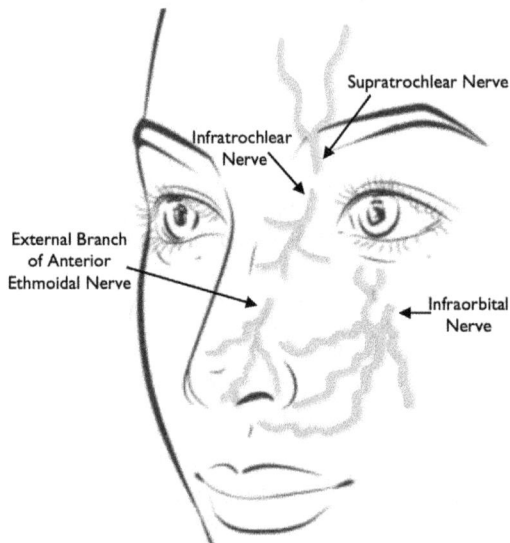

Fig. 1. Sensory nerve contributions to the external nose.

splints. Most of the postoperative pain is categorized as nociceptive pain, arising from tissue damage or trauma, but there are also elements of neuropathic pain, from direct nerve injury.[10,11] Historically, rhinoplasty patients have been given opioid medications in the immediate postoperative setting, to be used on an as-needed basis.[12,13] More recent trends, however, have advocated for greater discretion, and use of multimodal regimens, calling upon provider responsibility to help reduce unnecessary and potentially harmful narcotic prescriptions. Studies have shown a significant proportion of rhinoplasty patients use only 25% to 50% of their prescribed narcotics.[13–16] Some studies estimate 15% of patients do not require any postoperative narcotics at all, whereas only 3% of patients required a refill,[13] and almost all patients had excess opioids leftover.[17]

A multimodal regimen is helpful to target all aspects of the postoperative pain pathway. Typical medications include acetaminophen, nonsteroidal antiinflammatory drugs (NSAIDs), and opioids—targeting somatic and visceral nociceptive pain—and gabapentinoids—targeting neuropathic pain.[11] Gabapentin has its own risks including dizziness, nausea, and sedation; however, select studies have evaluated its role in reducing acute postoperative pain and have shown it to be very effective and well-tolerated in doses between 600 and 1800 mg per day, including for rhinoplasty and sinus surgery patients.[18–21] Traditionally, the use of NSAIDs has been cautioned in the postrhinoplasty setting, as the inhibition of the cyclooxygenase (COX)-1 pathway interferes with platelet function and theoretically increases risk of postoperative bleeding and ecchymosis with associated soft tissue swelling.[16,22] However, several prospective trials have found NSAIDs to be noninferior to opioids for postrhinoplasty pain control and without increased risk of complications such as bleeding or hematoma.[14,16,22–24] The equivocal effect of NSAID use on post-rhinoplasty bleeding risk implicates it should also not increase postoperative ecchymosis and swelling, but there is insufficient evidence in the literature thus far to support this. In some studies, a small proportion of patients (less than 10%) required escalation from NSAIDs to opioids. Additionally, celecoxib has been highlighted as a COX-2 selective NSAID that does not affect platelets, to be considered for use in the postoperative setting.[16,25] Overall caution for NSAIDs should still be regarded, for patients with additional bleeding risk factors, liver disease, kidney disease, or gastric ulcers.[16]

Importance of Postrhinoplasty Pain Management

The importance of carefully selecting a postrhinoplasty pain regimen cannot come at the cost of insufficient pain control. Appropriate postrhinoplasty pain control is crucial. Lack of such pain control can pose potential health risks, including hypertension, bleeding, endocrine and metabolic dysregulation, impaired immune function, thromboembolism, and anxiety.[26–28] It also significantly affects patient satisfaction and quality of life. For functional rhinoplasty in particular, poor pain control has been linked in several studies to decreased nasal breathing scores and worse patient-perceived functional benefits.[15,16] There are unavoidable variations between patients in terms of pain tolerance, and as such, escalation of certain regimens to include opioids should be considered, but the quantity could be limited for most individuals.

Special Considerations for Post-Rhinoplasty Pain

There are certain scenarios in which postoperative pain may be heightened for the rhinoplasty patient. The use of autologous rib grafts has been associated with breathing, mood, pain, and sleeping disturbances.[29] There is also evidence to suggest psychosocial factors may influence patient perceptions of postoperative pain.[30] Preoperative anxiety and depression have been associated with worse postoperative pain scores and increased opioid use in a variety of surgical subspecialties.[31,32] Few studies have specifically assessed the association of mental health in rhinoplasty pain perceptions; however, several report a higher incidence of psychosocial disorders in rhinoplasty patients, both functional and cosmetic, including anxiety, depression, body dysmorphia, and lower scores on mental and overall health questionnaires.[33–35]

Evidence suggests feelings of depression lowers pain thresholds and weakens immune systems, which can lead to additional complications.[36] The acute inflammation implicated in postoperative pain pathways may further exacerbate mental health and any preexisting vulnerabilities, leading to worse mood and pain experiences, both somatic and now combined with emotional pain.[30] In many instances, preoperative pain counseling has demonstrated a positive effect on postoperative pain scores for rhinoplasty patients, especially those with preexisting mental health symptoms.[29,30,37] This strategy should be regularly used and emphasized for patients who may have greater risks of pain sensitivity.

Guiding Recommendations

Several systematic reviews have commented on this topic, summarizing patient outcomes and experiences with different postrhinoplasty pain regimens.[13,16,24,38] The overarching consensus is to aim for a multimodal regimen, with non-narcotics as first-line agents (including acetaminophen, NSAIDs, and gabapentin), optimize preoperative local anesthetics, and reserve opioids for rescue moments or those requiring escalation. This should allow for a lower number of opioids prescribed. The American Academy of Otolaryngology-Head and Neck Surgery Foundation (AAO-HNSF) released a clinical practice guideline in 2021,[39] similarly emphasizing multimodal regimens, as well as the importance of preoperative pain counseling, and identifying patient-specific risk factors to reduce potential opioid harm. Large single- or multiinstitutional randomized clinical trials are necessary and currently underway, to better delineate whether nonnarcotics (eg, NSAIDs) carry any risks secondary to opioids (eg, bleeding).

PERIOPERATIVE ANTIBIOTICS IN FUNCTIONAL RHINOPLASTY
Risks and Sequelae

Another important consideration in functional rhinoplasty is infection prevention. Postrhinoplasty infections can lead to suboptimal healing, abnormal scar formation, patient dissatisfaction, discomfort, and worse functional outcomes.[40] Infections also pose risk of significant issues with cosmesis, such as saddle nose deformities.[41] Infections can include cellulitis, vestibulitis, septal abscess, or sinusitis.[42,43] The most feared complications are isolated reports of serious infectious extensions, such as cavernous sinus thrombosis, intracranial abscess, or meningitis.[44] The use of postoperative nasal packing or splints has historically been considered a risk factor for toxic shock syndrome, and as such, prophylactic antibiotics have been recommended while splints are in place.[43,45]

Although infection is considered a significant complication following rhinoplasty, its overall incidence remains low. It has been disparately reported as between 0% and 21% but generally less than 2% by most studies.[46–49] Many reports have not found a difference in postoperative complications regardless of antibiotic use, but most rhinoplasty surgeons continue to routinely prescribe antibiotics due to an abundance of caution, given the notable functional and aesthetic implications.[45,50] Peri-rhinoplasty antibiotics have generally been the accepted practice, rather than the exception.

Perioperative Antibiotics in Rhinoplasty

Perioperative antibiotics in functional rhinoplasty is typically broken into two categories—an intraoperative intravenous dose before incision and a postoperative oral course.[51] Several studies, including meta-analyses and prospective randomized controlled trials, have found no differences in the rate of postoperative infections between those with a single preincision intravenous dose and those with a combined postoperative oral course.[41,48,52,53] This is true even for patients with postoperative nasal packing and silastic septal splints.[52] Others have found the rate of postrhinoplasty infections and bacteremia to be very low in healthy patients even without any antibiotics at all.[48,51,54] The detriments of an oral course of antibiotics include gastrointestinal intolerance, nausea, pruritus, potential allergic or adverse events, higher health care costs, including greater medication costs to treat side effects, and greater risk of microbial resistance.[51,52] As such, most studies recommend just a single preoperative intravenous dose for prophylaxis in uncomplicated rhinoplasty cases.

There are certain situations with greater propensity for postoperative infections and complications. These situations include complex revision rhinoplasty, extensive septal reconstruction, external osteotomies, composite grafts, and alloplastic grafts or implants.[48,51] In these instances, antibiotics have demonstrated a benefit in decreasing postoperative rates of infection.[45,49,51] However, even in complex cases, a single preoperative intravenous dose may still be similarly sufficient to a combined postoperative oral course.[38,45,51,52]

Certain patient populations might also warrant special considerations. Those at higher risks include patients with prosthetic cardiac valves or additional endocarditis risk factors, and those with notable immunosuppression, such as prior organ transplant.[41,51,52] Most studies excluded these patient groups from their cohorts but recognize the implications and potential danger of bacteremia in these patients. In these specific circumstances, an additional postoperative course of oral antibiotics would be considered.

Clinical Practice Guidelines

Current World Health Organization statement on antibiotic prophylaxis in rhinoplasty recommends using a single intravenous dose before incision.[55] The Center for Disease Control and Prevention similarly recommends a single preoperative dose for rhinoplasty.[56] AAO-HNSF's clinical practice guidelines on rhinoplasty in 2017 acknowledged the potential benefit of antibiotics to minimize rhinoplasty infections, despite a low incidence, but recommended postoperative antibiotics, if any, to be used for less than 24 hours after surgery.[49] Exceptions would be revision or complex cases, implants, immunocompromised patients, concurrent medical indication (eg, rhinosinusitis), baseline methicillin-resistant *Staphylococcus aureus* colonization, and postoperative nasal packing (however, this was recommended against, even if septoplasty is performed).[49]

SUMMARY

A single intravenous dose of prophylactic antibiotics before incision is sufficient for most cases of uncomplicated functional rhinoplasty. Special considerations should be given for complex revision cases, use of allogenic or alloplastic grafts or implants, external osteotomies, or patients with immunosuppression, at risk for endocarditis, or with concurrent sinusitis. Given the low rate of postsurgical infections, further large multiinstitutional randomized clinical trials are necessary to confirm the benefit of antibiotics and the safety of reduced antibiotic use.

CLINICS CARE POINTS

- Consider using a multimodal pain regimen following rhinoplasty, of acetaminophen and NSAID combination first, to reduce the dependence on as-needed opioids as second-line therapy.
- Pre-rhinoplasty pain counseling should be discussed with all patients, especially those with anxiety, depression, or other psychosocial symptoms, to set expectations for postrhinoplasty healing and pain management.
- A single intravenous dose of prophylactic antibiotics before incision is recommended as sufficient for most functional rhinoplasty procedures in healthy patients.
- Additional postoperative oral course of antibiotics can be considered for complex revision cases, extensive septal reconstructions, or at-risk patients, such as those with immunosuppression or at risk for endocarditis.

DISCLOSURE

The authors have nothing to disclose.

REFERENCES

1. Heidekrueger PI, Juran S, Ehrl D, et al. Global aesthetic surgery statistics: a closer look. J Plast Surg Hand Surg 2017;51(4):270–4.
2. Friedman O, Cekic E, Gunel C. Functional rhinoplasty. Facial Plast Surg Clin North Am 2017;25(2):195–9.
3. Stewart MG, Witsell DL, Smith TL, et al. Development and validation of the Nasal Obstruction Symptom Evaluation (NOSE) Scale. Otolaryngol Head Neck Surg 2004;130(2):157–63.
4. Deconde AS, Mace JC, Bodner T, et al. SNOT-22 quality of life domains differentially predict treatment modality selection in chronic rhinosinusitis. Int Forum Allergy Rhinol 2014;4(12):972–9.
5. Shukla RH, Nemade SV, Shinde KJ. Comparison of visual analogue scale (VAS) and the Nasal Obstruction Symptom Evaluation (NOSE) score in evaluation of post septoplasty patients. World J Otorhinolaryngol Head Neck Surg 2020; 6(1):53.
6. Chen K, Zhou L. The effect of functional rhinoplasty on quality of life: a systematic review and meta-analysis. Aesthetic Plast Surg 2023;48(5):847–54.
7. Galarza-Paez L., Marston G. and Downs B.W., Anatomy, head and neck, nose, 2023, Statpearls Publishing, Treasure Island, FL, 1–16, Available at: https://www.ncbi.nlm.nih.gov/books/NBK532870/ (Accessed 7 April 2024).
8. Mistry RK, Al Khalili Y. Neuroanatomy, infratrochlear nerve. StatPearls. 2023. Available at: https://www.ncbi.nlm.nih.gov/books/NBK551696/. Accessed May 24, 2024.
9. Oneal RM, Beil J, Schlesinger J. Surgical anatomy of the nose. Otolaryngol Clin North Am 1999;32(1):145–81.
10. Armstrong SA, Herr MJ. Physiology, nociception. StatPearls. 2023. Available at: https://www.ncbi.nlm.nih.gov/books/NBK551562/. Accessed April 13, 2024.
11. Wick EC, Grant MC, Wu CL. Postoperative multimodal analgesia pain management with nonopioid analgesics and techniques: a review. JAMA Surg 2017; 152(7):691–7.

12. Sethi RKV, Lee LN, Quatela OE, et al. Opioid prescription patterns after rhinoplasty. JAMA Facial Plast Surg 2019;21(1):76.
13. Patel S, Sturm A, Bobian M, et al. Opioid use by patients after rhinoplasty. JAMA Facial Plast Surg 2018;20(1):24.
14. Marshall RV, Rivers NJ, Manickavel S, et al. Postoperative opioid use in rhinoplasty procedures: a standardized regimen. Facial Plast Surg 2021;37(1):110–6.
15. Gadkaree SK, Shaye DA, Occhiogrosso J, et al. Association between pain and patient satisfaction after rhinoplasty. JAMA Facial Plast Surg 2019;21(6):475.
16. Liu RH, Xu LJ, Lee LN. Opioid-sparing pain control after rhinoplasty: updated review of the literature. Facial Plast Surg 2023;39(6):674–8.
17. Sclafani AP, Kim M, Kjaer K, et al. Postoperative pain and analgesic requirements after septoplasty and rhinoplasty. Laryngoscope 2019;129(9):2020–5.
18. Fassoulaki A, Patris K, Sarantopoulos C, et al. The analgesic effect of gabapentin and mexiletine after breast surgery for cancer. Anesth Analg 2002;95(4):985–91.
19. Turan A, Memiş D, Karamanlioğlu B, et al. The analgesic effects of gabapentin in monitored anesthesia care for ear-nose-throat surgery. Anesth Analg 2004;99(2):375–8.
20. Chang CY, Challa CK, Shah J, et al. Gabapentin in acute postoperative pain management. BioMed Res Int 2014;2014.
21. Peng PWH, Wijeysundera DN, Li CCF. Use of gabapentin for perioperative pain control – A meta-analysis. Pain Res Manag : The Journal of the Canadian Pain Society 2007;12(2):85.
22. Frants A, Garber D, Lafer MP, et al. Prospective randomized trial comparing opioids versus nonsteroidal antiinflammatory drugs for postoperative analgesia in outpatient rhinoplasty. Plast Reconstr Surg 2021;147(1):56–62.
23. Justicz N, Gadkaree SK, Yamasaki A, et al. Defining typical acetaminophen and narcotic usage in the postoperative rhinoplasty patient. Laryngoscope 2021;131(1):48–53.
24. Shafiee A, Bahri RA, Mohammad TA, et al. Pain management following septorhinoplasty surgery: evidence from a systematic review. Eur Arch Oto-Rhino-Laryngol 2023;280(3):3931–52.
25. Newberry CI, McCrary HC, Cerrati EW. The efficacy of oral celecoxib following surgical rhinoplasty. Facial Plast Aesthet Med 2020;22(2):100–4. Available at: https://home.liebertpub.com/fpsam.
26. Wu CL, Naqibuddin M, Rowlingson AJ, et al. The effect of pain on health-related quality of life in the immediate postoperative period. Anesth Analg 2003;97(4):1078–85.
27. Baratta JL, Schwenk ES, Viscusi ER. Clinical consequences of inadequate pain relief. Plast Reconstr Surg 2014;134:15S–21S.
28. Joshi GP, Ogunnaike BO. Consequences of inadequate postoperative pain relief and chronic persistent postoperative pain. Anesthesiol Clin North Am 2005;23(1):21–36.
29. Wittekindt D, Wittekindt C, Schneider G, et al. Postoperative pain assessment after septorhinoplasty. Eur Arch Oto-Rhino-Laryngol 2012;269(6):1613–21.
30. Hariharan S. Do patient psychological factors influence postoperative pain? Pain Manag 2016;6(6):511–3.
31. Chambers MKM, Castaneda DM, Rivera-Pintado C, et al. Mental health disorders and pain modulation in orthopedic shoulder patients. JSES Int 2023;7(6):2523–7.
32. Gravani S, Matiatou M, Nikolaidis PT, et al. Anxiety and depression affect early postoperative pain dimensions after bariatric surgery. J Clin Med 2021;10(1):1–10.

33. Jones HE, Faulkner HR, Losken A. The psychological impact of aesthetic surgery: a mini-review. Aesthet Surg J Open Forum 2022;4.

34. Kucur C, Kuduban O, Ozturk A, et al. Psychological evaluation of patients seeking rhinoplasty. Eurasian J Med 2016;48(2):102.

35. Dey JK, Ishii M, Phillis M, et al. Body dysmorphic disorder in a facial plastic and reconstructive surgery clinic: measuring prevalence, assessing comorbidities, and validating a feasible screening instrument. JAMA Facial Plast Surg 2015; 17(2):137–43.

36. Ghoneim MM, O'Hara MW. Depression and postoperative complications: an overview. BMC Surg 2016;16(1).

37. Topan H, Mucuk S, Yontar Y. The effect of patient education prior to rhinoplasty surgery on anxiety, pain, and satisfaction levels. J Perianesth Nurs 2022;37(3): 374–9.

38. Nguyen BK, Yuhan BT, Folbe E, et al. perioperative analgesia for patients undergoing septoplasty and rhinoplasty: an evidence-based review. Laryngoscope 2019;129(6):E200–12.

39. Anne S, Mims JW, Tunkel DE, et al. Clinical practice guideline: opioid prescribing for analgesia after common otolaryngology operations. Otolaryngology-Head Neck Surg (Tokyo) 2021;164(2_suppl):S1–42.

40. Holt GR, Garner ET, McLarey D. Postoperative sequelae and complications of rhinoplasty. Otolaryngol Clin North Am 1987;20(4):853–76.

41. Benites C, Awan MU, Patel H, et al. An examination of antibiotic administration in septorhinoplasty: A systematic review and meta-analysis. Am J Otolaryngol 2024; 45(4):104333.

42. Layliev J, Gupta V, Kaoutzanis C, et al. Incidence and preoperative risk factors for major complications in aesthetic rhinoplasty: analysis of 4978 patients level of evidence: 2. Aesthetic Surg J 2017;37(7):757–67.

43. Cochran CS, Landecker A. Prevention and management of rhinoplasty complications. Plast Reconstr Surg 2008;122(2).

44. Haddad FS, Hubballa J, Zaytoun G, et al. Intracranial complications of submucous resection of the nasal septum. Am J Otolaryngol 1985;6(6):443–7.

45. Rettinger G. Risks and complications in rhinoplasty. GMS Curr Top Otorhinolaryngol Head Neck Surg 2007;6:14. Available at: http://pmc/articles/PMC3199839/. Accessed May 20, 2024.

46. Yoo DB, Peng GL, Azizzadeh B, et al. Microbiology and antibiotic prophylaxis in rhinoplasty: a review of 363 consecutive cases. JAMA Facial Plast Surg 2015; 17(1):23–7.

47. Layliev J, Gupta V, Kaoutzanis C, et al. Incidence and preoperative risk factors for major complications in aesthetic rhinoplasty: analysis of 4978 patients. Aesthetic Surg J 2017;37(7):757–67.

48. Nuyen B, Kandathil CK, Laimi K, et al. Evaluation of antibiotic prophylaxis in rhinoplasty: a systematic review and meta-analysis. JAMA Facial Plast Surg 2019; 21(1):12.

49. Ishii LE, Tollefson TT, Basura GJ, et al. Clinical practice guideline: improving nasal form and function after rhinoplasty. Otolaryngology-Head Neck Surg (Tokyo) 2017;156(2_suppl):S1–30.

50. Bouaoud J, Loustau M, Belloc JB. Functional and aesthetic factors associated with revision of rhinoplasty. Plast Reconstr Surg Glob Open 2018;6(9):e1884.

51. Kullar R, Frisenda J, Nassif PS. The more the merrier? should antibiotics be used for rhinoplasty and septorhinoplasty?—a review. Plast Reconstr Surg Glob Open 2018;6(10).

52. Rajan GP, Fergie N, Fischer U, et al. Antibiotic prophylaxis in septorhinoplasty? A prospective, randomized study. Plast Reconstr Surg 2005;116(7):1995–8.

53. Andrews PJ, East CA, Jayaraj SM, et al. Prophylactic vs postoperative antibiotic use in complex septorhinoplasty surgery: a prospective, randomized, single-blind trial comparing efficacy. Arch Facial Plast Surg 2006;8(2):84–7.

54. Slavin SA, Rees TD, Guy CL, et al. An investigation of bacteremia during rhinoplasty. Plast Reconstr Surg 1983;71(2):196–8.

55. Allegranzi B, Bischoff P, de Jonge S, et al. New WHO recommendations on pre-operative measures for surgical site infection prevention: an evidence-based global perspective. Lancet Infect Dis 2016;16(12):e276–87.

56. Berriós-Torres SI, Umscheid CA, Bratzler DW, et al. Centers for disease control and prevention guideline for the prevention of surgical site infection, 2017. JAMA Surg 2017;152(8):784–91.

Choosing the Best Graft Source in Nasal Valve Repair

Vivian Xu, MD[a], Uche Nwagu, MD[a], Eric Barbarite, MD[b],*

KEYWORDS

• Graft • Septum • Conchal • Costal • Cadaveric

KEY POINTS

- Choosing a graft source for nasal valve repair should be tailored to the individual patient's anatomic and functional concerns.
- Graft sources may be autologous or homologous, and these mainly include septal cartilage and/or bone, auricular cartilage, and costal cartilage.
- Knowledge of the advantages and disadvantages of each graft source is required to achieve the best outcome with the least patient morbidity.

INTRODUCTION

The patency and function of the nasal valves serve as a crucial determinant of nasal airflow. The nasal valve is divided into internal and external components, both of which warrant detailed examination when assessing a patient with nasal obstructive symptoms. Effective management of nasal valve deficiency depends on a patient-specific approach dictated by clinical history and anatomy.

Structural grafting plays an important role in the surgical correction of nasal obstruction, particularly in the setting of nasal valve deficiency. Internal nasal valve (INV) collapse is commonly corrected with spreader grafts, alar batten grafts, and lateral crural strut grafts, whereas external nasa valve (ENV) collapse is commonly corrected with lateral crural strut grafts and alar rim grafts.[1] Additional approaches to surgical correction of the nasal valve include suture techniques and cartilage scoring or trimming.[2]

When planning nasal valve repair, correct selection of graft source relies on a detailed history and physical examination. Clinical history specific to cartilage sourcing must include prior surgery or trauma to the head and neck or thoracic regions, as well as medical comorbidities such as those affecting cartilage strength. Clinical examination should include an external nasal analysis, anterior rhinoscopy, palpation

[a] Otolaryngology–Head and Neck Surgery, Thomas Jefferson University, 925 Chestnut Street, 6th Floor, Philadelphia, PA 19107, USA; [b] Otolaryngology–Head and Neck Surgery, Washington University in St. Louis, Saint Louis, MO, USA
* Corresponding author. 1044 N. Mason Drive, Suite L10, Creve Coeur, MO 63141.
E-mail address: barbarite@wustl.edu

Otolaryngol Clin N Am 58 (2025) 247–255
https://doi.org/10.1016/j.otc.2024.09.002
0030-6665/25/© 2024 Elsevier Inc. All rights reserved, including those for text and data mining, AI training, and similar technologies.

of septal cartilage strength and quantity, Cottle and/or modified Cottle maneuvers, and possible rigid endoscopy in the case of severe obstruction or comorbid sinus symptomatology.

Graft sources may be categorized broadly as autologous or homologous (cadaveric). Autologous grafts (autografts) are derived from the patient and may be obtained intranasally or extranasally. These include septal cartilage and/or bone, auricular cartilage, and costal cartilage. Cadaveric cartilage is a suitable option in the case of autologous graft scarcity, and these grafts eliminate the need for additional surgical harvesting procedures and the associated time under anesthesia. Cadaveric costal cartilage represents the most commonly utilized nonautologous graft in rhinoplasty. The following sections will describe in more detail the various sources of cartilage grafting for nasal valve repair along with their advantages and disadvantages.

INTRANASAL GRAFTS
Septal Cartilage and Perpendicular Plate

Nasal septal cartilage represents the most used graft source in rhinoplasty.[3] The nasal septum is comprised of the quadrangular cartilage anteriorly, which articulates with the bony perpendicular plate of the ethmoid superiorly, the vomer of the maxilla posteriorly, and the maxillary crest inferiorly.[4] Harvest of the quadrangular cartilage may be performed via an open septorhinoplasty or endonasal approaches using hemitransfixion, full transfixion, or Killian incisions. After the elevation of mucoperichondrial flaps and separation of the bony-cartilaginous junction, septal cartilage may be obtained. To maintain structural integrity of the nose and avoid destabilization of the septal L-strut, standard practice is to preserve at least 1 cm dorsal and caudal septal struts when planning cartilage harvest. However, the exact location of septal cartilage incisions is often dictated by the number of grafts required, as well as the need to excise obstructing septal elements such as deviations or spurs. Extracorporeal or modified extracorporeal septoplasty may be performed in cases of severe septal deviation in order to maximize material harvest while targeting obstruction along the critical aspects of the septal L-strut.[4,5]

When available, septal cartilage has many advantages. It may be easily harvested from the primary surgical site, and typically demonstrating strong integrity and thin profile. In cases of primary septorhinoplasty, there is often enough cartilage to accomplish nasal valve repair, which spares the morbidity of a second donor or cost of additional material. When harvesting cartilage for grafting of the nasal valve, it is generally best to obtain a straight piece of cartilage, and this can then be contoured and carved into desired shape while providing adequate structural support. The posterior portion of the cartilaginous septum is generally thicker, allowing for more bulk when designing grafts.[6] In the case of a deviated septal harvest, the graft may be secured in a way such that its natural curvature counteracts the direction of nasal valve narrowing.

The perpendicular plate of the ethmoid may also be harvested as a structural support graft.[7] This may be performed in isolation or in continuity with the quadrangular cartilage as a composite graft. For treatment of the nasal valves, perpendicular plate grafts have been employed as spreader grafts and caudal septal extension grafts. Holes typically must be fashioned in the bone with an 18-gauge needle or powered drill to allow the passage of suture through the graft. Relative to cartilage, the higher density of a bone graft allows greater distribution of stress and less nasal deformation.[8] Composite grafts are particularly useful when there is a limited amount of native septal cartilage, such as in ethnic rhinoplasty, or to limit other donor sites.[9]

The disadvantages of septal cartilage and bone grafts are primarily related to the availability of material. Size of harvest is limited by the need to preserve dorsal and columellar struts and can be further limited in the case of prior septoplasty, where little to no cartilage or bone may be available. Additionally, in cases of severe contour irregularity, designing grafts can be challenging due to deviation, memory, or inadequate structurally sound material.[6]

Cartilage-Sparing Techniques

Cartilage-sparing techniques are more conservative and consist of rearranging rather than harvesting intranasal cartilages. These approaches can be applied to both INV and ENV repair.

The auto-spreader graft is a common cartilage-sparing technique for INV repair that has been demonstrated to significantly improve Nasal Obstruction Symptoms Evaluation (NOSE) scores in patients undergoing combined functional and cosmetic rhinoplasty.[10] Yoo and colleagues described the technique as disarticulation of the ULCs from the septum, infolding of the medial dorsal aspect of the ULC after scoring, and resecuring to the dorsal septum with a horizontal mattress suture.[10] The success of the auto-spreader graft is dependent upon the shape and thickness of the ULC, which may vary by patient. If the cartilage is too thick, it may not be sufficient to cause a notable increase in airflow through the INV. Challenges may also be met with extension of the ULC inferiorly to the anterior septal angle, as the cartilage may be too short. In this case, additional cartilage graft may also be harvested to ensure extension of graft to anterior septal angle.[11]

The lateral crural turn-in technique can be used to enhance the aesthetic appearance of the nasal tip, while improving the function and patency of the ENV. It can be approached via open rhinoplasty or delivery approach and starts with adequate exposure of the lateral crura. A 6 to 8 mm margin from the caudal border of the LLC is marked, the scroll area disarticulated as well as nasal mucosa dissected off the cartilage. The cephalic portion is folded over and secured with mattress sutures.[12] This technique reinforces the lateral crus, restructuring and shaping it while widening the ENV. It allows for aesthetic tip improvements by medializing the tip-defining points, reducing tip volume, and increasing visual gain in tip position. It can be easily modified and can be combined with other grafts. This technique may be limited by the availability of lateral crural cartilage, especially in setting of revision rhinoplasty.[12,13] Additionally, the lateral crura must be left sufficiently wide to avoid inadequate structural stability and worsened valve narrowing.

EXTRANASAL GRAFTS

When the native nasal cartilage is insufficient for graft harvest, such as in instances of trauma, infection, or prior surgery, extranasal sources may be considered. Auricular conchal cartilage and costal cartilage have been widely described as favorable graft sources for nasal valve repair and rhinoplasty.

Auricular Conchal Cartilage

Auricular conchal cartilage is an easily obtainable graft material with minimal donor site morbidity.[14] The naturally curved contour of conchal cartilage offers a unique advantage in that it allows for reduced time spent on graft shaping, with improved ability to blend into the nasal tip, dorsum, and lateral nasal cartilages.[15] The most commonly utilized and proven use of conchal cartilage is the butterfly graft, which is placed superficial to the anterior septal angle and caudal edge of the ULC for dynamic nasal valve collapse.[16] However, conchal cartilage may also be used for spreader or strut grafting to the nasal valves when present in sufficient amount and appropriate contour.

Harvest of autologous conchal cartilage may be performed via a preauricular or postauricular incision. Various shapes and sizes of cartilage may be obtained from the cymba concha and cavum concha, with or without perichondrium. Care should be taken to preserve a portion of the posterior wall of the conchal cartilage, as over-resection of this area may cause medialization of the pinna and external deformity. Complete harvest of the concha may be performed, if necessary, though patients should be appropriately counseled preoperatively due to the potential aesthetic alteration.[6] Individuals with autoimmune disease, collagen vascular disease, or prior history of keloids may not be ideal candidates for auricular cartilage harvest.

Auricular cartilage may also be harvested as a composite graft, consisting of skin, subcutaneous tissue, and cartilage. These grafts are typically obtained from the cymba concha, however, wedge resection from the helical rim may also be performed. Composite grafts may be used to repair defects of the INV, nasal sill-ala junction, nasal vestibule, or external nasal ala and should be considered in cases of inadequate internal nasal lining. Failure to reconstruct the internal lining may result in suboptimal functional and aesthetic results due to graft exposure or extrusion, scar contracture, and distortion of the nasal framework or wound infection.[17] Composite grafts should be around 1 cm to maximize survival due to a high demand for vascular supply, although larger grafts have been described.[18] Grafts should be handled with care to avoid shearing skin from cartilage, and placement should be performed immediately following harvest to minimize extracorporeal ischemic time.[19,20] Toriumi and colleagues described an auricular composite graft survival rate of 93.7% ($n = 234$) using a perichondrial underlay technique, wherein a cuff of graft cartilage and perichondrium is overlapped with recipient site mucosa to promote graft revascularization.[20] Postoperative steroids and hyperbaric oxygen therapy have also been suggested to improve graft survival.[20,21] The donor site may be left to heal via secondary intention, closed primarily or skin grafted with low donor site morbidity.

The use of conchal cartilage for primary structural support is limited in some instances by its brittle nature.[6] For this reason, conchal cartilage has often been viewed as a salvage option or employed in conjunction with other techniques that provide strength. Conchal cartilage grafts may be subject to deformation or warping postimplantation. Higher rates are reported in perichondrium-containing grafts, particular those placed on the nasal dorsum.[15,22] To combat the potential for deformation, one may consider removal of perichondrium when grafting in a high-risk area such as the nasal dorsum. However, there are also benefits of leaving the perichondrium intact, such as a shorter time to graft assimilation and lower likelihood of graft migration.[23] Despite its limitations, conchal cartilage remains an excellent choice for nasal valve reconstruction in appropriately selected patients.

Autologous Costal Cartilage

Autologous costal cartilage (ACC) is the workhorse graft source for cases with insufficient native septal cartilage, such as revision rhinoplasty, or when major deficiencies must be corrected, as in traumatic or saddle nose deformities.[24] A great advantage of ACC lies in its versatility and ample supply available for grafting. ACC may be carved into many different shapes, thicknesses, or lengths while maintaining its pliability and strength. Additionally, it may be crushed or diced for onlay grafting. Harvest may be performed simultaneously with nasal work by a second surgeon to reduce operative time.[25]

Harvest is carried out via a single incision, roughly 2 to 4 cm in length, in the inframammary fold or overlying the costal cartilage of choice.[26] The fifth, sixth, or seventh costal cartilages are typically harvested and are the most suitably shaped for nasal grafting.[27] During harvest, care should be taken to not violate the underlying pleural space. It is good practice to perform a Valsalva maneuver with saline in the harvested wound bed prior to closure to ensure no air leak or bubbling that would suggest a pleural injury. Meticulous removal of any perichondrium and soft tissue should be performed prior to graft placement due to its chondrogenic potential. It should also be noted that ACC may become calcified with age, thus, caution should be taken when considering this type of graft in the older patient. Calcified cartilage may be more difficult to carve to the desired shape; however, it can also be advantageous as it is less prone to warping.[28]

One of the most cited disadvantages of ACC is graft warping.[29] Rates of warping described in literature are highly heterogeneous. Miranda and colleagues studied postoperative outcomes after rib graft septorhinoplasty and identified warping in 26% of their cohort.[26] Contrary to this, 2 meta-analyses of 1648 and 491 such patients found mean warping rates of 3.05% and 3.08%, respectively.[29,30] Time to graft distortion is also variable, ranging from minutes postharvest to weeks or months postoperatively.[31] Properly planned cross-sectional carving may help prevent warping. Concentric cutting demonstrates less warping as compared with eccentric techniques.[32] When inherent memory is unavoidable, multiple graft pieces may be sutured together such that their concave surfaces oppose and the distorting forces are neutralized.[33] Once suitably carved, proper fixation of the graft material aims to prevent in situ changes postoperatively. Gunter and colleagues demonstrated that rigid graft fixation with wire resulted in significantly less warping, however, multiple cases of postoperative wire extrusion were also noted.[34]

ACC can be associated with donor site morbidity. A large meta-analysis including 20 studies identified the following rates of donor site complication: 1.45% wound infection, 1.53% contour irregularity, 2.08% hypertrophic scar.[30] Overall, rates of long-term donor site complications are low.[29] Committeri and colleagues recommended leaving the perichondrium intact at the donor site to facilitate chondrogenesis and minimize risk of chest wall deformity.[35] Others opt to fill the harvested space with fat or unused cartilage.[36] Pneumothorax represents both the most feared and the rarest complication after costal cartilage harvest, with observed rates of 0% to 0.1%.[29,30] When diagnosed, often with chest radiograph, inpatient admission for further monitoring and/or intervention may be warranted. In the event of iatrogenic pleural tear (0.6%), this can be primarily repaired at the time of injury.[37]

Donor site pain from costal cartilage harvest may be significant, particularly with movement.[38] Both static and dynamic donor site pain may be minimized by performing a muscle-sparing dissection.[38] In this technique, the rectus abdominis muscle is opened bluntly parallel to the orientation of its fibers, thereby eliminating the need to cut through muscle to gain exposure of the underlying rib. Some surgeons prefer to perform intercostal nerve block and/or leave an indwelling catheter at the donor site through which to infused topical local anesthetic.[39] This is well tolerated and has been associated with decreased pain scores postoperatively.

Homologous (Cadaveric) Costal Cartilage

Homologous, or cadaveric, costal cartilage (HCC) provides an alternative to ACC with many similar advantages. Cadaveric sourcing may offer ample quantity of cartilage stock, while eliminating the risks associated with donor site morbidity and additional time under anesthesia. Cost analyses have demonstrated a similar cost ceiling between autologous and cadaveric grafting in the setting of outpatient primary and revision rhinoplasty.[40] However, the upper limit of cost is nearly doubled for autologous graft harvest when considering admission for monitoring, pain or pneumothorax.

Multiple forms of homologous costal cartilage exist based on processing technique. Irradiated homologous costal cartilage (IHCC) is the most widely available and commonly used. IHCC is processed by exposing the cartilage to 30 to 40 kGy of γ radiation to remove all donor cells, as well as major histocompatibility antigens to limit the graft-versus-host response.[41,42] Hesitation among many in adopting cadaveric cartilage as a graft source stems from fear of infection and resorption over time, as radiation treatment has been shown to decrease chondrocyte viability and collagen fiber content of the cartilage.[42] Early studies found significant rates of infection and resorption of IHCC grafts utilized for reconstruction of various head and neck defects.[43] However, the literature is varied in its evidence, with more recent studies and meta-analyses demonstrating low rates of infection and graft resorption.[44,45] In patients undergoing nasal surgery, no difference has been found between ACC and IHCC grafts when examining warping, resorption, contour deformity, infection, or revision surgery.[45,46]

Concerns over infection and warping of IHCC lead to the implementation of fresh frozen costal cartilage (FFCC). Fresh frozen cartilage differs from IHCC in that it is debrided of any soft tissue, treated with surfactant to remove the blood, lipid, and cellular components, then decontaminated with antibiotic. It is then sealed in a sterile container and preserved in frozen conditions (-40°C to -80°C) to be later thawed when ready for use. The avoidance of harsh processing techniques results in a lower propensity for FFCC warping, however, this preparation also results in lesser availability compared with IHCC.[47] Studies have shown comparable objective and subjective aesthetic results between autologous and FFCC.[48] Furthermore, compared with irradiated costal cartilage, FFCC demonstrates similar or improved rates of infection, warping, resorption, and rates of revision surgery.[47,48] At this time, there is no gold standard form of costal cartilage, and the use is largely provider-dependent and institution-dependent.

SUMMARY

Nasal valve compromise is a common cause of symptomatic nasal obstruction. Nasal valve repair typically involves the use of structural grafting, with a wide array of graft sources and techniques available. The optimal graft source for nasal valve repair is determined by patient history and examination, which dictate material availability and surgical goals. Additionally in play are physician skill and comfort level with techniques to repair the nasal valve. As such, it is difficult to standardize the correct graft material for nasal valve repair. Instead, the approach to sourcing graft material should be tailored to each individual patient's anatomic and functional concerns. More than one cartilage source is often available, and it is incumbent upon the surgeon to have knowledge of the advantages and disadvantages of each to achieve the best outcome with least patient morbidity.

CLINICS CARE POINTS

- Nasal septal cartilage is the most commonly used graft material in rhinoplasty.
- In cases of insufficient nasal septal cartilage, costal cartilage is typically preferred.

- Autologous costal cartilage is the gold standard for extranasal graft material, however cadaveric costal cartilage may be indicated in certain contexts.
- The use of cadaveric cartilage is shown to be safe and effective.

DISCLOSURE

None.

REFERENCES

1. Toriumi DM. Discussion: evaluation of validity and specificity of the Cottle maneuver in diagnosis of nasal valve collapse. Plast Reconstr Surg 2020;146(2):281–2.
2. Rasic I, Pegan A, Kosec A, et al. Use of intranasal flaring suture for dysfunctional nasal valve repair. JAMA Facial Plast Surg 2015;17(6):462–3.
3. Gunther S, Guyuron B. Economizing the septal cartilage for grafts during rhinoplasty, 40 Years' experience. Aesthetic Plast Surg 2021;45(1):224–8.
4. Most SP, Rudy SF. Septoplasty: basic and advanced techniques. Facial Plast Surg Clin North Am 2017;25(2):161–9.
5. Most SP. Anterior septal reconstruction: outcomes after a modified extracorporeal septoplasty technique. Arch Facial Plast Surg 2006;8(3):202–7.
6. Sajjadian A, Rubinstein R, Naghshineh N. Current status of grafts and implants in rhinoplasty: part I. Autologous grafts. Plast Reconstr Surg 2010;125(2):40e–9e.
7. An Y, Yang X, Xue H, et al. Inferior portion of the perpendicular plate of the ethmoid as a suitable grafting material in rhinoplasty and septoplasty procedures. J Plast Reconstr Aesthet Surg 2018;71(11):1664–78.
8. An Y, Shu F, Zhen Y, et al. The ethmoid bone is the ideal graft to strengthen nasal septum L-strut among different grafts: an evaluation based on finite element analysis. J Plast Reconstr Aesthet Surg 2022;75(11):4304–11.
9. Wang J, Li B, Wang Q, et al. A modified technique in rhinoplasty: a septal extension graft complex using septal cartilage, ethmoid bone, and auricular cartilage. Aesthet Surg J 2023;43(2):125–36.
10. Yoo S, Most SP. Nasal airway preservation using the autospreader technique: analysis of outcomes using a disease-specific quality-of-life instrument. Arch Facial Plast Surg 2011;13(4):231–3.
11. Manavbaşi YI, Kerem H, Başaran I. The role of upper lateral cartilage in correcting dorsal irregularities: section 2. The suture bridging cephalic extension of upper lateral cartilages. Aesthetic Plast Surg 2013;37(1):29–33.
12. Tellioglu AT, Cimen K. Turn-in folding of the cephalic portion of the lateral crus to support the alar rim in rhinoplasty. Aesthetic Plast Surg 2007;31(3):306–10.
13. Apaydin F. Lateral crural turn-in flap in functional rhinoplasty. Arch Facial Plast Surg 2012;14(2):93–6.
14. Stucker FJ, Hoasjoe DK. Nasal reconstruction with conchal cartilage. Correcting valve and lateral nasal collapse. Arch Otolaryngol Head Neck Surg 1994;120(6):653–8.
15. Toriumi DM. Autogenous grafts are worth the extra time. Arch Otolaryngol Head Neck Surg 2000;126(4):562–4.
16. Barrett DM, Casanueva FJ, Cook TA. Management of the nasal valve. Facial Plast Surg Clin North Am 2016;24(3):219–34.
17. Weber SM, Wang TD. Options for internal lining in nasal reconstruction. Facial plastic surgery clinics of North America 2011;19(1):163–73.

18. Zhang AY, Meine JG. Flaps and grafts reconstruction. Dermatol Clin 2011;29(2): 217–30.
19. Lu GN, Tawfik O, Sykes K, et al. Association of skin and cartilage variables with composite graft healing in a rabbit model. JAMA facial plastic surgery 2019; 21(1):44–9.
20. Toriumi DM, Kao R, Vandenberg T, et al. Auricular composite graft survival in rhinoplasty. Facial plastic surgery & aesthetic medicine 2023;25(1):6–15.
21. Harbison JM, Kriet JD, Humphrey CD. Improving outcomes for composite grafts in nasal reconstruction. Curr Opin Otolaryngol Head Neck Surg 2012;20(4): 267–73.
22. Parker Porter J. Grafts in rhinoplasty: alloplastic vs. autogenous. Arch Otolaryngol Head Neck Surg 2000;126(4):558–61.
23. Stucker FJ, Lian T, Karen M. Management of the keel nose and associated valve collapse. Arch Otolaryngol Head Neck Surg 2002;128(7):842–6.
24. Skoog T, Johansson SH. [New articular cartilage from transplanted perichondrium]. Lakartidningen 1975;72(17):1789–92.
25. Nelson M, Gaball C. Technique to reduce time, pain, and risk in costal cartilage harvest. JAMA Facial Plast Surg 2017;19(4):333–4.
26. Miranda N, Larocca CG, Aponte C. Rhinoplasty using autologous costal cartilage. Facial Plast Surg 2013;29(3):184–92.
27. Bender-Heine AN, Zdilla MJ, Russell ML, et al. Optimal costal cartilage graft selection according to cartilage shape: anatomical considerations for rhinoplasty. Facial Plast Surg 2017;33(6):670–4.
28. Balaji SM. Costal cartilage nasal augmentation rhinoplasty: study on warping. Ann Maxillofac Surg 2013;3(1):20–4.
29. Wee JH, Park MH, Oh S, et al. Complications associated with autologous rib cartilage use in rhinoplasty: a meta-analysis. JAMA Facial Plast Surg 2015;17(1): 49–55.
30. Chen H, Wang X, Deng Y. Complications associated with autologous costal cartilage used in rhinoplasty: an updated meta-analysis. Aesthetic Plast Surg 2023; 47(1):304–12.
31. Harris S, Pan Y, Peterson R, et al. Cartilage warping: an experimental model. Plast Reconstr Surg 1993;92(5):912–5.
32. Kim DW, Shah AR, Toriumi DM. Concentric and eccentric carved costal cartilage: a comparison of warping. Arch Facial Plast Surg 2006;8(1):42–6.
33. Agrawal KS, Bachhav M, Shrotriya R. Namaste (counterbalancing) technique: Overcoming warping in costal cartilage. Indian J Plast Surg 2015;48(2):123–8.
34. Gunter JP, Clark CP, Friedman RM. Internal stabilization of autogenous rib cartilage grafts in rhinoplasty: a barrier to cartilage warping. Plast Reconstr Surg 1997;100(1):161–9.
35. Committeri U, Arena A, Carraturo E, et al. Minimally invasive harvesting technique for costal cartilage graft: donor site, morbidity and aesthetic outcomes. J Clin Med 2023;12(10). https://doi.org/10.3390/jcm12103424.
36. Moon BJ, Lee HJ, Jang YJ. Outcomes following rhinoplasty using autologous costal cartilage. Arch Facial Plast Surg 2012;14(3):175–80.
37. Varadharajan K, Sethukumar P, Anwar M, et al. Complications associated with the use of autologous costal cartilage in rhinoplasty: a systematic review. Aesthet Surg J 2015;35(6):644–52.
38. Özücer B, Dinç ME, Paltura C, et al. Association of autologous costal cartilage harvesting technique with donor-site pain in patients undergoing rhinoplasty. JAMA Facial Plast Surg 2018;20(2):136–40.

39. Guoyu J, Tao W, Xi Y. Application of methylene blue combined with ropivacaine intercostal nerve block in postoperative analgesia of autologous costal cartilage augmentation rhinoplasty. Anaesthesiologie 2022;71(Suppl 2):233–9.

40. Starr NC, Creel L, Harryman C, et al. Cost utility analysis of costal cartilage autografts and human cadaveric allografts in rhinoplasty. Ann Otol Rhinol Laryngol 2022;131(10):1123–9.

41. Kadakia N, Nguyen C, Motakef S, et al. Is irradiated homologous costal cartilage reliable? A meta-analysis of complication rates in rhinoplasty. Plast Surg (Oakv). 2022;30(3):212–21.

42. Wee JH, Mun SJ, Na WS, et al. Autologous vs irradiated homologous costal cartilage as graft material in rhinoplasty. JAMA Facial Plast Surg 2017;19(3):183–8.

43. Welling DB, Maves MD, Schuller DE, et al. Irradiated homologous cartilage grafts. Long-term results. Arch Otolaryngol Head Neck Surg 1988;114(3):291–5.

44. Kridel RW, Ashoori F, Liu ES, et al. Long-term use and follow-up of irradiated homologous costal cartilage grafts in the nose. Arch Facial Plast Surg 2009;11(6):378–94.

45. Adams WP, Rohrich RJ, Gunter JP, et al. The rate of warping in irradiated and nonirradiated homograft rib cartilage: a controlled comparison and clinical implications. Plast Reconstr Surg 1999;103(1):265–70.

46. Vila PM, Jeanpierre LM, Rizzi CJ, et al. Comparison of autologous vs homologous costal cartilage grafts in dorsal augmentation rhinoplasty: a systematic review and meta-analysis. JAMA Otolaryngol Head Neck Surg 2020;146(4):347–54.

47. Mohan R, Shanmuga Krishnan RR, Rohrich RJ. Role of fresh frozen cartilage in revision rhinoplasty. Plast Reconstr Surg 2019;144(3):614–22.

48. Kadhum M, Khan K, Al-Ghanim K, et al. Fresh frozen cartilage in rhinoplasty surgery: a systematic review of outcomes. Aesthetic Plast Surg 2024. https://doi.org/10.1007/s00266-024-03977-4.

Evaluation and Management of the External Nasal Valve

Lane B. Donaldson, MD[a],*, William Mason, MD[a],
Lamont R. Jones, MD, MBA[b,c,d]

KEYWORDS

- External nasal valve • Nasal obstruction • Caudal septum • Rhinoplasty

KEY POINTS

- Evaluation of external nasal valve dysfunction is dependent upon a thorough history and physical examination.
- It is important to be familiar with nonsurgical and surgical options for the management of external nasal valve dysfunction.
- The benefits of treating external nasal valve dysfunction to improve symptoms and quality of life should be weighed against the risk of worsening nasal obstruction and creating external deformities.

INTRODUCTION

The external nasal valve (ENV) is classically defined as the anatomic region bounded by the caudal septum, alar rim, medial crura of the lower lateral cartilage (LLC), and nasal sill at the level of the nasal vestibule inferior to the lobule (**Fig. 1**). However, various authors have described different boundaries.[1] Spielmann and colleagues[2] define the ENV as bounded by the septum, premaxilla, and medial and lateral crura of the LLC, whereas Khosh and colleagues[3] define the ENV as bounded by the caudal edge of the upper lateral cartilage (ULC) superolaterally, the piriform aperture and fibrofatty tissues of the ala laterally, and the nasal floor. The surgeon should recognize that different definitions of the ENV exist, but ultimately it is most important to be specific in the anatomic description of where the pathology exists when examining a patient with ENV dysfunction as this has significant impact on the surgical and nonsurgical options available for the treatment.

[a] Department of Otolaryngology–Head and Neck Surgery, Henry Ford Hospital, 2799 West Grand Boulevard K-8, Detroit, MI 48202, USA; [b] Department of Otolaryngology–Head and Neck Surgery, Division of Facial Plastic and Reconstructive Surgery, Henry Ford Hospital, 2799 West Grand Boulevard K-8, Detroit, MI 48202, USA; [c] Department of Surgery, Michigan State University, 4660 South Hagadorn Road, Suite #620, East Lansing, MI 48823, USA; [d] Wayne State University School of Medicine, 540 East Canfield Street, Detroit, MI 48201, USA
* Corresponding author. 11423 6th Street, Detroit, MI 48226.
E-mail address: ldonald9@hfhs.org

Otolaryngol Clin N Am 58 (2025) 257–268
https://doi.org/10.1016/j.otc.2024.07.015
oto.theclinics.com

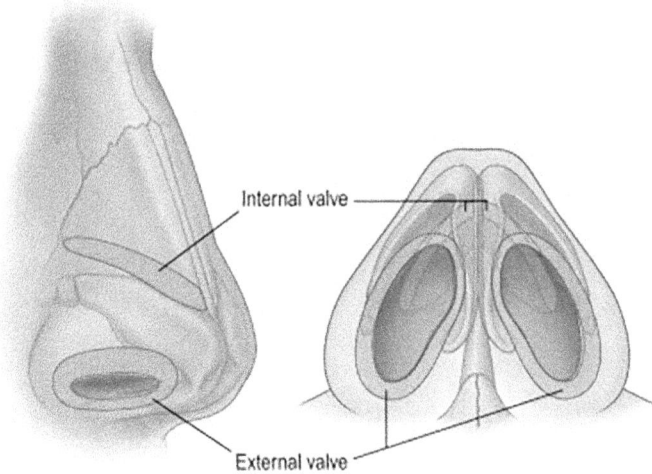

Fig. 1. Internal and external nasal valves. External nasal valve formed by the lower lateral cartilage medial and lateral crura with associated alar rim soft tissue and the nasal sill. (*From* Losee JE, Hopper R, Neligan PC. Plastic Surgery. 5th Ed. Elsevier; 2024. Fig 20.9.)

DISCUSSION
Evaluation

History
Patients with external nasal valve dysfunction (eNVD) will typically present with a chief complaint of nasal obstruction. This is a highly subjective complaint that can be caused by a myriad of pathologies.[4] Therefore, a thorough history is required to help determine the contribution of eNVD to the obstruction, to identify other nasal structural abnormalities or diseases, and rule out potentially serious sinonasal pathologies.

A range of anatomic, physiologic, neurologic, and iatrogenic factors can contribute to nasal obstruction, and as such, the obstruction may be multifactorial in origin. In order to determine the etiology, Fraser and Kelly[5] suggest 11 points to be evaluated when obtaining a history: (1) sidedness of symptoms, (2) duration, (3) seasonal/diurnal variation, (4) associated sinonasal symptoms, (5) change in smell, (6) additional medical problems, (7) prior surgery or trauma, (8) medications, (9) drug, tobacco, and alcohol use, (10) pregnancy, and (11) occupation. It can also be useful to ascertain whether the use of commercially available external nasal dilators/strips reduce or alleviate symptoms. Other commonly associated symptoms of eNVD beyond nasal obstruction are typically a result of turbulent airflow. Examples include recurrent epistaxis, nasal crusting or dryness, increased snoring, compensatory rhinorrhea, among other pathologies.

Relevant anatomy
Much controversy exists regarding the terminology and anatomic boundaries of the ENV. The nasal valve region was first described in 1903 by Mink as the narrow opening formed between the ULC and the nasal septum, typically a 10° to 15° angle in Europeans (wider in other ethnic groups), which is the region of maximum nasal resistance.[6] Unsurprisingly, this region is, therefore, important physiologically. The definition has since evolved with further subclassifications. In 2000, Shaida and

Kenyon[7] proposed 2 nasal valve mechanisms, an internal and an external, separated by the caudal border of the ULC and the cephalic boarder of the LLC.

The ENV is, therefore, bounded medially by the columella/caudal septum and medial crus of the LLC, laterally by the lateral crus of the LLC and the associated fibro-fatty tissue of the wing of the nose, and posteriorly by the nasal vestibule/sill (see **Fig. 1**). Functionally, these components join to form a tube, redirecting air and creating laminar flow within the nasal cavity. The tissue within the nasal valve also contains thermoreceptors, which contribute to the sensation of nasal breathing.[8,9]

Physical examination

For patients presenting with nasal obstruction, when considering eNVD, you must first rule out other sources or contributors of their symptoms (inferior turbinate hypertrophy, nasal polyps, and so forth). Performing physical examinations both before and after application of a nasal decongestant can often be helpful. Once other sources have been sufficiently identified, a more focused physical examination can be performed to evaluate eNVD as a primary source or contributor. Both a static and dynamic physical examination should be performed, as structural abnormalities of the various anatomic support structures can lead to alterations in both.

In terms of static physical examination, the single most important variable in nasal airflow is the diameter of the nasal passage. The average diameter in adults is typically reported to be 10 to 12 mm, with variation in the size and orientation of the nostril existing among various ethnic groups.[10] The long axis is typically oriented vertically (leptorrhine) in those of European descent, horizontally (platyrrhine) in those of African descent, and obliquely (mesorrhine) in those of Asian descent.[11] This orientation becomes important with aging, as more cephalically oriented cartilage will tend to weaken and droop more significantly over time. Also if cephalic malposition exists or cartilages are oriented significantly vertically, they will not be positioned appropriately to support the lateral portion of the valve, which can result in severe lateral external valve collapse. As shown by Morgan and colleagues, differences also exist in cross-sectional area secondary to differences in the width of the piriform aperture.[12] These considerations are important cosmetically, as well as functionally, as changes in cross-sectional area of the nostril will greatly impact actual and perceived nasal airflow.[12]

Various pathologies can reduce the size of this opening and result in nasal obstruction, such as a significant caudal septal deviation (**Fig. 2**). Additionally, the LLC can become deformed at its junction with the septum because of trauma or prior surgery, webs of scarred mucosa can form between the septum and the lateral nasal wall, or the nasal tip can demonstrate significant ptosis. All of these pathologies are readily visible on static physical examination.

To perform a dynamic physical examination, the physician will have the patient breathe in normally, followed by deeply, through the nose. The ENV is then inspected for any dynamic collapse of the lateral nasal wall. Simply seeing collapse, however, is not enough to conclude that this is the cause of the patient's nasal obstruction, as during normal physiology there is some degree of lateral wall collapse during inspiration due to the Bernoulli principle (though typically the rigidity of the nasal cartilages works to resist significant collapse).[8] Therefore, adjunct tests such as the Cottle or modified Cottle maneuver can be helpful in determining if the collapse contributes significantly to their obstruction.

The Cottle maneuver is performed by gently pulling the cheek laterally on the side being tested in order to open the nasal valve.[13] The modified Cottle maneuver is performed by using the back of a cotton tip applicator to elevate and laterally displace the LLC (**Fig. 3**). When performing these maneuvers, it is important to note that the physician should not elevate the lateral cartilage further laterally than would be possible to

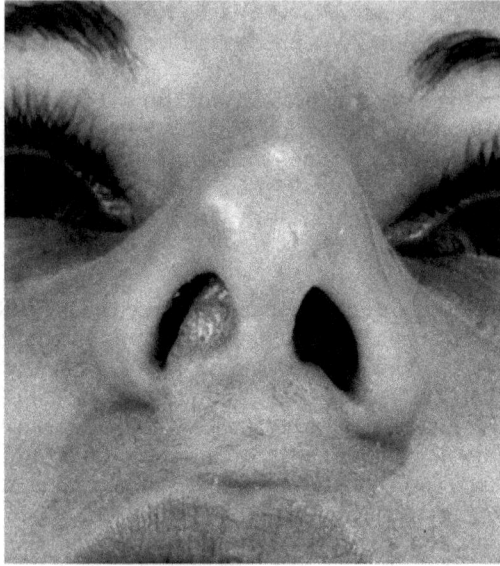

Fig. 2. Caudal septal deviation. (*From* Dorafshar AH, Rodriguez ED, Manson PN. Facial Trauma Surgery: From Primary Repair to Reconstruction. Elsevier; 2020. Fig 3.6.19.)

obtain surgically or nonsurgically. Subjective improvement in nasal airflow, along with an audible improvement in airflow, is considered a positive test and indicates that the patient may benefit from the treatment of eNVD.[14] While these tests are classically taught, there are much conflicting data regarding the validity and efficacy of the tests, and no studies to date have confirmed the association between a positive Cottle maneuver and the need for nasal valve repair.[15]

Additional adjunct testing such as anterior rhinomanometry, acoustic rhinometry, and rhinoresistometry have also been described in various studies.[16–19] These tests function to objectively assess nasal airflow and cross-sectional area of the nasal cavity. While these tests can be used to help diagnose nasal obstruction, their utility is limited when compared to nasal endoscopy, which is widely available, inexpensive, and well tolerated. These techniques have greater utility in measuring response to medical or surgical treatment of obstruction[16] and for providing objective data for research studies.

Despite the lack of randomized control trials, the American Academy of Otolaryngology—Head and Neck Surgery has reached a consensus regarding the utility of various physical examination findings when assessing nasal valve dysfunction. These include the subjective improvement of nasal airflow during a Cottle maneuver, the visible collapse of the nasal wall/alar rim during inspiration and increased nasal obstruction during deep inspiration. There was also consensus, however, that there was no gold standard test to diagnose eNVD.[20] Therefore, it is up to the clinician to combine findings from a thorough history and physical examination in order to diagnose and determine the best therapeutic option for eNVD.

Management

Nonsurgical

Treatment of the ENV can be broadly divided into surgical and nonsurgical in nature. In patients who are poor candidates for surgery, or those who wish to pursue nonsurgical

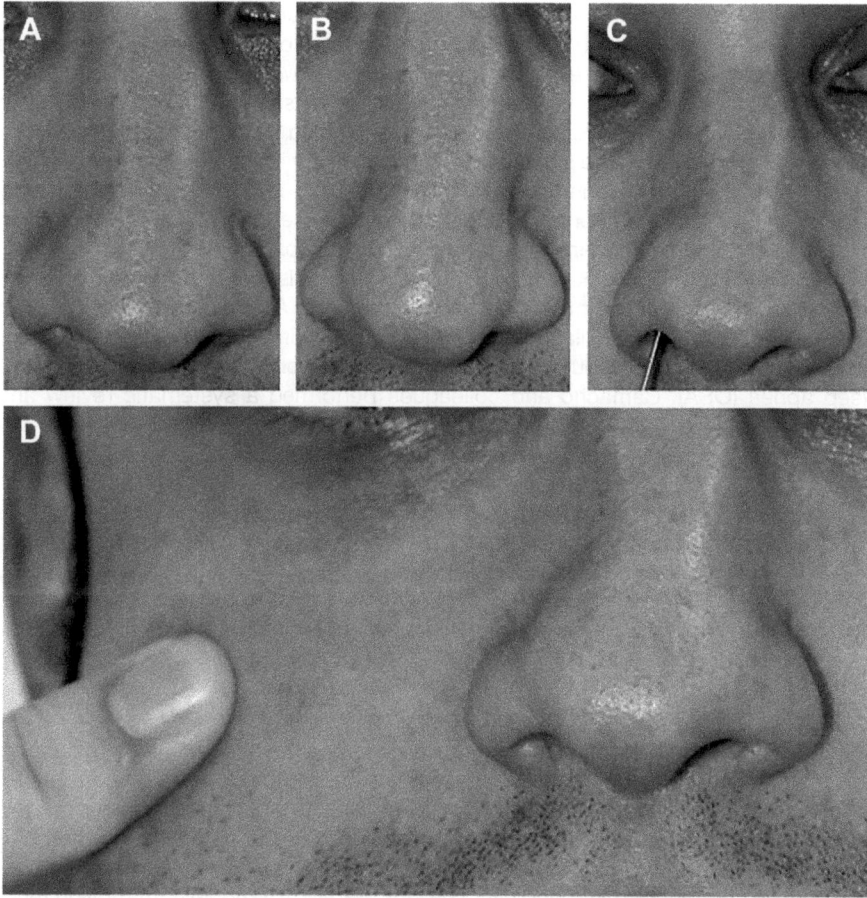

Fig. 3. Cottle maneuver: Anterior view of nose at rest (A) and with inspiration (B). Modified Cottle maneuver (C) and traditional Cottle maneuver (D) are performed. (*From* Massa ST, Farhood Z, Walen SG. Evidence-Based Clinical Practice in Otolaryngology. Elsevier; 2018. Fig. 6.2.)

management initially, several options are at the disposal of the surgeon.[21] When offering nonsurgical options, it is important that patients are aware of the pros, such as avoidance of surgery and immediate results, and cons, including cost, need for compliance, and local complications. Inexpensive commercial devices such as Breathe Right strips (GlaxoSmithKline, 980 Great West Road, Brentford, Middlesex, TW8 9GS, UK) can be purchased over the counter and work by expanding the lateral nasal wall. Several studies have demonstrated that these external dilators can improve several functional nasal breathing parameters such as increased inspiratory and expiratory nasal airflow and reduced nasal resistance.[3,22–24] The external dilators attach to the skin via medical grade adhesive and tend to be well tolerated with minimal skin irritation.[20]

Internal nasal dilators are an additional nonsurgical option that work by stenting the vestibule open. Multiple devices exist such as the Nasanita (by Siemens & Co, Germany) and Nozovent (by Pharmacure Health Care AB, Sweden). Riechelmann and colleagues investigated the efficacy of Nasanita and found a significant decrease in ENV size, as measured with computer assisted nasal base planimetry, in patients with alar collapse as compared to healthy controls.[25] However, both groups reported improved sense of nasal patency and notably alar collapse was completely abolished in the treatment group.[25] Lekakis and colleagues studied the impact of multiple internal nasal dilators as well as a single external nasal dilator on nasal valve compromise. Interestingly, their study found a statistically significant improvement in peak nasal inspiratory flow for all 3 internal devices, but not for the external device. However, all devices did improve patient-reported nasal obstruction scores.[26]

When offering a nonsurgical option to manage ENV, it is also important to know the underlying condition or symptom that is being targeted. As described earlier, certain external and internal nasal dilators are effective at reducing subjective nasal obstruction and improving airflow, but this does not extend to conditions such as obstructive sleep apnea (OSA). Camacho and colleagues performed a systematic review and meta-analysis to evaluate the efficacy of internal and external nasal dilators in the treatment of OSA and found no significant change in apnea-hypopnea index (AHI) scores in 12 of 14 studies.[27] Two studies showed a decrease in AHI with internal nasal dilators, but this was not curative of their OSA. Interestingly, nasal dilators may reduce the pressure required for continuous positive airway pressure (CPAP) use, which can help with patient tolerance of their CPAP devices.[28] Finally, the analysis performed by Camacho and colleagues revealed minimal improvement in snoring index with external nasal dilators, but a more significant improvement in the snoring index with internal nasal dilators.[27]

Surgical

Surgical management of the ENV depends on knowing the anatomic area of concern and the functional and cosmetic impact. The caudal septum is often responsible for nasal obstruction at the ENV level because of trauma or congenital abnormalities. However, the caudal septum is generally considered the most difficult portion of a septoplasty, and excision should be done with caution. Correction of caudal septum deviation can be broadly classified into 2 groups: cartilage remodeling/removing techniques or cartilage reconstruction techniques and can be performed with either endonasal or open approaches.[29]

When eNVD is associated with a long and deviated caudal septum, conservative resection of the deviation can open the ENV and avoid loss of tip support or avoid columellar abnormalities. Relaxing incisions along the concave side of the cartilage, alone or in combination with Mustardé sutures tied to the convex side, can help straighten the septum and fix it into position[29] (**Fig. 4**). In addition, a piece of bony septum can be secured to and straighten the deviated caudal septum.[30] Occasionally, a small amount of inferior caudal septum must be resected to accommodate appropriate vertical height[21] and allow it to be sutured to the anterior nasal spine. The swinging door technique is often described to correct deviations of the caudal septum laterally and off the midline of the maxillary crest. In this technique, the posterior septal angle is dissected from the maxillary crest and a space created between the mucosa on the contralateral side of the maxillary crest. The caudal septum is then placed on the opposite side of the crest using the maxillary crest as a door stop to keep it in place (**Fig. 5**). When using this technique, care should be taken not to cause narrowing of the contralateral ENV. In certain cases, the caudal septum can be repositioned into a groove along the contralateral side of the nasal spine and sutured to it without needing to excise excess cartilage.[21,29] The tongue-in-groove technique can be useful for a long caudal septum. Once the caudal septum is fixed to the midline, the medial crura

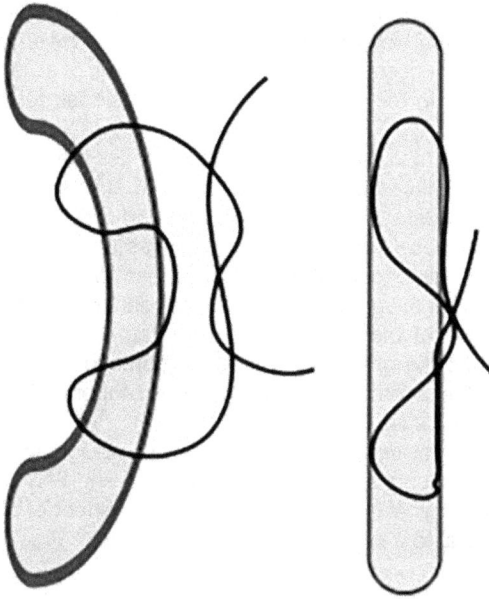

Fig. 4. Mustardé suture through septal cartilage: Knot placed on convex side that will then straighten septum when secured.

bilaterally are sutured to the caudal edge of the septum providing additional strength to the medial crura–septum complex and serving to define tip rotation and projection.[29]

In cases where the caudal septum is absent/deficient, or lacking in support, and cannot be properly repositioned or reinforced, cartilage reconstructive techniques should be pursued. An option is to use septal cartilage as a graft. When resecting cartilage, it is important to preserve an L-strut of 10 to 15 mm both caudally and dorsally to minimize the risk of complications such as saddle nose deformity.[31,32] If the caudal edge cannot be preserved, the harvested graft can be affixed to the nasal spine caudally and the remaining L-strut dorsally with polydioxane suture, thereby

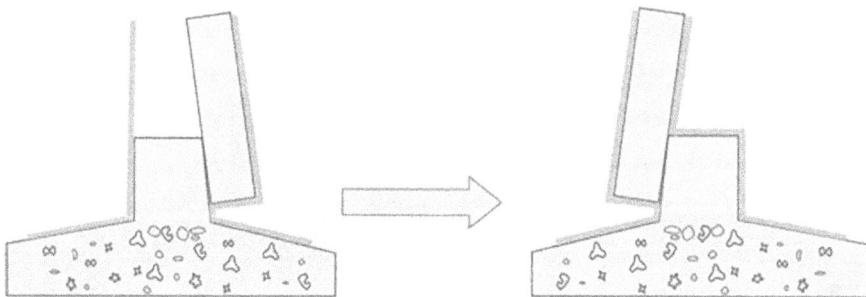

Fig. 5. Swinging door technique. Septum deviated off the maxillary crest to the left. Pink represents mucosa. Septum is then placed on the opposite side of the maxillary crest after a mucosal pocket is created, and the crest is utilized as a stop door to keep the septum in place.

recreating the caudal septum and L-strut. When there is insufficient or inadequate septal cartilage for grafting, extracorporeal techniques can be employed. These often use polydioxane plates or costal cartilage, either cadaveric or autograft, to reconstruct the L-strut with fixation to the anterior nasal spine, residual dorsal cartilage, and/or nasal bones.

Numerous techniques have been described to address the lateral wall insufficiency (LWI) component of ENV incompetency or obstruction. Batten grafts can be fashioned from harvested septal, costal, or conchal cartilage and are used to address LWI both at the level of internal nasal valve and ENV either as an overlay or underlay where maximal sidewall collapse occurs (**Fig. 6**). To address LWI at the level of the ENV, it is recommended to place the graft in line with or caudal to the lateral crus at the lateral half or two-thirds point of the crus.[33,34] Disadvantages to the batten graft include external fullness where the graft resides that is cosmetically displeasing as well as the possibility for LWI exacerbation if the graft is improperly placed.[1] Additionally, a poorly placed graft can cause nasal obstruction.

Alar rim grafts were first described by Troell and colleagues[34] in 2000 as a novel method to provide additional support at the nasal rim and ENV. Cartilage grafts are tunneled, through a marginal incision, along the inner aspect of the alar rim from the pyriform aperture lateral to a point medial to the nasal tip[35] (**Fig. 7**). As demonstrated

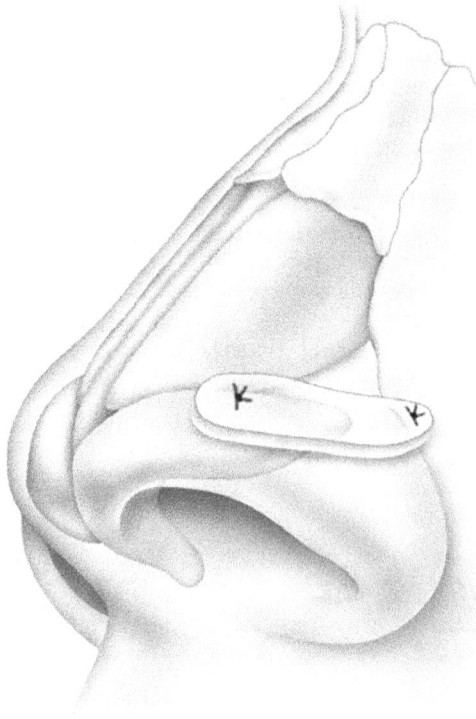

Fig. 6. Alar batten graft (onlay) extending from lateral half of lateral crus to pyriform aperture. (*From* Messina-Doucet, MT. Sleep Apnea and Snoring: Surgical and Non-Surgical Therapy. 2nd Ed. Elsevier; 2020. Fig. 23.5.)

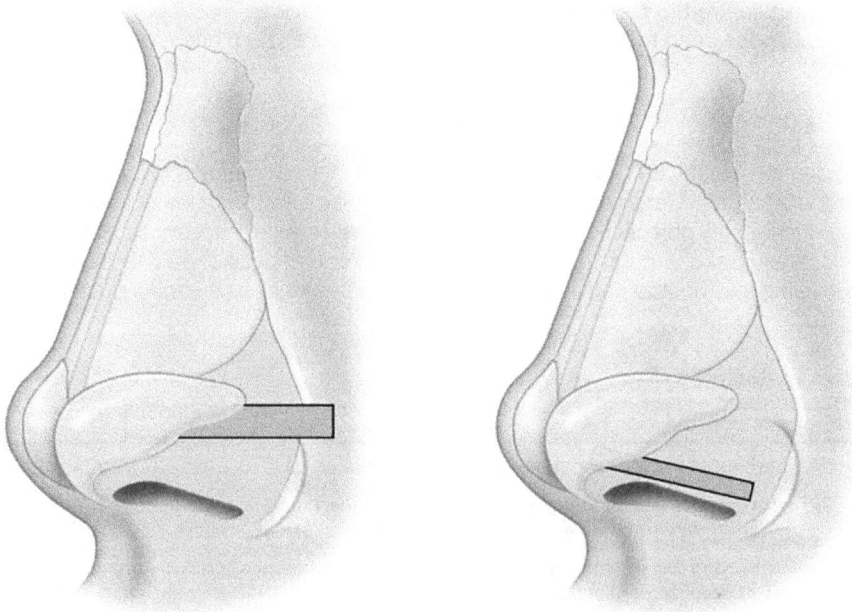

Fig. 7. Left panel demonstrating lateral crural strut graft (underlay). Right panel demonstrating alar rim graft. (*From* Moubayed SP, Most SP. Evaluation and Management of the Nasal Airway. Clin Plast Surg. 2022 Jan;49(1):23-31. Fig. 3.)

by Guyuron and colleagues, an alar rim graft is often a component of a rhinoplasty with their analysis showing 565 patients out of the 1427 analyzed who underwent nose reconstruction or rhinoplasty receiving an alar rim graft.[36] It is unlikely that the ENV compromise would solely be due to collapse/insufficiency of the alar rim, but the results from Guyuron and colleagues do show widening of the nostril with employment of this technique, thus increasing cross-sectional area.[36] These findings are also supported by Boahene and Hilger who analyzed 150 patients undergoing rhinoplasty, with 31 receiving alar rim grafts.[37] Of these 31 patients, 8 received an alar rim graft for dynamic collapse at the alar margin and noted improvement in ENV dysfunction postoperatively.[37] Like batten grafts, disadvantages to the alar grafts include external fullness in addition to poorly placed grafts causing nasal obstruction or nostril asymmetry.

Many methods to modify the lateral crus alone exist in addressing LWI. Malposition of the lateral crura can be cephalic due to the long axis of the lateral crus, or sagittal due to the short axis of the lateral crus.[33] According to Hamilton,[32] the goal when correcting a sagittal malposition is to position the caudal border of the lateral crus to a height equal to that of the cephalic border, thus ensuring the short axis is perpendicular to the septum. Regarding correction of long axis or cephalic malposition, this is often addressed with lateral crural strut graft reinforcement and suture fixation more caudally.[33] Lateral crural strut grafts are typically harvested from septal cartilage and can be placed as an overlay or underlay between the cartilage and vestibular skin/mucosa and project beyond the lateral crus cephalic edge (see **Fig. 7**). The result is reinforcement of the lateral crus thereby stiffening the crus and preventing LWI.[1,33,34] Apaydin describes lateral crural repositioning, whereby naturally concave lateral crura that lead to LWI can be dissected free from surrounding soft tissue, divided vertically near the dome, flipped over and thus creating a convex appearance, and again sutured to the dome.[34] A modification of this is to resect both lateral crura and transpose each to the contralateral side and suture into place after flipping each over.[34]

SUMMARY

The definition of the ENV can be variable and associated disease pathologies complex and multifactorial. Careful evaluation and detailed discussion with the patient are paramount to identify objective and subjective concerns. Multiple nonsurgical and surgical options exist and should be tailored to each patient's specific needs. Preoperative counseling and postoperative follow-up are important to ensure each patient obtains the desired result.

CLINICS CARE POINTS

- The anatomy of the ENV and the resultant etiology of eNVD is complex and multifactorial.
- The workup of eNVD should focus on evaluating the multiple contributing factors and incorporating patient goals.
- Nonsurgical and surgical management options for the treatment of eNVD exist and the risks/benefits of each should be explained to patients.
- The surgical treatment of eNVD should address the specific affected subsite(s) keeping in mind cosmetic outcomes.

DISCLOSURE

The authors have nothing to disclose.

REFERENCES

1. Barrett DM, Casanueva FJ, Cook TA. Management of the nasal valve. Facial Plast Surg Clin North Am 2016;24:219–34.
2. Spielmann PM, White PS, Hussain SS. Surgical techniques for the treatment of nasal valve collapse: a systematic review. Laryngoscope 2009;119:1281–90.
3. Khosh MM, Jen A, Honrado C, et al. Nasal valve reconstruction: experience in 53 consecutive patients. Arch Facial Plast Surg 2004;6:167–71.
4. Osborn JL, Sacks R. Chapter 2: Nasal obstruction. Am J Rhinol Allergy 2013; 27(Suppl 1):S7–8.
5. Fraser L, Kelly G. An evidence-based approach to the management of the adult with nasal obstruction. Clin Otolaryngol 2009;34:151–5.
6. Mink PJ. Le nez comme voie respiratorie. Press Otolaryngol Belg; 1903. p. 481–96.
7. Shaida AM, Kenyon GS. The nasal valves: changes in anatomy and physiology in normal subjects. Rhinology 2000;38:7–12.
8. Nigro CE, Nigro JF, Mion O, et al. Nasal valve: anatomy and physiology. Braz J Otorhinolaryngol 2009;75:305–10.
9. Sulsenti G, Palma P. [The nasal valve area: structure, function, clinical aspects and treatment. Sulsenti's technic for correction of valve deformities]. Acta Otorhinolaryngol Ital 1989;9(Suppl 22):1–25.

10. Schriever VA, Hummel T, Lundström JN, et al. Size of nostril opening as a measure of intranasal volume. Physiol Behav 2013;110-111:3–5.
11. Ohki M, Naito K, Cole P. Dimensions and resistances of the human nose: racial differences. Laryngoscope 1991;101:276–8.
12. Morgan NJ, MacGregor FB, Birchall MA, et al. Racial differences in nasal fossa dimensions determined by acoustic rhinometry. Rhinology 1995;33:224–8.
13. Tikanto J, Pirila T. Effects of the Cottle's maneuver on the nasal valve as assessed by acoustic rhinometry. Am J Rhinol 2007;21:456–9.
14. Das A, Spiegel JH. Evaluation of validity and specificity of the cottle maneuver in diagnosis of nasal valve collapse. Plast Reconstr Surg 2020;146:277–80.
15. Bonaparte JP, Campbell R. A prospective cohort study assessing the clinical utility of the Cottle maneuver in nasal septal surgery. J Otolaryngol Head Neck Surg 2018;47:45.
16. Fisher EW, Lund VJ, Scadding GK. Acoustic rhinometry in rhinological practice: discussion paper. J R Soc Med 1994;87:411–3.
17. Hilberg O, Jackson AC, Swift DL, et al. Acoustic rhinometry: evaluation of nasal cavity geometry by acoustic reflection. J Appl Physiol (1985) 1989;66:295–303.
18. Mlynski G, Low J. [Rhinoresistometry–a further development of rhinomanometry]. Laryngo-Rhino-Otol 1993;72:608–10.
19. Kern EB. Rhinomanometry. Otolaryngol Clin North Am 1973;6:863–74.
20. Rhee JS, Weaver EM, Park SS, et al. Clinical consensus statement: Diagnosis and management of nasal valve compromise. Otolaryngol Head Neck Surg 2010;143:48–59.
21. Hamilton GS 3rd. The external nasal valve. Facial Plast Surg Clin North Am 2017;25:179–94.
22. Gehring JM, Garlick SR, Wheatley JR, et al. Nasal resistance and flow resistive work of nasal breathing during exercise: effects of a nasal dilator strip. J Appl Physiol (1985) 2000;89:1114–22.
23. Kirkness JP, Wheatley JR, Amis TC. Nasal airflow dynamics: mechanisms and responses associated with an external nasal dilator strip. Eur Respir J 2000;15:929–36.
24. Ward J, Ciesla R, Becker W, et al. Randomized trials of nasal patency and dermal tolerability with external nasal dilators in healthy volunteers. Allergy Rhinol (Providence) 2018;9. 2152656718796740.
25. Riechelmann H, Karow E, DiDio D, et al. External nasal valve collapse - a case-control and interventional study employing a novel internal nasal dilator (Nasanita). Rhinology 2010;48:183–8.
26. Lekakis G, Dekimpe E, Steelant B, et al. Managing nasal valve compromise patients with nasal dilators: objective vs. subjective parameters. Rhinology 2016;54:348–54.
27. Camacho M, Malu OO. Kram YAet al. Nasal Dilators (Breathe Right Strips and No-Zovent) for Snoring and OSA: A Systematic Review and Meta-Analysis. Pulm Med 2016;2016:4841310.
28. Schonhofer B, Kerl J, Suchi S, et al. Effect of nasal valve dilation on effective CPAP level in obstructive sleep apnea. Respir Med 2003;97:1001–5.
29. Cobo R, Caldas A. Caudal septum surgery techniques reviewed. Curr Opin Otolaryngol Head Neck Surg 2017;25:4–11.
30. Gelidan AG. Technique to fix the stubborn deviated caudal septum with an internal bone graft splint. Plast Reconstr Surg Glob Open 2021 Dec 20;9(12):e3921.

31. Russell MD, Kangelaris GT. Comparison of L-strut preservation in endonasal and endoscopic septoplasty: a cadaveric study. Int Forum Allergy Rhinol 2014;4: 147–50.
32. Mowlavi A, Masouem S, Kalkanis J, et al. Septal cartilage defined: implications for nasal dynamics and rhinoplasty. Plast Reconstr Surg 2006;117:2171–4.
33. Hamilton GS 3rd. Form and function of the nasal tip: reorienting and reshaping the lateral crus. Facial Plast Surg 2016;32:49–58.
34. Apaydin F. Nasal valve surgery. Facial Plast Surg 2011;27:179–91.
35. Troell RJ, Powell NB, Riley RW, et al. Evaluation of a new procedure for nasal alar rim and valve collapse: nasal alar rim reconstruction. Otolaryngol Head Neck Surg 2000;122:204–11.
36. Guyuron B, Bigdeli Y, Sajjadian A. Dynamics of the alar rim graft. Plast Reconstr Surg 2015;135:981–6.
37. Boahene KD, Hilger PA. Alar rim grafting in rhinoplasty: indications, technique, and outcomes. Arch Facial Plast Surg 2009;11:285–9.

Evaluation and Management of Lateral Wall Insufficiency

Monica K. Rossi Meyer, MD, Sam P. Most, MD*

KEYWORDS

- Lateral wall insufficiency • Rhinoplasty • Functional rhinoplasty
- Nasal valve collapse

KEY POINTS

- Nasal airway obstruction can have inflammatory and structural etiologies and proper treatment depends on accurate diagnosis.
- Lateral wall insufficiency (LWI) is best evaluated during normal inspiration and further characterized with use of the modified Cottle maneuver.
- Patient-reported outcome measures are a vital part of the evaluation of patients with lateral wall insufficiency.
- Several different surgical techniques have been described for treatment of lateral wall insufficiency and while no consensus exists, there is strong evidence to support use of lateral crural strut grafts and alar rim grafts to correct dynamic valve collapse.
- Minimally invasive treatments of LWI have been reported but require careful patient selection for successful use.

INTRODUCTION

Nasal airway obstruction is characterized as the sensation of insufficient airflow or difficulty breathing through the nose.[1] Nasal obstruction is very common, and its etiology can be multifactorial with both inflammatory and structural contributions. Most inflammatory causes of nasal obstruction will improve with medical management alone while surgery is applied to patients with structural deficiencies.[2] Structural deficiencies can generally be classified as fixed or dynamic as they apply to the involved nasal anatomy. The external nasal valve (ENV) is formed by the caudal septum, medial crura of the alar cartilages, alar rim, and nasal sill and serves as the entry point to the nasal airway.[3] Caudal septal deviations account for approximately 5% to 8% of all patterns of septal deviation and produce a much greater symptomatic nasal obstruction than posterior septal deviations.[4–6] Bernoulli effect can cause a dynamic ENV collapse

Division of Facial Plastic and Reconstructive Surgery, Department of Otolaryngology–Head and Neck Surgery, Stanford University School of Medicine, 801 Welch Road, Stanford, CA 94305, USA
* Corresponding author.
E-mail address: smost@stanford.edu

Otolaryngol Clin N Am 58 (2025) 269–278
https://doi.org/10.1016/j.otc.2024.07.027
0030-6665/25/© 2024 Elsevier Inc. All rights are reserved, including those for text and data mining, AI training, and similar technologies.
oto.theclinics.com

secondary to contralateral caudal septal deviation which is usually corrected with caudal septoplasty. Dynamic collapse of the ENV can also be attributed to a congenitally weak lateral nasal wall, iatrogenic weakening following rhinoplasty with lower lateral cartilage resection, or a severely ptotic nasal tip.[3,7] The internal nasal valve (INV) is bound by the nasal sidewall, upper lateral cartilage, and inferior turbinate laterally, septum medially, and nasal floor inferiorly. The cross-sectional area of the INV is the most restrictive to air flow and therefore is a major contributor to nasal airway obstruction.[8] Static narrowing of the INV can be congenital or iatrogenic due to midvault destabilization after dorsal hump reduction in primary rhinoplasty.[9] Dynamic collapse of the INV can occur due to congenital and iatrogenic causes and is now defined along with dynamic ENV collapse as lateral wall insufficiency.[10]

The term lateral wall insufficiency (LWI) was coined by the senior author to describe dynamic lateral wall movement with inspiration, and may occur both normally and in the pathologic state.[11] Furthermore, the senior author recognized 2 primary zones of LWI, with Zone 1 referring to the dynamic movement of the nasal sidewall at the level of the upper lateral cartilage and scroll region, while Zone 2 describes the region at the level of the ala between the upper and lower lateral cartilages and is roughly equivalent to previously described external nasal valve collapse (**Fig. 1**).[10,12]

Evaluation of Lateral Wall Insufficiency

Eliciting a focused yet thorough patient history is the first step in identifying the etiology of nasal obstruction. Onset and duration of the patient's nasal airway obstruction are important to obtain for example, post-traumatic, post-operative, recent environmental

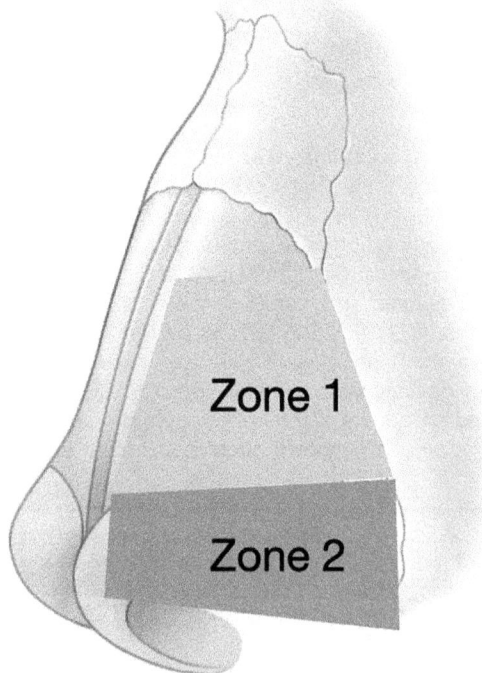

Fig. 1. Zone 1 (*upper zone*) corresponds to dynamic internal nasal valve collapse. Zone 2 (*lower zone*) corresponds to previously described external nasal valve collapse.

changes, and chronicity. Additionally, noting the laterality of symptoms is important as unilateral obstruction is highly suggestive of anatomic causes, albeit bilateral obstruction does not exclude anatomic conditions.[13] Aggravating or alleviating factors, and determining efficacy of nasal medications such as nasal steroid sprays or nasal decongestants can also help narrow the differential. If a patient is being considered for surgery, comorbidities and personal history should also be included to help guide operative counseling.

Evaluation of LWI is done by observing the nasal vestibule and assessing the position of the lateral nasal sidewall at rest and degree of lateral nasal sidewall motion with normal inspiration.[11] Examination of the nasal vestibule should determine if columellar deviation is present as this may suggest an underlying caudal septal deviation. The area(s) of inward motion during inspiration are then noted. Two important notes on examination: first, this must be done without a speculum. Second, inspiration must be at normal levels—supranormal (ie, fast or labored) inhalation causes some degree of collapse in most all patients. Third, the examiner should identify any volitional muscle closure movement, which many patients exhibit (ie, downward motion of the levator labii superioris alaeque nasalis musculature). In each zone, LWI is graded according to the distance the nasal wall moves toward the septum (grade 0 is no movement, grade 1 is 1%–33%, grade 2 is 34%–66%, and grade 3 is 67%–100%). Zone 1 collapse is more often idiopathic and can be attributed to age, trauma, or hereditary. Zone 2 collapse occurs more inferiorly and is more often iatrogenic.[11] The modified Cottle maneuver is then performed by placing an ear curette or wooden end of a cotton-tip applicator into the nose and providing stabilization and then lateralization of the lateral nasal wall during inspiration. In cases of static collapse, improvement with inspiration on the obstructed side with lateralization and an identifiable source of obstruction, for example, caudal septal deviation may indicate surgical correction.[7] In cases of dynamic collapse, both stabilization and lateralization of the nasal side wall are tested during inspiration and can determine if surgical correction of the source of collapse is achievable.[2] The original Cottle maneuver—lateral distraction of the cheek during normal inspiration—should not be used as it has been shown to have low construct validity.[14]

Several objective anatomic and physiologic measures of the nasal airway exist: acoustic rhinometry, sinonasal imaging, rhinomanometry, nasal peak inspiratory flow, and computational fluid dynamics,[15] However, a strong correlation between these measures and patient's subjective complaint of nasal obstruction has not yet been established.[16–20] Therefore, there is currently no gold standard objective test for nasal airway obstruction.[3] Patient-reported outcome measures (PROMs) evaluate the subjective experience of the patient and the patient's self-reported assessment of treatment efficacy without interpretation from the physician.[15] Both the nasal valve compromise and rhinoplasty clinical practice guidelines recommend the routine use of PROMs in nasal surgical patients.[3,21]

When the nasal valve is the source of nasal obstruction, operative correction can potentially result in alteration of the external nasal appearance.[2] Therefore, a combined functional and cosmetic PROM should be administered both before and after surgery to assess the change in both components. The Standardized Cosemesis and Health Nasal Outcomes Survey (SCHNOS) is a one such validated PROM.[22] Additionally, the survey's minimal clinically important difference was determined and found to be clinically significant in its ability to assess both the obstructive and cosmetic concerns of rhinoplasty patients.[22] The Nasal Obstruction and Septoplasty Effectiveness (NOSE) score is a validated 5-question disease-specific questionnaire based on a 4-point scale with raw scores multiplied by 5 and reported as a range from 0 to 100 (mild: 5–25, moderate:

30–50, severe: 55–75, extreme: >80).[23] It has been shown to be a reliable, sensitive evaluation of nasal obstruction and was originally validated in patients undergoing septoplasty surgery and is often reported in studies of functional rhinoplasty.[24–28] However, since any rhinoplasty may alter function or esthetics, the obstruction-focused NOSE questionnaire does not adequately monitor rhinoplasty patients, be they functional, esthetic, or both. Other rhinoplasty-related PROMs include the Rhinoplasty Outcomes Evaluation, Functional Rhinoplasty Outcomes Inventory, Rhinoplasty Health Inventory Nasal Outcomes (RHINO) scale, and Esthetic Rhinoplasty Scale, all of which are examples of combined functional and cosmetic PROMs but have not been validated or characterized as extensively as the SCHNOS.[29]

Treatment of Lateral Wall Insufficiency

Multiple techniques have been described in the treatment of LWI but there is no widely adopted approach. The American Academy of Otolaryngology-Head and Neck Surgery has previously published a consensus statement based on a panel of functional rhinoplasty experts regarding diagnosis and management of nasal valve collapse.[8] Importantly, they concluded that treating the lateral nasal wall and alar rim are distinct entities from procedures that correct a deviated nasal septum or inferior turbinate hypertrophy. Additionally, the consensus statement makes note that in certain cases, nasal strips can be used therapeutically in patients with nasal valve collapse. The statement then concludes that the use of PROMs is more valuable than objective measures underscoring the fact that no gold standard objective test exists for nasal airway obstruction.

Proper treatment of LWI starts with correct identification of the underlying deficiency. Zone 1 LWI is typically caused by weakness of the upper lateral cartilage attachment to the pyriform aperture and is common in the aging population. Several surgical techniques have been described for the treatment of internal nasal valve stenosis and collapse. Destabilization of the midvault and subsequent zone 1 LWI can occur after dorsal hump reduction in primary rhinoplasty.[30] In this situation, spreader grafts or autospreader flaps are a good treatment option to support the INV. The autospreader technique involves making a flap based on the upper lateral cartilages (ULC) and is best suited in the reductive rhinoplasty setting.[9] Whereas, spreader grafts are carved from harvested cartilage and secured between the ULC and septum.[30,31] The butterfly graft is another approach to correcting an iatrogenically weakened internal nasal valve whereby a conchal cartilage graft spans the supratip area and inserts under the cephalic edge of the lower lateral cartilages (LLC) and supporting the caudal edge of the INV.[32] While the butterfly graft is effective, it does increase the tip width on frontal view which can be undesirable for some patients.[33] Lateral crural strut grafts (LCSG) or bone-anchored sutures have also been described to treat zone 1 LWI with the senior author (SPM) favoring the former.[34,35] The LCSG is placed underneath the LLC and extends to the pyriform aperture. Its position can vary from more cephalic to more caudal with a cephalic orientation better suited for treatment of zone 1 LWI. Functionally, it strengthens and straightens the LLC thus improving airway **Fig. 2**.[36,37]

Zone 2 LWI may also occur in cases of excessive cephalic orientation of the lower lateral cartilages, weak alar soft tissue, or it can be iatrogenic from resection of the LLC during rhinoplasty. Alar batten grafts were first introduced by Tardy to address both internal and external nasal valve incompetence.[38] The grafts are a curvilinear shape and placed into a precise pocket at the point of maximal lateral wall collapse or supra-alar pinching but similar to the butterfly graft, will create a visible fullness at the site of the graft.[39] Therefore, zone 2 collapse is best treated with structural support such as free or articulated rim grafts, or an inferiorly placed lateral crural strut graft.[35]

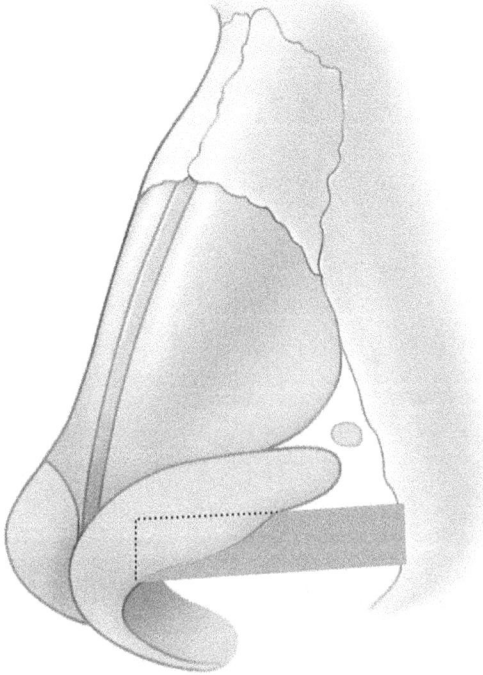

Fig. 2. Lateral crural strut graft (LCSG). LCSG is placed underneath the lower lateral cartilage (LLC) and extends laterally over the pyriform aperture. It functions to strengthen and straighten the LLC contributing to both functional support of zone 1 and improved tip aesthetics.

Alar rim grafts were first reported by Troell and colleagues to demonstrate a 94.4% improvement in nasal obstruction from nasal valve collapse.[40] Alar rim grafts are now a common technique used to correct zone 2 LWI but they also serve to advance the ala caudally, widen the nostril, and elongate a short nostril.[41] Articulated rim grafts (ARG) were first described by Davis and colleagues and are a variation of the alar rim graft. ARGs differ from the free-floating alar rim grafts in that they are secured to the nasal tip above the lower lateral cartilage.[42] Esthetically, ARGs provide a highlight that extends to the tip, an advantage over the free-floating alar rim graft. Underlay articulated rim grafts (uARGs) or extended alar contour grafts are a variation on ARGs.[43] The senior author (SPM) positions uARGs below the domal cartilages, secures them with sutures, and then places them into soft tissue pockets at the alar margins (**Fig. 3**). The grafts may be advantageous in thin skinned patients with cartilage predominant tips in which overlay ARGs may be more visible.[37] Esthetically, the uARG creates a highlight along the rim margin, eliminating tip to lobule discrepancy and functionally they add support to zone 2.

The LCSG and alar rim graft are the 2 preferred techniques of the senior author for treatment of zone 1 and zone 2 LWI, respectively. Vaezeafshar and colleagues evaluated 44 patients who underwent open septorhinoplasty to repair dynamic valve collapse and compared them to age-matched and sex-matched controls undergoing cosmetic rhinoplasty. Zone 2 collapse was treated with alar rim grafts and zone 1 collapse was treated with LCSG. The authors found objective and subjective

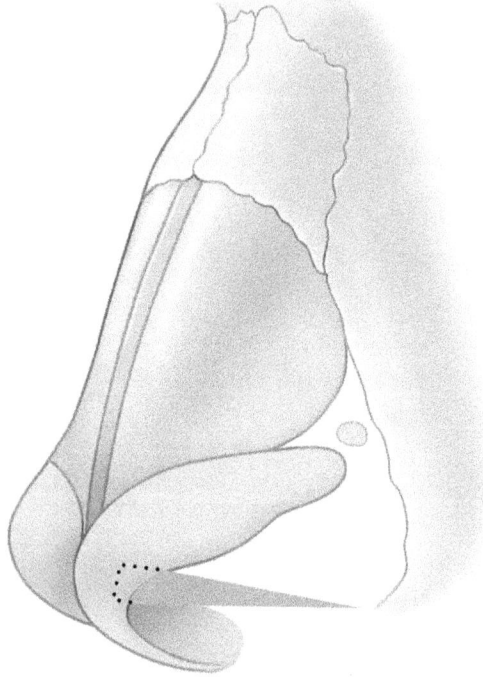

Fig. 3. Underlay articulated rim graft. Variation of an articulated rim graft that is secured underneath the dome of the LLCs and placed into soft tissue pocket at the alar margins. Functions to support zone 2 in cases of lateral wall insufficiency and provide an esthetic highlight along the rim margin.

improvements in the nasal airway after LWI repair with significant improvement in the LWI grades post-operatively and stable on long-term follow-up.[35] In another study, Barham and colleagues compared LCSG with cephalic turn-in of the lateral crura to correct external nasal valve dysfunction. They concluded that both techniques were effective in improving objective and subjective measures with the LCSG group demonstrating significant reductions in NOSE scores post-operatively.[44]

Alloplastic materials have also been explored as options for treatment of LWI. Non-absorbale implants made from expanded polytetrafloroethylene[45] and high-density porous polyethylene[46] have been inserted into the soft tissues of the lateral nasal walls to improve stiffness. However, these have not gained wide acceptance due to increased risk of infection, extrusion, and possible need for revision.[47] San Nicolo and colleagues introduced a bioabsorbable implant as a minimally invasive treatment option for nasal obstruction caused by LWI.[48] The implant is a 70:30 blend of poly (L-lactide) and poly (D-lactide) placed via an endonasal approach to the nasal sidewall parallel to the dorsum. The implant sits over the nasal bone and extends caudally to support the soft tissues of the area corresponding to the upper and lower lateral cartilages.[48] The implant functions to stabilize and not lateralize the nasal sidewall; therefore, careful examination using the modified cottle technique should be employed to determine patient candidacy.[49] In-human studies have demonstrated the potential for the implant to improve the nasal obstruction symptoms from 6 to 24 months,[50,51]; however, an incidence of 13.2% and 16.5% of device-related complications including infection, hematoma, inflammation, and mandatory device retrieval were also re-ported.[52] Thus, more clinical trials are needed to determine its overall effectiveness.[49]

SUMMARY

It is important to recognize lateral wall insufficiency (LWI) as an independent cause of nasal airway obstruction. A thorough history that includes PROMs and physical exam-ination provides the functional rhinoplasty surgeon with the diagnosis; treatment can then be tailored to the specific cause. While multiple approaches to treatment of LWI exist, the senior author prefers to treat zone 1 LWI with lateral crural strut grafts and zone 2 with alar rim grafts because of their robust functional outcomes and esthetic superiority over other described operative techniques. In addition to being used as a pre-operative grading system, LWI has been shown to correlate well with PROMs and is a reliable indicator of subjective improvement after surgery.[35]

CLINICS CARE POINTS

- Evaluation of lateral wall insufficiency (LWI) starts with a focused history to rule out other etiologies of nasal obstruction.
- Examination of LWI should be performed without a nasal speculum and during normal inspiration.
- During the exam, it is also important to determine if lateralization or stabilization of the lateral nasal side wall improves the obstruction.
- The approach to surgically treating Zone 1 LWI depends on the etiology; lateral crural strut grafts are a great option for supporting the caudal edge of the internal nasal valve.
- Zone 2 LWI corresponds to the area of external nasal valve collapse and is best treated with articulated rim grafts; the underlay technique is great for patients with thin skin or cartilage predominant tips.

DISCLOSURES

The authors have no financial or funding contributions to disclose.

REFERENCES

1. Mohan S, Fuller JC, Ford SF, et al. Diagnostic and therapeutic management of nasal airway obstruction: advances in diagnosis and treatment. JAMA Facial Plastic Surgery 2018;20:409–18.
2. Moubayed S, Most SP. Evaluation and management of the nasal airway. Clin Plast Surg 2022;49(1):23–31.
3. Rhee JS, Weaver EM, Park SS, et al. Clinical consensus statement: diagnosis and management of nasal valve compromise. Otolaryngol Head Neck Surg 2010;143: 48–59.
4. Grymer L, Holberg O, Elbrond O, et al. Acoustic rhinometry: evaluation of the nasal cavity with septal deviations, before and after septoplasty. Laryngoscope 1989;99:1180–7.
5. Guyuron B, Uzzo CD, Schull H. A practical classification of septonasal deviation and an effective guide to septal surgery. Plast Reconstr Surg 1999;104:2202–9.

6. SedwicK J, Lopez AB, Gajewski BJ, et al. Caudal septoplasty for treatment of septal deviation: aesthetic and functional correction of the nasal base. Arch Facial Plast Surg 2005;7:158–62.

7. Rudy S, Moubayed SP, Most SP. Lateral wall insufficiency after sepatl reconstruction. Facial Plast Surg 2017;33:451–2.

8. Rhee JS, Arganbright JM, McMullin BT, et al. Evidence supporting functional rhinoplasty or nasal valve repair: a 25 year systematic review. Otolaryngol Head Neck Surg 2008;139:10–20.

9. Saedi B, Amali A, Gharavis V, et al. Spreader flaps do not change early functional outcomes in reduction rhinoplasty: a randomized control trial. Am J Rhinol Allergy 2014;28:70–4.

10. Tsao G, Fijalkowski N, Most SP. Validation of a grading system for lateral nasal wall insufficiency. Allergy Rhinology 2013;4(2):e66–8.

11. Most SP. Trends in functional rhinoplasty. Arch Facial Plast Surg 2008;10(6):410–3.

12. Most SP. Comparing methods for repair of the external nasal valve one more step toward a unified view of lateral wall insufficiency. JAMA Facial Plastic Surgery 2015;17(5):345–6.

13. Valero A, Navarro AM, Del Cuvillo A, et al. Position paper on nasal obstruction: evaluation and treatment. J Investig Allergol Clin Immunol 2018;28:67–90.

14. Das A, Spiegel J. Evaluation oof validity and specificity of the cottle maneuver in diagnosis of nasal valve collapse. Plast Reconstr Surg 2020;146:277–80.

15. Spataro E, Most SP. Measruing nasal obstruction. POtolaryngol Clin North Am 2018;51:883–95.

16. Fairley J, Durham LH, Ell SR. Correlation of subjective sensation of nasal patency with nasal inspiratory peak flow rate. Clin Otolaryngol Allied Sci 1993;18:19–22.

17. Hirschberg A. Correlation between objective and subjective assessments of nasal patency. ORL J Otorhinolarngol Relat Spec 1998;60:206–11.

18. Lam DJ, Weaver EM. Comparison of anatomic, physiological, and subjective measures of the nasal airway. Am J Rhinol 2006;20:463–70.

19. Sipila J, Suonpaa J, Silvoniemi P, et al. Correlations between subjective sensation of nasal patency and rhinomanometry in both unilateral and total nasal assessment. ORL J Otorhinolarngol Relat Spec 1995;57:260–3.

20. Wang D, Raza MT, Goh DY, et al. Acoustic rhinometry in nasal allergen challenge study: which dimensional measures are meaningful? Clin Exp Allergy 2004;34:1093–8.

21. Ishii L, Tollefson TT, Basura GJ, et al. Clinical practice guideline: improving nasal form and function after rhinoplasty executive summary. Otolaryngol Head Neck Surg 2017;2017(156):205–19.

22. Kandathil C, Saltychev M, Abdelwahab M, et al. Minimal clinically important difference of the standardized cosmesis and health nasal outcomes survey. Aesthetic Surg J 2019;39(8):837–40.

23. Stewart MG, Witsell DL, Smith TL, et al. Development and validation of the nasal obstruction symptom evaluation (NOSE) scale. Otolaryngol Head Neck Surg 2004;130(4):157–63.

24. Stewart MG, Smith TL, Weaver EM, et al. Outcomes after nasal septoplasty: results from the nasal obstruction septoplasty effectiveness (NOSE) study. Otolaryngol Head Neck Surg 2004;130:283–90.

25. Rhee JS, Poetker DM, Smith TL, et al. Nasal valve surgery improves disease-specific quality of life. Laryngoscope 2005;115(3):437–40.

26. Most SP. Analysis of outcomes after functional rhinoplasty using a disease- specific quality-of-life instrument. Arch Facial Plast Surg 2006;8(5):306–9.
27. Rhee JS, Sullivan CD, Frank DO, et al. A systematic review of patient-reported nasal obstruction scores: defining normative and symptomatic ranges in surgical patients. JAMA Facial Plast Surg 2014;16(3):219–25.
28. Lipan MJ, Most SP. Development of a severity classification system for subjective nasal obstruction. JAMA Facial Plast Surg 2013;15(5):358–61.
29. Barone M, Cogliandro A, DiStefano N, et al. A systematic review of patient-reported outcome measures after rhinoplasty. Eur Arch Otorhinolaryngol 2017; 274(4):1807–11.
30. Rudy S, Moubayed SP, Most SP. Midvault reconstruction in primary rhinoplasty. Facial Plast Surg 2017;33(2):133–8.
31. Sheen J. Spreader graft: a method of reconstructing the roof of the middle nasal vault following rhinoplasty. Plast Reconstr Surg 1984;73(2):230–9.
32. Clark JM, Cook TA. The 'butterfly' graft in functional secondary rhinoplasty. Laryngoscope 2002;112(11):1917–25.
33. Chaiet SR, Marcus BC. Nasal tip volume analysis after butterfly graft. Ann Plast Surg 2014;72(1):9–12.
34. Roofe S, Most SP. Placement of lateral nasal suspension suture via an external rhinoplasty approach. Arch Facial Plast Surg 2007;9:214–6.
35. Vaezeafshar R, Moubayed SP, Most SP. Repair of lateral wall insufficiency. JAMA Facial Plast Surg 2018;20:111–5.
36. Gunther J, Friedman RM. Lateral crural strut graft: technique and clinical applications in rhinoplasty. Plast Reconstr Surg 1997;99:934–52.
37. Most S. Altering nasal tip volume and geometry. In: Comprehensive rhinoplasty: structural & preservation concepts. St Louis (MO): Quality Medical Publishing Inc; 2023. p. 280–6.
38. Tardy ME, Garner ET. Inspiratory nasal obstruction secondary to alar and nasal valve collapse: technique for repair using autologous cartilage. Operative Tech Otolaryngol Head Neck Surg 1990;1:215–8.
39. Toriumi D, Josen J, Weinberger M, et al. Use of alar batten grafts for correction of nasal valve collapse. Arch Otolaryngol Head Neck Surg 1997;123(8):802–8.
40. Troell RJ, Riley RW, Li KK. Evaluation of a new procedure for alar rim and valve collapse. Otolaryngol Head Neck Surg 2000;122(2):204–11.
41. Guyuron B, Bigdeli Y, Sajjadian A. Dynamics of the alar rim graft. Plast Reconstr Surg 2015;135(4):981–6.
42. Ballin AC, Chance E, Davis RE, et al. The articulated alar rim graft: reengineering the conventional alar rim graft for improved contour and support. Facial Plast Surg 2016;32(4):384–97.
43. Cochran CS, Sieber DA. Extended alar contour grafts: an evolution of the lateral crural strut graft techinque in rhinoplasty. Plast Reconstr Surg 2017;140: 559e–67e.
44. Barhan HP, Christensen J, Sacks R, et al. Costal cartilage lateral crural strut grafts vs. cephalic crural turn-in for correction of external nasal valve dysfunction. JAMA Facial Plast Surg 2015;17(5):340–5.
45. Winkler AA, Soler ZM, Leong PL, et al. Complications associated with alloplastic implants in rhinoplasty. Arch Facial Plast Surg 2012;14(6):437–41.
46. Ramakrishnan JB, Danner CJ, Yee SW. The use of porous polyethylene implants to correct nasal valve collapse. Otolaryngol Head Neck Surg 2007;136(3): 357–61.

47. Berghaus A. Implants for reconstructive surgery of the nose and ears. GMS Curr Top Otorhinolaryngol Head Neck Surg 2007;6:Doc06.
48. San Nicoló M, Stelter K, Sadick H, et al. Absorbable implant to treat nasal valve collapse. Facial Plast Surg 2017;332:233–40.
49. Sanan A, Most SP. A bioabsorbable lateral nasal wall stent for dynamic nasal valve collapse: a review. Facial Plast Surg Clin North Am 2019;27(3):367–71.
50. San Nicoló M, Stelter K, Sadick H, et al. 2-Year follow-up study of an absorbable implant to treat nasal valve collapse. Facial Plast Surg 2018;34(5):545–50.
51. Stolovitzky P, Sidle DM, Ow RA, et al. A prospective study for treatment of nasal valve collapse due to lateral wall insufficiency: Outcomes using a bioabsorbable implant. Laryngoscope 2018;128(11):2483–9.
52. Kim D, Lee HH, Kim SH, et al. Effectiveness of using a bioabsorbable implant (Latera) to treat nasal valve collapse in patients with nasal obstruction: systemic review and meta-analysis. Int Forum Allergy Rhinol 2020;10(6):719–25.

Indications and Evolution of the Butterfly Graft in Nasal Valve Repair

Tyler M. Rist, MD[a], J. Madison Clark, MD[b],*

KEYWORDS

- Butterfly graft • Nasal valve repair • Internal nasal valve • Nasal airway obstruction
- Nasal valve compromise • Rhinoplasty

KEY POINTS

- Persistent nasal airway obstruction due to nasal valve compromise is common, and spreader grafts are the historic gold standard for repair.
- The butterfly graft is an alternative method for nasal valve repair, and the modern surgical technique has evolved over the past 20+ years.
- There is growing objective evidence that proves butterfly grafts are as efficacious as, if not superior to, spreader grafts at repairing nasal valve compromise without unwanted esthetic concerns.

▶ Video content accompanies this article at http://www.oto.theclinics.com.

NASAL AIRWAY OBSTRUCTION AND THE INTERNAL NASAL VALVES

Most head and neck surgeons are trained to address straightforward anatomic deformities of the septum and turbinates, and these procedures remain some of the most commonly performed otolaryngologic procedures today.[1] Still, many studies report high rates of nasal obstruction after primary nasal surgery.[2–5] It is common, in our experience, to see revision nasal surgery patients with persistent nasal obstruction related to inadequately addressed nasal valve compromise (NVC) despite adequate correction of septal deviation and inferior turbinate hypertrophy.

Classically, the internal nasal valve (INV) is defined as the space among the dorsal septum, the caudal edge of the upper lateral cartilage (ULC), and the head of the inferior turbinate.[6] This area is described as the narrowest portion of the upper airway and accounts for approximately 50% of nasal airway resistance.[7] Nasal airway obstruction

[a] Department of Otolaryngology, University of North Carolina, Chapel Hill, NC, USA; [b] Division of Facial Plastic and Reconstructive Surgery, University of North Carolina, Chapel Hill, NC, USA
* Corresponding author. 170 Manning Drive, Campus box #7070, Chapel Hill, NC, 27599.
E-mail address: madison_clark@med.unc.edu

Otolaryngol Clin N Am 58 (2025) 279–293
https://doi.org/10.1016/j.otc.2024.07.026
oto.theclinics.com

(NAO) at the INV is further compounded by static nasal valve stenosis and/or dynamic collapse. This area is prone to dynamic collapse due to the combination of lateral wall insufficiency (weak ULCs) and decreased pressure with increased laminar airflow (the Bernoulli effect).

The senior author further subdivides the INV into a superior and inferior corridor and focuses evaluation on each of the 4 quadrants[8] (**Fig. 1**). The goals of INV repair are to treat all 4 quadrants by eliminating areas of obstruction and/or dynamic collapse. In patients with NAO following primary nasal surgery, we find that most often the superior corridor was incompletely treated.

A complete review of surgical techniques to repair NVC is beyond the scope of this article and is summarized elsewhere.[9] The senior author has extensive experience with the butterfly graft (BFG) and is convinced that it is superior to spreader grafts (SGs) in appropriately selected patients (**Fig. 2**). This study is intended to convince the reader to incorporate the BFG in their surgical armamentarium. The rest of this section will provide a detailed description of the proper utilization of the BFG and summarize current literature to prove its efficacy in repairing the superior corridor of the INV.

THE BUTTERFLY GRAFT

The BFG was originally described in 2002 by Clark and Cook as a conchal cartilage onlay graft used in revision rhinoplasty to repair the INV.[10] This description of the BFG was inspired by previous grafts described in Germany[11] and by Stucker and Hoasjoe.[12] While the technique has evolved since this description in 2002, the same basic principle of the graft remains—supporting the native ULCs to resist collapse from inspiratory airflow through the valve and acting as an intrinsic spring to physically increase the angle between the dorsal septum and ULC.[13] Multiple studies have since demonstrated the efficacy of the BFG in patients with both primary and revision rhinoplasty.[10,14–17] A detailed description of the current surgical technique used by the

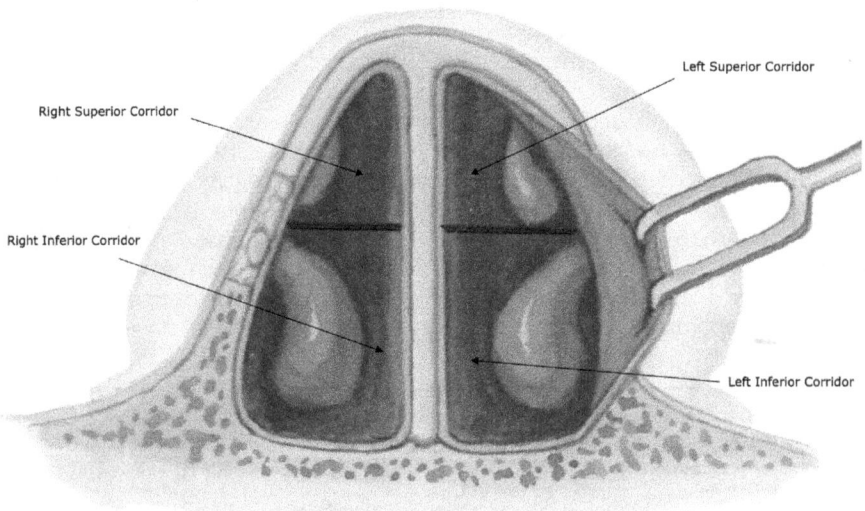

Fig. 1. Black line drawn horizontally through the superior attachment of the inferior turbinate divides the superior corridor from the inferior corridor.

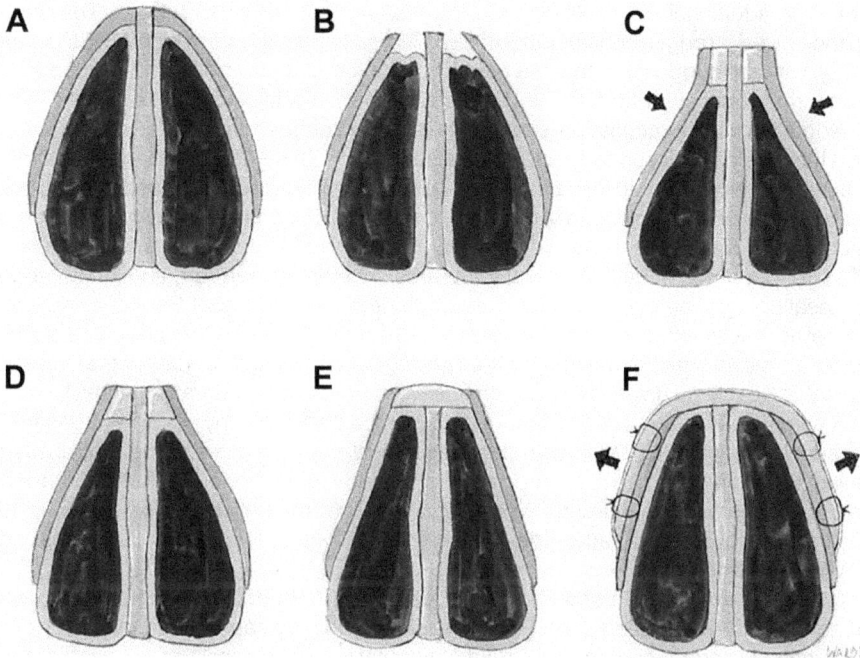

Fig. 2. (*A*) Cross-sectional image through the INV showing the positions of the septum (*brown*), nasal mucosa (*pink*), and ULCs (lavender). (*B*) Cross-sectional image showing release of the ULCs from the dorsal septum. (*C, D*) Cross-sectional image showing SGs (*blue*) in position between the ULCs and the dorsal septum. Note how these can cause narrowing of the valve angle (*arrows*) if sutured or structured inappropriately. Appropriate placement of the graft with a trapezoidal cross-section allows for a more physiologic reconstruction. (*E*) Cross-sectional image showing a dorsal onlay graft that widens the midvault but does not add tension to the ULCs. (*F*) Cross-sectional image showing an onlay BFG (*blue*) that opens the ULCs, prevents collapse, and adds tension to the lateral nasal sidewalls.

senior author after more than 20 years of experience and the evolution of this technique is described later in this section.

EVALUATION OF A PATIENT WITH NASAL AIRWAY OBSTRUCTION AND INDICATIONS FOR A BUTTERFLY GRAFT

As with most patient encounters, evaluation of NAO starts with a detailed history. Focus is directed toward any prior nasal trauma or surgery and contribution of mucosal disease. Relief of NAO with the use of external nasal dilators or intranasal cones can support the diagnosis of NVC but also has particular significance pertaining to candidacy for a BFG—in fact, the BFG is often described to patients as an internal or implanted nasal dilator.[13]

A significant portion of time should be targeted at a deeper understanding of how the NAO impairs daily living for each patient. Validated patient-reported outcome measures (PROMs) are vital in this process; the most commonly used PROMs include the Nasal Obstruction and Septoplasty Effectiveness Scale (NOSE)[18] or Standardized Cosmesis and Health Nasal (SCHNOS)[19] questionnaires. A lack of correlation between PROMs and/or patient perception and objective findings is not disqualifying but indicates the need for additional counseling regarding realistic patient expectations. The senior author gives stronger consideration to BFG in patients with very high NOSE scores (>70), with the supposition that the functional impairment may be "worth" the potential tradeoff of slight supratip fullness. This is, of course, discussed with the patient.

A detailed nasal examination follows the history. A comprehensive external nasal analysis has been well described in literature elsewhere.[20] This external nasal analysis must follow a systemic method for each patient so subtle findings are not missed, for example, dorsal hump or overprojection of the entire dorsum, lateral crural concavity, lateral crural recurvature, or a very narrow middle vault. Palpation of the nose offers critical clues to the strength of the underlying nasal structures, inherent tip support, and length/shape of nasal bones. The palpable shape, strength, and recoil of the ULCs at the mid-vault can give crucial information supporting a decision to reinforce this area with a BFG. For example, in patients with palpably strong ULCs, but stenotic apices of the INV, sub-dorsal SGs may be given stronger consideration (to minimize supratip fullness).

A dynamic evaluation of the nasal valves can be performed by asking the patient to inhale normally first and then with deep vigor, further giving clues to the propensity of collapse at different subsites. A positive modified Cottle maneuver further supports the diagnosis of NVC. An enthusiastic reaction from the patient during the modified Cottle maneuver encourages the surgeon about potential surgical outcomes with INV repair using the BFG.

Intranasal examination should then be performed with dedicated attention to all 4 quadrants of every patient (see **Fig. 1**). Nasal endoscopy can be extremely helpful in evaluating the superior corridor without manipulation with a nasal speculum and offers a deeper assessment of the nasal airway and areas such as the middle meatus and nasopharynx to ensure that no underlying sinonasal pathology is overlooked (**Fig. 3**).

Often, patients will have a multifactorial etiology of their NAO, and the patient must understand that any surgical intervention performed will not correct underlying mucosal pathologies. If present, mucosal contribution to NAO should be medically optimized prior to proceeding with surgery, although joint surgery with functional endoscopic sinus surgery is performed when indicated.

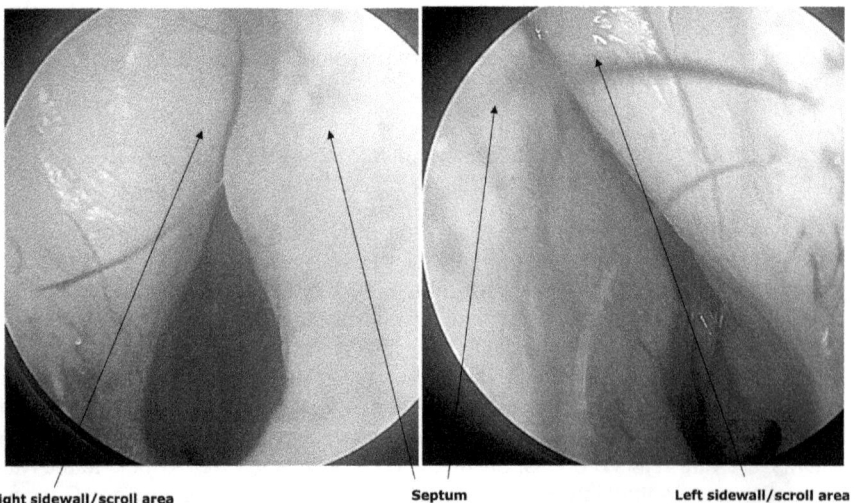

Right sidewall/scroll area   Septum   Left sidewall/scroll area

Fig. 3. Preoperative view of the superior corridors using 0° Hopkins rod (leaving the nostril undisturbed).

Once the surgeon has been satisfied that the patient has INV compromise amenable to repair with a BFG, standard surgical counseling is performed including a detailed description of the surgery, a short video animation of the technique, and before and after photographs that clearly demonstrate the expected increased supratip fullness postoperatively.

THE MODERN-DAY BUTTERFLY GRAFT

In its most simplistic form, the BFG is a conchal cartilage onlay graft that is fulcrumed on the dorsal septum and the caudal margins of the graft are sutured to the caudal margins of the ULCs. Since its original description,[10] the graft has evolved with several nuanced modifications by the senior author and others.[16] The following description describes the current surgical technique (Video 1 summarizing endonasal placement of BFG).

Harvest of Conchal Cartilage

An area of the concha cavum is targeted for the graft—most often from the left ear so the harvest can occur simultaneously with other nasal work (**Fig. 4**). Generally, approximately 2.2 x 1.2 cm of cartilage is harvested. Local anesthesia is first infiltrated into the conchal cartilage (in a supraperichondrial plane anteriorly and a subcutaneous plane posteriorly). A scalpel is then used to make an incision just inside the antihelix through the skin only. The anterior dissection is performed in a supraperichondrial plane since a true subpericondrial plan causes the elastic cartilage to fracture. The posterior dissection keeps the more robust perichondrium attached to the overlying cartilage

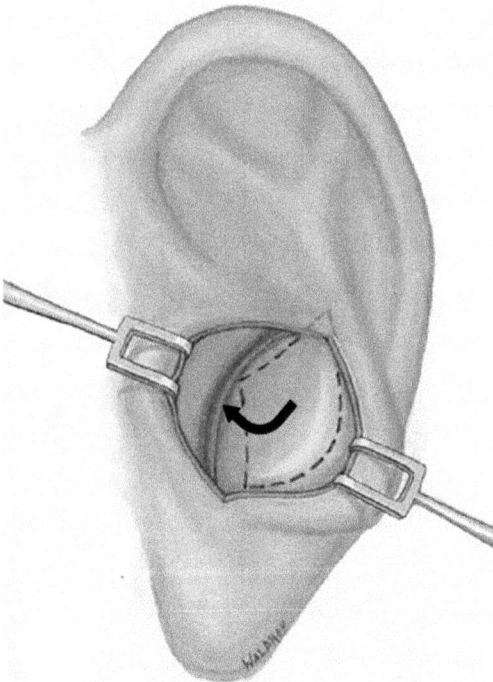

Fig. 4. Left ear with skin elevated over the conchal bowl. Dotted line showing where the graft is harvested from—immediately posterior to the tragus and inferior to the helical root. Care is taken to preserve the perichondrium on the graft.

(the convex side of the cartilage). The cuts are made with the scalpel using the "off-hand" fingers to feel the "shadow" of the blade while cutting. The cartilage piece is gently retracted with Adson Brown forceps, while Metz scissors are used to harvest the intact graft. It is then placed in sterile normal saline for use later in the case. Hemostasis is obtained, the ear incision is then closed with a 5-0 FAG on a PC-1 needle, and a Telfa bolster is placed for one night to prevent hematoma formation.

Carving of the Cartilage Graft

Each graft must be carefully customized to that patient. First, the cartilage is carefully examined for any inherent deformities or fractures. The graft is gently flexed to evaluate the strength and pliability of the cartilage. Inherent flexion points of the cartilage are noted and incorporated into the graft design. The edges of the cartilage are carefully carved to create a beveled surface on the cephalic edge and to fit precisely in the space created at the anterior septal angle (to be described later). Care is taken during this process to preserve the adherent posterior perichondrium. A small cuff of the posterior perichondrium extends past the borders of the cartilaginous portion of the graft to aid with post-placement camouflage. On average, the final size of the graft is approximately 18 x 9 mm but varies according to patient-specific factors. If necessary, gentle softening of portions of the graft can be performed with Adson Brown forceps to slightly adjust stiffer flexion points for each patient. A marking pen is used to make a dot on each side of the most caudal edge of the graft (used to guide placement symmetry; **Fig. 5**). All additional cartilage is saved in sterile normal saline to be potentially used later for minced cartilage grafts.

Preparation for Graft Placement

The graft itself can be placed through a closed endonasal versus an open approach, but in both cases, the final graft should be designed to sit with its caudal edge at the

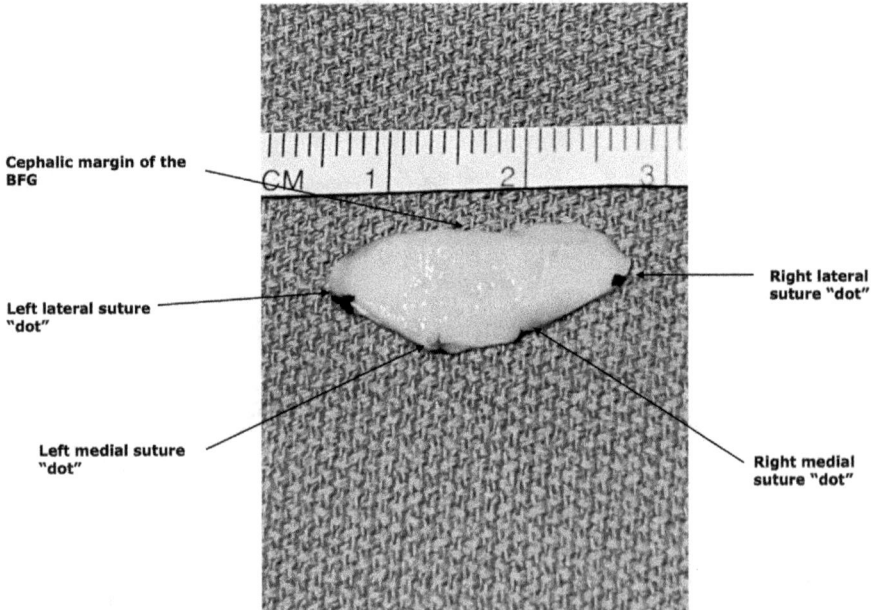

Fig. 5. Intraoperative ventral view of the BFG prior to inset. The 4 purple "dots" are to guide placement of the 5-0 PDS sutures.

scroll area as caudal as possible to minimize visibility of the graft. All other procedures including septoplasty, osteotomies, dorsal hump reduction (dorsal preservation is the senior author's favored approach), placement of other cartilage grafts, and inferior turbinate reduction are performed before placement of the BFG. Reduction of the dorsal projection is considered in all patients who are overly dorsally projected (especially tension nose deformity), but in patients with dorsal underprojection (platyrrhine nose), increase in tip projection serves to improve or maintain dorsal profile esthetics. In nearly all cases, a depression is then surgically created at the anterior septal angle to precisely match the shape of the graft (**Fig. 6**). This also releases the ULCs from the dorsal septum. The release is often carried cephalically to allow the ULC orientation to move more horizontally at the apex of the INV (**Fig. 7**).

Placement of the Graft

The graft is then placed to fit precisely within the previously designed dorsal defect. Careful inspection is performed, and appropriate trimming/adjustments are made (**Fig. 8**). After satisfactory size and shape are achieved, the graft is secured. 5-0 Polydioxanone suture on a P-2 needle is used to place a suture through the medial caudal edge of the ULC to the graft on each side at the dot made at the caudal margin of the graft (**Fig. 9**). The skin is redraped, and the graft position is assessed. If satisfactory, then a third suture is placed as lateral as possible, closing the space that exists between the lateral ULC and the BFG (**Fig. 10**). The graft is usually displaced by the placement of the third suture, so the contralateral edge of the graft is retrieved through the intercartilaginous (IC) incision and repositioned so that the fourth suture is placed as lateral as possible, again closing the space between the ULC and BFG. Any lateral fullness is addressed in situ to ensure satisfactory external contour. Although seldom necessary, camouflage grafts, including minced cartilage onlay grafts, are used to hide any step-offs. The intranasal incisions are closed with 5-0 chromic sutures on a P-2 needle, and the dorsum is supported by paper tape and a thermoplastic splint.

Approach for Placement

The senior author prefers to place the graft via an endonasal approach in all cases, even cases where an open approach is used (ie, extracorporeal septoplasty or significant tip modifications). An IC incision is made bilaterally, and the superficial musculoaponeurotic system is elevated to the rhinion before subperiosteal dissection is performed cephalically to the nasion. Frequently, if there is overprojection of the dorsum, a let-down type of dorsal preservation rhinoplasty without lateral keystone release will have already been performed. This creates an iatrogenically thicker skin and soft tissue envelope aiding in camouflage of the graft. In the dorsal preservation rhinoplasty cases, the subperiosteal dissection is not performed unless the bony cap requires reduction. The graft is then placed in the precise endonasal pocket and secured in place as discussed in the previous section. If an open approach is used, incisions are closed before the IC incisions are made and the graft is then placed in the usual manner through the endonasal approach.

Postoperative Care

All patients are seen on postoperative day one, and the Telfa bolster is removed from the ear. The nasal passageways are suctioned, and nasal irrigations and steroids are initiated and continued for 3 months.

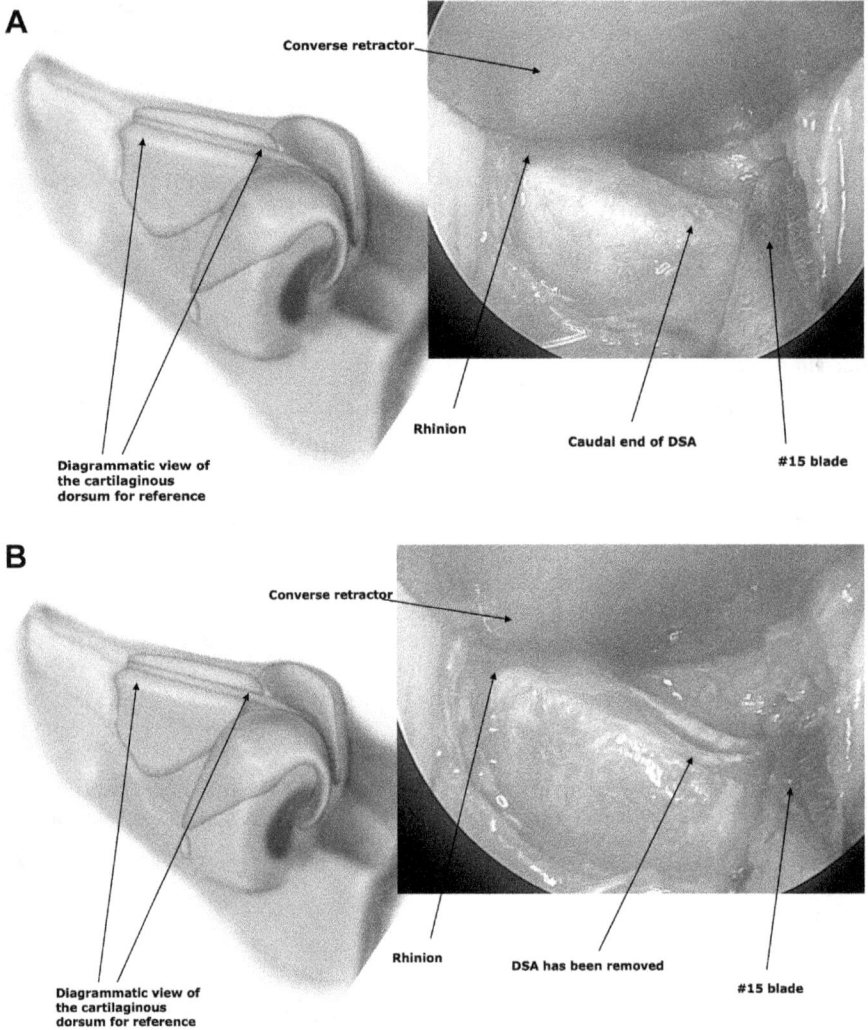

Fig. 6. (*A*) Intraoperative endonasal view of the cartilaginous dorsum through the right IC incision. (*B*) Intraoperative endonasal view of the cartilaginous dorsum through the right IC incision. The DSA has been resected to accommodate the BFG. DSA, dorsal septal/ULC articulation.

EVOLUTION OF THE BUTTERFLY GRAFT

Since originally described in 2002,[10] the BFG has undergone several subtle but critical changes that contribute to its overall success.

First, the importance of keeping the perichondrium attached to both sides of the graft is paramount. The anterior perichondrium, while not as robust as the posterior perichondrium, preserves the integrity of the cartilage during harvest and precise carving of the final graft. The posterior perichondrium is designed to overhang the cartilage edges after carving and is critical in camouflaging the graft. The perichondrium also provides robust anchoring for the polydioxanone suture (PDS) sutures used to secure the graft in place.

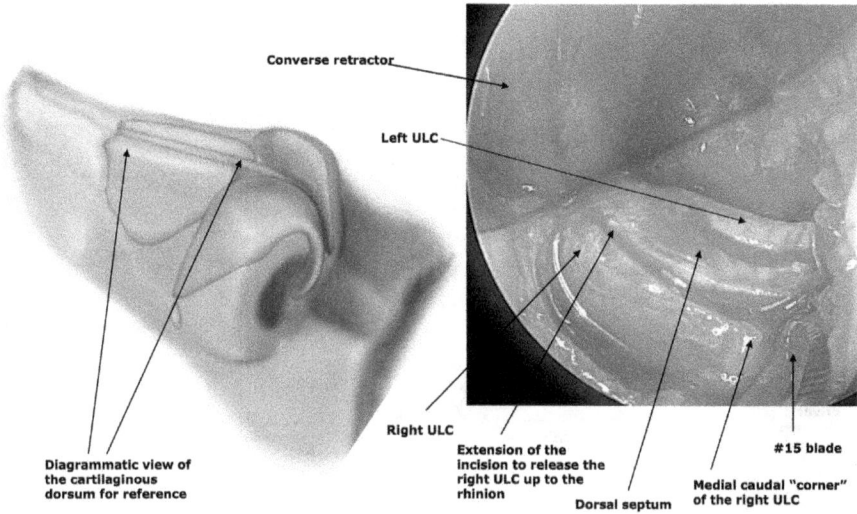

Fig. 7. Intraoperative endonasal view of the cartilaginous dorsum through the right IC incision. DSA has been removed and incisions extended cephalad to the rhinion for full ULC release.

With repetition and experience, the surgeon better understands that portions of the graft are amenable to aggressive carving to be able to fully customize it to each patient's surrounding nasal structure and overlying skin texture/thickness. The senior author has found that the most critical aspect of carving is shaving the peripheral cartilaginous edges at an angle to ensure a smooth transition from the graft to native

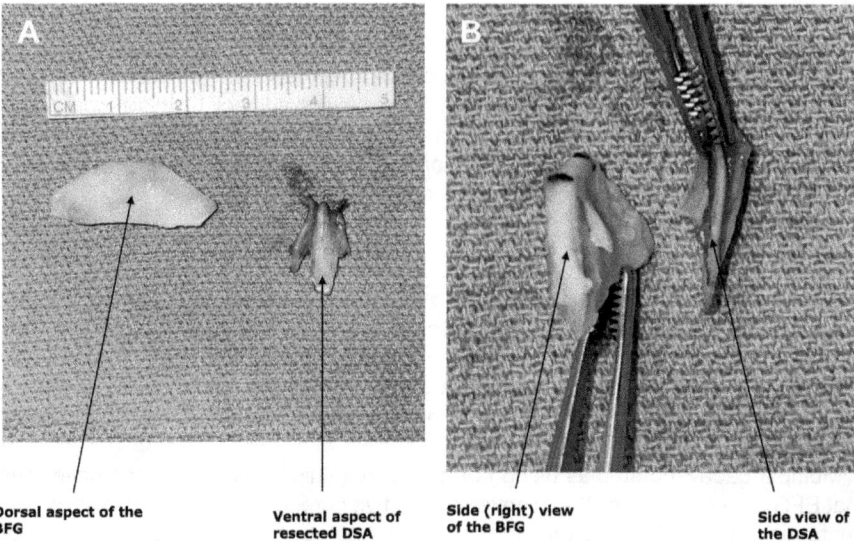

Fig. 8. (A, B) Intraoperative views of the BFG prior to inset. The goal is to match resected portion of the DSA and the dimensions of the BFG to create a "perfect fit" at the inset of the BFG.

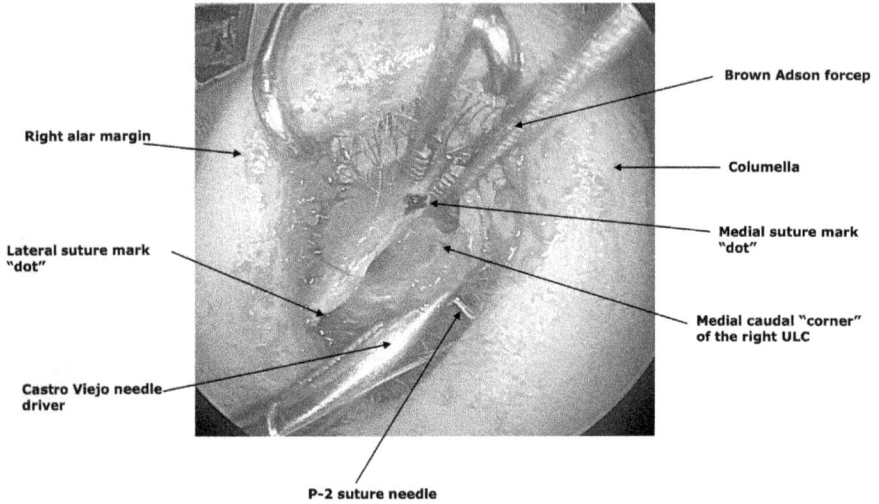

Fig. 9. Intraoperative endonasal view of the inset of the right side of the BFG. The first suture is placed through the medial caudal "corner" of the ULC, affixing it to the medial suture mark "dot."

cartilages (see **Fig. 8**). The lateral aspects of the graft can be aggressively contoured without compromising functionality as long as the posterior perichondrium remains intact for suturing to the ULCs.

While it may seem counterintuitive, it is critical to ensure that the ULCs are completely released from the dorsal septum, especially with vertically oriented ULCs. While this initially destabilizes the INV, this maneuver allows the native cartilages greater mobility in relation to the dorsal septum that is utilized to further expand the narrowed INV angle. The ULCs are then secured to the BFG to create a more horizontal orientation (more obtuse apical valve angle) and to prevent future nasal collapse (**Fig. 11**).

The senior author has fully integrated dorsal preservation rhinoplasty into his practice and has found that the BFG fits as an excellent adjunct to this technique. As mentioned previously, dorsal preservation rhinoplasty naturally creates skin and soft tissue relative thickness at the supratip along with a small supratip depression that accommodates a BFG well when using the described technique.

EFFICACY OF THE BUTTERFLY GRAFT

Growing evidence proves that BFGs are as effective, if not superior in many ways, to SGs. SGs address static INV compromise by displacing the ULC laterally and, depending on shape and suture placement, may increase the angle at the apex of the INV. The BFG not only widens this angle to improve static collapse but also adds additional strength to the lateral nasal wall that resists dynamic collapse[13] (see **Fig. 2**).

Multiple cadaveric studies using computational fluid dynamic metrics have found that BFGs are superior to SGs in several objective categories.[21–23] Initial studies using anatomic optical coherence tomography—a technology that can obtain dynamic volumetric imaging of the airways—have also suggested equivalent objective measures between spreader and BFG.[24] More studies directly comparing the 2 techniques using patient-reported outcomes are needed, but a single surgeon review demonstrated

A

Brown Adson forcep

Right alar margin

Columella

Lateral suture mark "dot"

Lateral caudal border of the right ULC

Castro Viejo needle driver

P-2 suture needle

B

Dorsal aspect of the BFG

Right alar margin

Columella

Cephalic margin of the BFG

Caudal margin of the right ULC

Castro Viejo needle driver

Caudal margin of the BFG

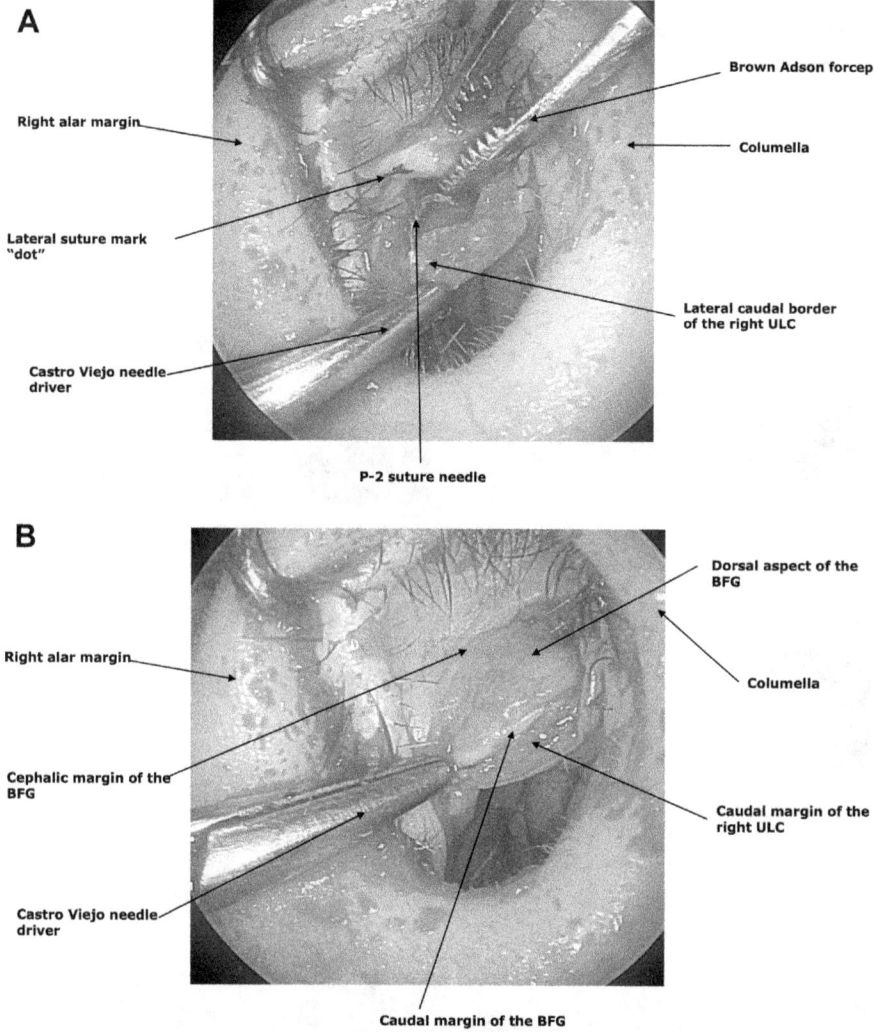

Fig. 10. (*A*) Intraoperative endonasal view of the inset of the right side of the BFG. The third suture is placed through the lateral caudal border of the right ULC, affixing it to the lateral suture mark "dot." (*B*) Intraoperative endonasal view of the inset of the right side of the BFG. The caudal margin of the right ULC is affixed to the caudal margin of the right side of the BFG.

equivalent patient-reported improvement in nasal obstruction (improved breathing was reported in 90% with the BFG vs 83.3% with SGs).[15] Further comparative research needs to be conducted, but BFGs seem to be, at a minimum, as effective as SGs.

ESTHETICS OF THE BUTTERFLY GRAFT

The chief argument against the BFG causing hesitation for implementation is its tendency to widen the tip and add slight width/fullness to the supratip. While the graft does tend to increase the width of the nose slightly (by 6.4%),[25] there is evidence

A

Right sidewall/scroll
area (location of IC
incision)

Septum

Closure of the right
IC incision

Significant increased
width at the apical
angle of the INV

Septum

B

Septum

Left sidewall/scroll
area (location of IC
incision)

Septum

Significant increased
width at the apical
angle of the INV

Closure of the left IC
incision

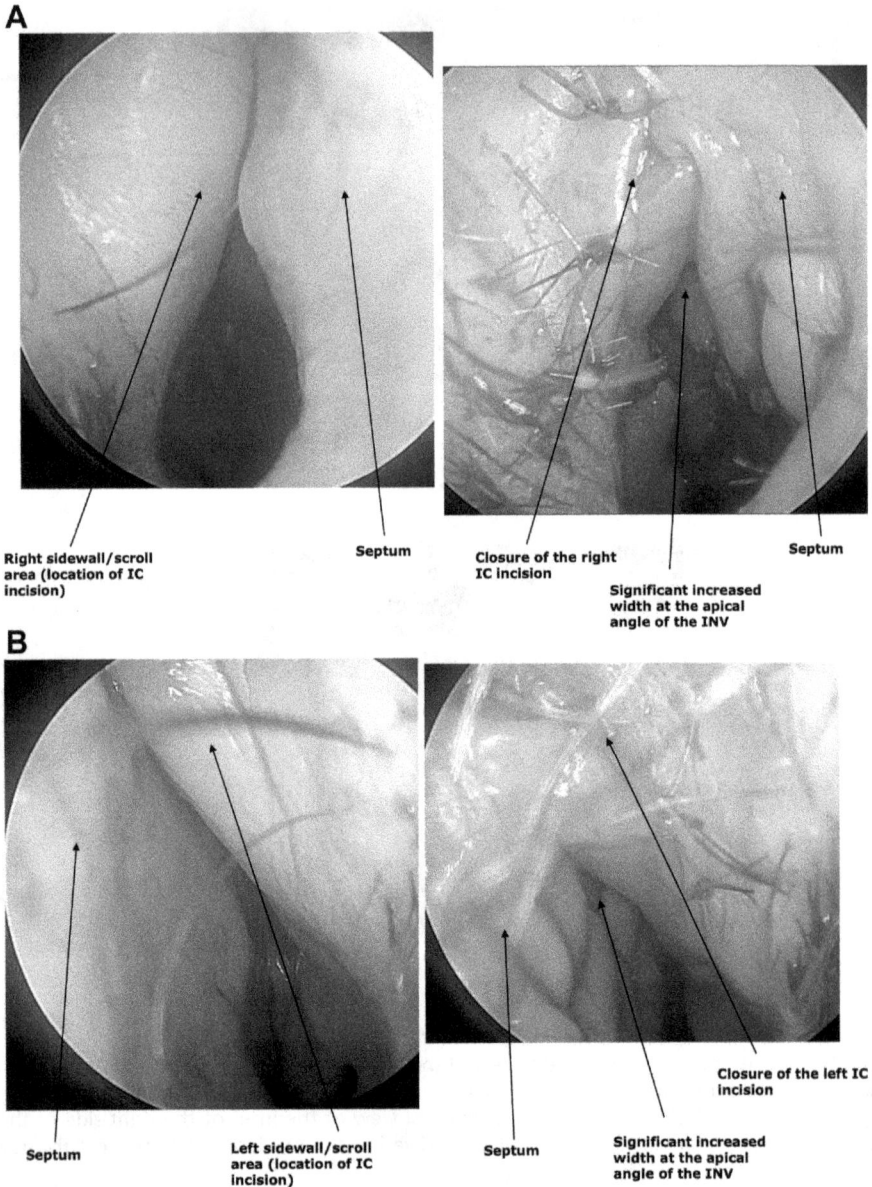

Fig. 11. (*A*) Preop view (*left*) and immediate postop view (*right*) of the right superior corridor using 0° Hopkins rod (leaving the nostril undisturbed). (*B*) Preop view (*left*) and immediate postop view (*right*) of the left superior corridor using 0° Hopkins rod (leaving the nostril undisturbed).

that SGs similarly widen the nose.[26–28] There are several reports that this subtle change in appearance is not bothersome or noticeable to the vast majority of the population. A study by Loyo and colleagues[16] in 2016 showed that medical students could not reliability select patients who had a history of a modified BFG from a collection of randomized postoperative photographs even after prompting to look for the graft. A study by Mims and colleagues[8] was designed to compare preoperative and postoperative changes in patients who underwent SGs and BFG but queried laypeople instead of medical professionals. Results demonstrated that the casual observer believed that the postoperative attractiveness of patients with a BFG was unchanged. Furthermore, observers who selected the supratip as being the least attractive region of the nose indicated that this region was similar between both the BFG and the SG groups. The senior author has also reported that this small change in appearance occasionally led to the desire for secondary contouring (2.7% among 374 patients). Although the initial experience is limited to a small number of patients, secondary contouring is a simple procedure that improves cosmesis and does not compromise the functional outcomes (Varman, Miller, Clark. Secondary contouring for the butterfly graft: Improving form and preserving function. Unpublished, 2024). With the aforementioned modifications, the BFG can be implemented in most patients who present for correction of NVC.

SUMMARY

The BFG is a reliable and robust method to repair the INV. With several modifications to the original surgical description as described earlier, the esthetic concerns regarding the visibility of the BFG are becoming less of a reason for patient dissatisfaction. There is growing evidence suggesting that the BFG may be superior to SGs in appropriately selected patients.

CLINICS CARE POINTS

- There are many proposed surgical techniques for repair of nasal valve compromise.
- The butterfly graft is one such method that both reinforces and adds tension the upper lateral cartilages to prevent nasal valve compromise during inspiration.
- Slight modifiations to the shape and placement of the butterfly graft have limited previous objections to use of the graft.
- Objective evidence has demonstrated that butterfly grafts are as efficacious as, if not superior to, spreader grafts.

DISCLOSURE

J. M. Clark—No relevant disclosures. T.M. Rist—No relevant disclosures.

SUPPLEMENTARY DATA

Supplementary data to this article can be found online at https://doi.org/10.1016/j.otc.2024.07.026.

REFERENCES

1. Dominguez JL, Ederaine SA, Haglin JM, et al. Medicare reimbursement trends for facility performed otolaryngology procedures: 2000-2019. Laryngoscope 2021; 131(3):496–501.
2. Yu K, Kim A, Pearlman SJ. Functional and aesthetic concerns of patients seeking revision rhinoplasty. Arch Facial Plast Surg 2010;12(5):291–7.

3. Vian HNK, Berger CAS, Barra DC, et al. Revision rhinoplasty: physician-patient aesthetic and functional evaluation. Braz J Otorhinolaryngol 2018;84(6):736–43.

4. Tsang CLN, Nguyen T, Sivesind T, et al. Long-term patient related outcome measures of septoplasty: a systematic review. EuroArch ORL 2018;275:1039–48.

5. Alsubeeh NA, AlSaqr MA, Alkarzae M, et al. Prevalence of considering revision rhinoplasty in Saudi patients and its associated factors. Maxillofac Plast Reconstr Surg 2019;41(1):59.

6. Rhee JS, Weaver EM, Park SS, et al. Clinical consensus statement: Diagnosis and management of nasal valve compromise. Otolaryngol Head Neck Surg 2010; 143(1):48–59.

7. Schlosser RJ, Park SS. Surgery for the dysfunctional nasal valve. Cadaveric analysis and clinical outcomes. Arch Facial Plast Surg 1999;1(2):105–10.

8. Mims MM, Shockley WW, Clark JM. Casual observers' perception on the aesthetics of the butterfly graft. Laryngoscope 2023;133(10):2578–83.

9. Sinkler MA, Wehrle CJ, Elphingstone JW, et al. Surgical management of the internal nasal valve: a review of surgical approaches. Aesthetic Plast Surg 2021;45(3): 1127–36.

10. Clark JM, Cook TA. The 'butterfly' graft in functional secondary rhinoplasty. Laryngoscope 2002;112(11):1917–25.

11. Walter C. The use of composite grafts in the head and neck region. Otolaryngol Head Neck Surg 1977;4:7–10.

12. Stucker FJ, Hoasjoe DK. Nasal reconstruction with conchal cartilage. Correcting valve and lateral nasal collapse. Arch Otolaryngol Head Neck Surg 1994;120(6): 653–8.

13. Clark JM. Does the butterfly graft really work? Current otorhinolaryngology reports 2022;10(2):148–54. New York: Springer US.

14. Friedman O, Cook TA. Conchal cartilage butterfly graft in primary functional rhinoplasty. Laryngoscope 2009;119(2):255–62.

15. Stacey DH, Cook TA, Marcus BC. Correlation of internal nasal valve stenosis: a single surgeon comparison of butterfly versus traditional spreader grafts. Ann Plast Surg 2009;63(3):280–4.

16. Loyo M, Gerecci D, Mace JC, et al. Modifications to the butterfly graft used to treat nasal obstruction and assessment of visibility. JAMA Facial Plast Surg 2016 1;18(6):436–40.

17. Howard BE, Madison Clark J. Evolution of the butterfly graft technique: 15-year review of 500 cases with expanding indications. Laryngoscope 2019;129(S1): S1–10.

18. Stewart MG, Witsell DL, Smith TL, et al. Development and validation of the Nasal Obstruction Symptom Evaluation (NOSE) scale. Otolaryngol Head Neck Surg 2004;130(2):157–63.

19. Moubayed SP, Ioannidis JPA, Saltychev M, et al. The 10-Item Standardized Cosmesis and Health Nasal Outcomes Survey (SCHNOS) for Functional and Cosmetic Rhinoplasty. JAMA Facial Plast Surg 2018 1;20(1):37–42.

20. Anthony P. Sclafani. Rhinoplasty : The Experts' Reference. Thieme. 2014. Available at: https://search.ebscohost.com/login.aspx?direct=true&AuthType=shib& db=e025xna&AN=956186&site=ehost-live. Accessed April 11, 2024.

21. Shadfar S, Shockley WW, Fleischman GM, et al. Characterization of postoperative changes in nasal airflow using a cadaveric computational fluid dynamics model: supporting the internal nasal valve. JAMA Facial Plast Surg 2014;16(5):319–27.

22. Brandon BM, Austin GK, Fleischman G, et al. Comparison of airflow between spreader grafts and butterfly grafts using computational flow dynamics in a cadaveric model. JAMA Facial Plast Surg 2018 1;20(3):215–21.

23. Brandon BM, Stepp WH, Basu S, et al. Nasal airflow changes with bioabsorbable implant, butterfly, and spreader grafts. Laryngoscope 2020;130(12):E817–23.

24. Waters CM, Stepp WH, Conduff J, et al. Anatomic Optical Coherence Tomography (aOCT) for Evaluation of the Internal Nasal Valve. Laryngoscope 2022; 132(11):2148–56.

25. Chaiet SR, Marcus BC. Nasal tip volume analysis after butterfly graft. Ann Plast Surg 2014;72(1):9–12. Erratum in: Ann Plast Surg. 2014 Apr;72(4):490. PMID: 23241767.

26. Ingels KJ, Orhan KS, van Heerbeek N. The effect of spreader grafts on nasal dorsal width in patients with nasal valve insufficiency. Arch Facial Plast Surg 2008; 10(5):354–6.

27. Fuller JC, Levesque PA, Lindsay RW. Analysis of patient-perceived nasal appearance evaluations following functional septorhinoplasty with spreader graft placement. JAMA Facial Plast Surg 2019 1;21(4):305–11.

28. Weitzman RE, Gadkaree SK, Justicz NS, et al. Patient-perceived nasal appearance after septorhinoplasty with spreader versus extended spreader graft. Laryngoscope 2021;131(4):765–72.

Closed Treatment of the Internal Nasal Valve

Carley Boyce, MD[a], Alyssa K. Ovaitt, MD[a], Laura Hetzler, MD[a,b,*]

KEYWORDS

- Internal nasal valve • Repair of nasal valve • Endonasal rhinoplasty
- Nasal obstruction • Spreader grafts • Rhinoplasty

KEY POINTS

- The internal nasal valve is a key component of nasal surgery and can be addressed via endonasal and traditional open approaches.
- The mainstay of closed treatment is the spreader graft, but batten grafts, butterfly grafts, and suspension suturing may also be considered. Careful planning of incisions and meticulous technique are the keys to these techniques.
- Candidate selection is critical to a successful outcome. Nonsurgical management must also be considered for patients who are not good candidates for surgery, or do not wish to pursue surgical management.
- Septoplasty and inferior turbinate reduction, while not addressed in this article, are helpful additions to the treatment of the nasal valve.

▶ Video content accompanies this article at http://www.oto.theclinics.com.

INTRODUCTION

The internal nasal valve has long been a target of airway improvement during nasal reconstruction and rhinoplasty. The internal valve is the narrowest part of the nasal airway, subject to both static and dynamic stenosis.[1,2] This area is defined by the septum, the upper lateral cartilage, the inferior turbinate, and the nasal floor.[1–3] It follows that the narrow internal nasal valve would be prone to collapse, given increased resistance and tendency for collapse, as described by Poisseuille's law.[1] In addition to a patient's natural anatomic form, avulsion of the upper lateral cartilage following trauma, septal deviations or septal trauma, large inferior turbinates, and weak cartilage or lateral nasal sidewalls can all contribute to clinical symptoms.[1]

While the internal nasal valve is often a target of open surgical maneuvers, endonasal or closed approaches are also available. These techniques are applicable to a

[a] Department of Otolaryngology-Head and Neck Surgery, Louisiana State University Health Sciences Center, New Orleans, LA, USA; [b] Our Lady of the Lake Regional Medical Center, Baton Rouge, LA, USA
* Corresponding author. 10222 Jefferson Highway, Baton Rouge, LA 70809.
E-mail address: lhetzl@lsuhsc.edu

Otolaryngol Clin N Am 58 (2025) 295–302
https://doi.org/10.1016/j.otc.2024.08.012
oto.theclinics.com
0030-6665/25/© 2024 Elsevier Inc. All rights reserved, including those for text and data mining, AI training, and similar technologies.

wide array of practices, as adjuncts in endonasal cosmetic rhinoplasty or preservation rhinoplasty, and as a component of standard septoplasty in the correct surgical candidate. While the definition of the ideal surgical candidate is not always clear given the subjectivity of nasal obstruction, Cottle and modified Cottle maneuvers are traditionally employed to assess symptomatic changes with manipulation of the internal nasal valve.[1,3,4] Others define internal nasal valve stenosis as a valve area less than 15°.[2] Some patients have obvious midvault narrowing externally, which can guide therapy in some cases.[2,3]

The advantages of closed repair are obvious, with less trauma to the internal nasal valve, less opportunity for risk of cosmetic change or even deformity, reduced postoperative swelling, and lack of external scar.[4,5] The operative time may also be shortened, without the need to open the nose simply to add spreaders or other grafts.[5] It should be noted that the learning curve can be steep when adopting these new techniques, as they do not allow as much visualization or control as an open approach. Securing grafts must also be completed via creation of tight pockets or suturing, which are often not amenable to multiple attempts and have fewer opportunities for correction of error.[2,5] The approaches may also require additional modification beyond a standard septoplasty or endonasal rhinoplasty approach.

Many options exist to address the nasal valve. Spreader graft placement has been the mainstay of treatment for many years. Like the open technique, unilateral or bilateral spreader grafts can be crafted from septal, auricular, or rib cartilage and placed between the septum and upper lateral cartilage to widen or blunt the nasal valve area.[1-8] Additional techniques include butterfly and alar batten grafts, although these are often criticized for becoming visible or palpable after surgery, particularly in thin skinned individuals,[9,10] Other options include scar release and suturing techniques.

Finally, while not addressed in this writing, excellent technique in septoplasty and inferior turbinate reduction are important components that can contribute to the enlargement of the internal nasal valve area and thus, improvement in nasal obstruction. Radiofrequency ablation techniques and injectable implants to address the nasal valve are not discussed here but remain options for non-surgical candidates, as are medical therapies and nasal cones/stents.[1,4,11]

DISCUSSION

Many techniques have been used and adapted to address a narrow internal nasal valve. Spreader grafts are arguably the most established player in internal nasal valve reconstruction, along with their role in correction of midvault asymmetries. First described by Sheen in 1984, the grafts are placed in a sub-mucoperichondrial plane between the dorsal nasal septum and the medial wall of the upper lateral cartilage.[12]

As in a traditional open approach, the spreader graft increases the cross-sectional area of the internal nasal valve and thus, the mid-vault. These grafts are cut into a rectangular shape and may be used unilaterally or bilaterally. Grafts typically measure 2 to 3 cm long and 3 to 5 mm wide/tall, with a thickness of approximately 1.5 to 2 mm.[2,11] It does require a donor source of cartilage. The nasal septum is typically preferred, although rib and conchal cartilage may also be used, with limitations of shape and size.[11] Cadaveric cartilage remains an additional option, particularly during revision rhinoplasty where harvestable cartilage may be sparse.[13] Auto-spreader flaps have also been described endonasally, although present a unique challenge when compared with an open approach.[5,14]

Endonasal spreader placement typically accompanies a standard septoplasty via Killian or hemitransfixion incision. This can be completed within the septoplasty incision itself (**Fig. 1**), or using a separate, small, and superior incision (**Fig. 2**). With either technique, a bridge of mucopericondrium is left between the 2 dissection pockets, so the graft is held in place while avoiding additional suturing intranasally. The pocket is created superiorly, just caudal to the caudal border of the upper lateral cartilage on the dorsal septum, just as tall as the cottle elevator itself (**Fig. 3**). This pocket is precisely created for the graft(s), and a spreader is placed within (Video 1). Preservation of a bridge of mucoperichondrium beneath the graft and "above" the septoplasty is critical, although it is possible to employ suturing for additional security of the graft(s) if needed.[2] If bilateral spreaders are desired, the contralateral pocket can be created by dissecting over the caudal septum to make a small and similar pocket with the cottle, or by making another small incision on the opposite side. The creation of the pocket itself is then as described earlier

Given the separate pocket superiorly, visibility may be somewhat reduced during the septoplasty. A patient with a low septal deviation is particularly well-suited, as there is ample room for removal of septal cartilage below and creation of pocket for the spreader above. Endonasal spreader grafts may also be used in an isolated valve obstruction or revision cases, where the septum may not need to be addressed. This then negates the need for a septoplasty incision altogether. Regardless of technique, closure of the incision(s) is typically performed with 5-0 chromic gut suture to avoid extrusion of the graft(s).

After graft placement, the middle third of the nose may appear wider, particularly in patients with thin skin, which may be an undesirable; however, there are cases where a wider nasal dorsum may be favorable, specifically those with a narrow middle vault or mild asymmetries.[1,15] Endonasal spreader grafts offer a balanced solution to both cosmetic and functional nasal concerns, by strengthening or widening of a weakened valve area, while maintaining the integrity of the natural nasal framework.

Although considered a mainstay to treat external nasal valve collapse, alar batten grafts can also support the internal nasal valve when positioned at the junction of

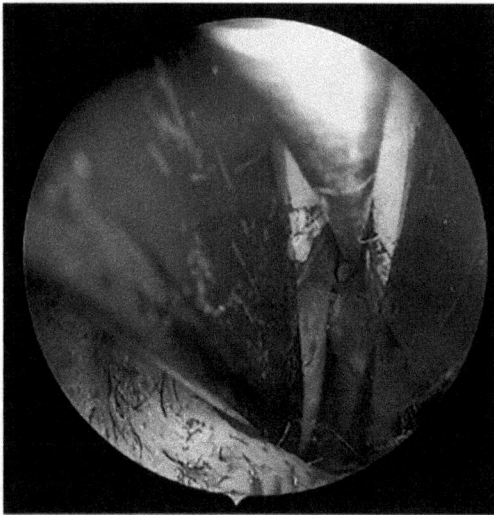

Fig. 1. An endoscopic view of the pocket described earlier with a bridge of mucoperichondrium beneath the graft and above the septoplasty plane. The same incision (here, Killian incision) is used to access both areas. The cottle is shown within the spreader pocket.

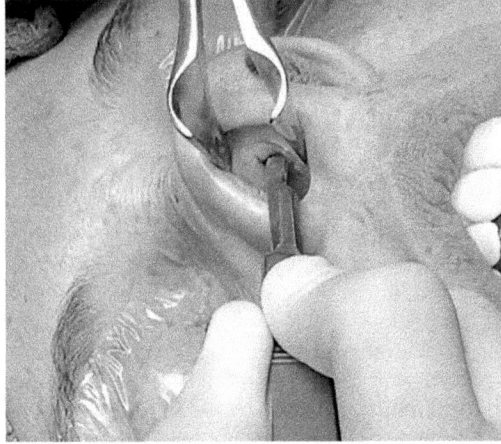

Fig. 2. A right-sided incision used to create a pocket for an endonasal spreader graft. A separate incision is used for each side. The incision is around the size of the 15 blade, and allows access for a cottle to dissect the pocket itself. (*Image Courtesy:* Celeste Gary, M.D.)

the upper lateral cartilages and lower lateral cartilages (scroll region).[3] The main goal is to provide structural support to the collapsed region of the lateral nasal wall, usually near the caudal edge of the upper lateral cartilage and the cephalic part of the lateral crura. Alar batten grafts are highly adaptable and can be utilized for both external nasal valve and internal nasal valve support. These grafts are typically 10 to 15 mm in length and 4 to 8 mm in width. They are placed in a subcutaneous pocket to enhance the lateral nasal wall. The grafts are strategically positioned at the point of maximal lateral wall collapse, extending from the piriform aperture to the junction of the middle and lateral third of the lateral crura (**Fig. 4**).[16]

A small inter-cartilaginous incision is made, corresponding to areas of supra-alar pinching, with the convex surface of the graft facing laterally.[3] Correct placement of

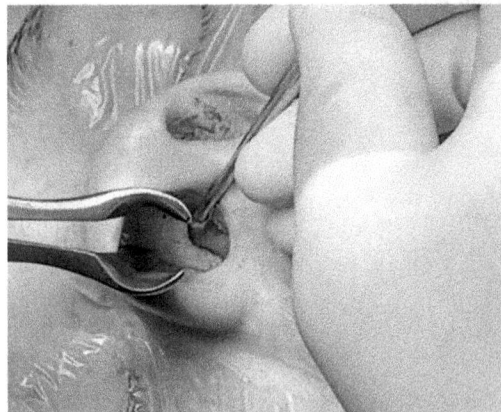

Fig. 3. Creation of a pocket for a spreader graft in the sub-mucoperichondrial plane. The cottle is used to create the precise pocket, which is the size of the cottle elevator itself, parallel to the nasal dorsum. Note the incision is created at the caudal edge of the upper lateral cartilage, at the highest visible point of the dorsal septum. (*Image Courtesy:* Celeste Gary, M.D.)

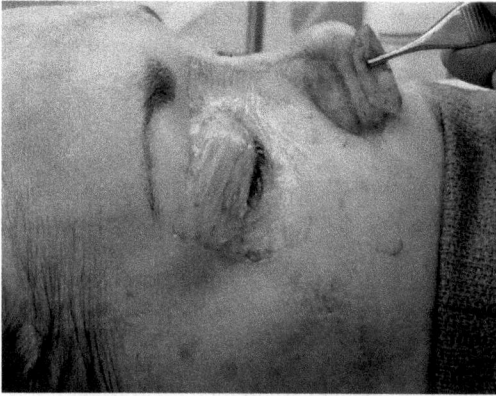

Fig. 4. Marker has been used to show area of internal nasal valve collapse along the inferior nasal sidewall and alar crease. An intracartilagenous incision is created for insertion of the visualized batten graft in this area.

these grafts is crucial to resist negative inspiratory forces. The subcutaneous pocket for the graft must be appropriately sized: too large a pocket can lead to graft sliding, while too small a pocket can cause the graft to curl. Proper placement eliminates the need for suture fixation and prevents migration. As with spreader grafts, patients should be counseled beforehand on this possible fullness where form may be sacrificed for improved function. In addition to nasal widening, alar batten grafts can efface the alar crease in some patients, as well as have a more visible or bulbous appearance, particularly in those with thin skin.[16–18]

In 1964, Hage introduced the butterfly graft.[19] This technique addresses both static and dynamic internal nasal valve obstructions in primary and secondary rhinoplasty. Butterfly grafts commonly utilize conchal cartilage, which is chosen for its naturally concave shape. In this procedure, the convex side of the cartilage is positioned upward toward the skin. Taking advantage of the natural shape, the nasal valve is suspended and opened, while the strength of the cartilage provides the necessary stabilization of the internal nasal valve.[1]

The butterfly graft is inserted through bilateral intercartilaginous incisions. The skin over the nasal dorsum is undermined and the graft positioned into a pocket over the nasal dorsum. The graft is carefully wedged into the appropriate position, deep to the cephalic edge of the lower lateral cartilages or with the caudal edge placed beneath the cephalic border of the lateral crura. This precise placement ensures that the internal nasal valve is effectively lifted, enhancing airflow and correcting obstruction.[20,21] The cartilage aids in maintaining the desired position and stability of the internal nasal valve, thereby improving nasal function and overall patient outcomes.

One of the main criticisms of the butterfly graft technique is the potential visibility of the graft along the supratip, which can lead to a less satisfactory esthetic outcome. The graft can create a noticeable contour irregularity in the nasal profile, particularly in patients with thin soft tissue envelopes.[5] Despite this drawback, the functional benefit of improved nasal airflow and valve stabilization often outweigh esthetic concerns.

Suturing is an alternative to spreader, batten, and butterfly graft placement for correcting internal nasal valve collapse. Flaring sutures are used to support, and in some cases, change the shape of the internal nasal valve. Mattress suturing can be strategically used to create more room intranasally. Sutures can be placed in a mattress fashion in both caudal and medial upper lateral cartilages, spanning across the nasal dorsum. When tied, this will support and suspend the upper lateral cartilages laterally and open the internal nasal valve.[1] This technique increases the angle of the valve and can impact both static and dynamic collapse.[21]

If even more vertical lift is required, suspension suturing technique may be implemented; however, it does require a second incision site and cannot be completed by intranasal incision alone. Suspension of these sutures is achieved through a transconjunctival or infraorbital approach with a screw, plate, or hole drilled into the bone.[22,23] Although rare, complications such as increased scleral show and ectropion have been recorded in the literature.[24] The longevity of these sutures and their stability has also been questioned in the literature due to the development of laxity in the sutures over time.[25] While durability may be questioned, this method offers a cartilage-sparing technique and decreased donor-site morbidity.

In secondary surgery, intranasal scarring may need to be addressed. Z-plasty is a well-known technique, often used on the skin to improve the appearance of scar via lengthening and reorientation. As such, it has also been described to treat intranasal cicatricial scarring at the junction of the medial upper lateral cartilage and the dorsal septum.[1] This scarring is often from previous nasal surgery. Similar to its employment in scar revision, triangular mucosal flaps are raised and reoriented to release and lengthen the scar itself.[1,5] In some cases, the caudal border of the upper lateral cartilages may need to be resected to facilitate proper rotation of the flaps. In a series by Dutton and Neidich, 12 patients who underwent intranasal Z-plasty were reported to have both objective improvements, confirmed on nasal endoscopy, as well as subjective improvement in nasal airway symptoms.[26]

Spreader grafts are commonly used for internal nasal valve stenosis, particularly if minimal change in nasal appearance is desired. Avoidance of the transcolumellar incision in endonasal techniques often allows for quicker surgery with less associated morbidity or risk of change in nasal appearance. The advantages of endonasal placement are clear, but all of the described techniques can still lead to cosmetic changes and/or increased nasal fullness. This may be desirable in some cases, but patients must be aware that the external aspect of the nose may be altered postoperatively. Suture techniques are another option if cartilage is not readily available. Z-plasty is indicated for patients with cicatricial scarring between the septum and upper lateral cartilages, where the mucosa causes alterations of the normal internal nasal valve angle. This may be particularly useful in revision rhinoplasty, to correct iatrogenic scarring from previous nasal surgery. While all are individually effective, these techniques may also be combined to maximize benefit.

SUMMARY

The internal nasal valve is a key part of nasal surgery, and its treatment can be approached through both endonasal and traditional open techniques. Spreader grafts have remained the cornerstone of valve treatment, but other options like batten grafts, butterfly grafts, flaring and suspension suturing, and Z-plasty can be utilized as well. If not necessary for other reasons, these can be completed endonasally and the nose need not be opened. Often, combining methods such as spreader grafts with batten or butterfly grafts can address multiple structural issues simultaneously, leading to more effective and durable results.

Despite the technical challenges, particularly with graft placement and/or suture fixation with reduced visibility, these procedures offer substantial benefit in terms of improved nasal airflow and valve stabilization. The closed approach produces less trauma to nasal structures and reduces the risk of visible scarring, making it a favorable option for many patients. Each technique requires meticulous planning, especially in terms of incision placement, to ensure optimal outcomes and minimize complications.

Overall, while each technique has its advantages and drawbacks, the key to effective nasal valve surgery lies in a personalized approach tailored to the patient's needs. This ensures both functional and esthetic outcomes are maximized, leading to improved patient satisfaction. The ongoing evolution of these techniques, combined with meticulous surgical planning and patient education, continues to enhance the field of nasal surgery, offering a variety of options to improve quality of life for patients with nasal valve collapse.

CLINICS CARE POINTS

- Minimized Trauma and Reduced Operative Time: Endonasal techniques offer a more conservative approach to the internal nasal valve, without the need to open the nose. This can shorten operative times and reduce the risk of external changes and scarring, when compared to traditional open methods.

- Precise Graft Placement and Visualization Challenges: Closed approaches require precise creation of tight pockets for grafts with reduced visualization, necessitating meticulous planning.

- Combining Techniques for Optimal Outcomes: Multiple techniques can be combined to address structural issues simultaneously, enhancing both functional and esthetic results.

- Personalized Surgical Planning: Understanding each patient's unique needs is essential for the identification of appropriate surgical candidates, and thus, successful outcomes.

DISCLOSURE

The authors have nothing to disclose.

SUPPLEMENTARY DATA

Supplementary data related to this article can be found online at https://doi.org/10.1016/j.otc.2024.08.012.

REFERENCES

1. Becker DG, Ransom E, Guy C, et al. Surgical treatment of nasal obstruction in rhinoplasty. Aesthetic Surg J 2010;30(3):347–80.
2. Samaha M, Rassouli A. Spreader graft placement in endonasal rhinoplasty: technique and a review of 100 cases. Plast Surg (Oakv) 2015;23(4):252–4.
3. Irene C, Perez-Garcia M. Management of the internal nasal valve. Rhinoplasty Archive; 2020. Available at: https://www.rhinoplastyarchive.com/articles/midvault-internal-nasal-valve/management-of-the-internal-nasal-valve. Accessed June 10, 2024.
4. André RF, Paun SH, Vuyk HD. Endonasal spreader graft placement as treatment for internal nasal valve insufficiency: no need to divide the upper lateral cartilages from the septum. Arch Facial Plast Surg 2004;6(1):36–40.
5. Go BC, Frost A, Friedman O. Addressing the nasal valves: the endonasal approach. Facial Plast Surg 2022;38(1):57–65.

6. Erickson B, Hurowitz R, Jeffery C, et al. Acoustic rhinometry and video endoscopic scoring to evaluate postoperative outcomes in endonasal spreader graft surgery with septoplasty and turbinoplasty for nasal valve collapse. J Otolaryngol Head Neck Surg 2016;45:2.

7. Kaya E, Catli T, Soken H, et al. A novel technique for spreader graft placement without dorsum resection during septoplasty. J Laryngol Otol 2015;129(10):1025–7.

8. Talmadge J, High R, Heckman WW. Comparative outcomes in functional rhinoplasty with open vs endonasal spreader graft placement. Ann Plast Surg 2018;80(5):468–71.

9. Brownlee BP, Hassoun A, Parikh A, et al. Cadaveric assessment of the butterfly graft in rhinoplasty. Laryngoscope 2024;134(4):1638–41.

10. Cervelli V, Spallone D, Bottini JD, et al. Alar batten cartilage graft: treatment of internal and external nasal valve collapse. Aesthetic Plast Surg 2009;33(4):625–34.

11. Teymoortash A, Fasunla JA, Sazgar AA. The value of spreader grafts in rhinoplasty: a critical review. Eur Arch Oto-Rhino-Laryngol 2012;269(5):1411–6.

12. Sheen JH. Spreader graft. Plast Reconstr Surg 1984;73(2):230–7.

13. Pfaff MJ, Bertrand AA, Lipman KJ, et al. Cadaveric costal cartilage grafts in rhinoplasty and septorhinoplasty: a systematic review and meta-analysis of patient-reported functional outcomes and complications. J Craniofac Surg 2021;32(6):1990–3.

14. Byrd HS, Meade RA, Gonyon DL. Using the autospreader flap in primary rhinoplasty. Plast Reconstr Surg 2007;119(6):1897–902.

15. Toriumi DM. Management of the middle nasal vault in rhinoplasty. Operat Tech Plast Reconstr Surg 1995;2(1):16–30.

16. Toriumi DM, Josen J, Weinberger M, et al. Use of alar batten grafts for correction of nasal valve collapse. Arch Otolaryngol Head Neck Surg 1997;123(8):802–8.

17. Khosh MM, Jen A, Honrado C, et al. Nasal valve reconstruction: experience in 53 consecutive patients. Arch Facial Plast Surg 2004;6(3):167–71.

18. Brenner MJ, Hilger PA. Grafting in rhinoplasty. Facial Plast Surg Clin North Am 2009;17(1):91–vii.

19. Hage J. Collapsed alae strengthened by conchal cartilage (the butterfly cartilage graft). Br J Plast Surg 1965;18:92–6.

20. Clark JM, Cook TA. The 'butterfly' graft in functional secondary rhinoplasty. Laryngoscope 2002;112(11):1917–25.

21. Ballert JA, Park SS. Functional considerations in revision rhinoplasty. Facial Plast Surg 2008;24(3):348–57.

22. Paniello RC. Nasal valve suspension. An effective treatment for nasal valve collapse. Arch Otolaryngol Head Neck Surg 1996;122(12):1342–6.

23. Friedman M, Ibrahim H, Syed Z. Nasal valve suspension: an improved, simplified technique for nasal valve collapse. Laryngoscope 2003;113(2):381–5.

24. Barrett DM, Casanueva FJ, Cook TA. Management of the nasal valve. Facial Plast Surg Clin North Am 2016;24(3):219–34.

25. Nuara MJ, Mobley SR. Nasal valve suspension revisited. Laryngoscope 2007;117(12):2100–6.

26. Dutton JM, Neidich MJ. Intranasal Z-plasty for internal nasal valve collapse. Arch Facial Plast Surg 2008;10(3):164–8.

Evaluation and Treatment of Nasal Valve Compromise in non-Caucasian Rhinoplasty

Max Feng, MD[a], Jennifer Fuller, MD[a,b],
Adeeb Derakhshan, MD[b,c],*

KEYWORDS

- Functional rhinoplasty • Nasal valve compromise • Nasal obstruction
- Non-caucasian rhinoplasty • Ethnic rhinoplasty

KEY POINTS

- A deeper appreciation of the anatomic differences amongst various ethnicities can help maintain ethnic congruency and optimize outcomes in functional rhinoplasty.
- During the preoperative evaluation, it is important to perform a thorough nasofacial analysis and understand how a patient's ethnic and cultural background may influence their perception of beauty.
- An open approach allows for direct visualization and intraoperative assessment of the osseocartilaginous framework, which is often difficult to appreciate due to the thicker and more sebaceous skin and soft tissue envelope.
- Establishing strong tip support is essential and serves as the foundation from which other grafts are built upon.

INTRODUCTION

Neoclassical canons of facial analysis, introduced by the ancient Greeks, have had a profound influence on modern beauty standards. Many of the nasal esthetic ideals described in the literature are based on the Caucasian nose, which have been identified in patients of northern European descent.[1–5] However, ethnic and racial diversity is projected to rapidly increase in the next several decades in the United States.[6] The degree of diversity in patients presenting with nasal obstruction in evaluation for functional rhinoplasty will likely follow suit. Thus, it is valuable for rhinoplasty surgeons to

[a] Department of Otolaryngology—Head & Neck Surgery, Loma Linda University Health, Loma Linda, CA 92354, USA; [b] Division of Facial Plastic and Reconstructive Surgery, Department of Otolaryngology—Head & Neck Surgery, Loma Linda University Health, Loma Linda, CA, USA; [c] Department of Otolaryngology—Head & Neck Surgery, Loma Linda University Health, 11234 Anderson Street, Room 2586A, Loma Linda, CA 92354, USA
* Corresponding author. 11234 Anderson Street, Room 2586A, Loma Linda, CA 92354.
E-mail address: ADerakhshan@llu.edu

Otolaryngol Clin N Am 58 (2025) 303–313
https://doi.org/10.1016/j.otc.2024.07.021
0030-6665/25/© 2024 Elsevier Inc. All rights are reserved, including those for text and data mining, AI training, and similar technologies.

oto.theclinics.com

have a deeper understanding of nasal anatomic variances amongst different ethnicities.

Functional rhinoplasty invariably impacts patient perception of nasal esthetics despite not being the primary surgical focus.[7] As cosmetic changes often occur as a result of addressing functional issues, a thorough knowledge of anatomic differences is crucial to ensuring such alterations are aligned with patients' expectations. Understanding these differences will allow the rhinoplasty surgeon to evaluate each nose individually, address problematic areas, and maintain ethnic congruence with surgery.

The purpose of this review is to define common anatomic variances amongst different ethnicities, review preoperative evaluation pearls, and highlight surgical considerations in the treatment of nasal valve compromise for non-Caucasian functional rhinoplasty.

ANATOMIC DIFFERENCES AMONGST ETHNICITIES

Though frequently used interchangeably, several differences exist between the terms *race* and *ethnicity*. *Race* is an objective term that includes people who share the same heritage and possess similar physical characteristics. *Ethnicity* is a subjective term that refers to a group an individual most readily identifies with and feels connected to. Although an individual may appear to belong to a certain racial group, their own experience of ethnic identity, self-image, and beauty constructs can vastly differ. Conversely, *culture* refers to a set of shared beliefs, values, social practices, or conventions of a group and can include many diverse racial and ethnic backgrounds. Thus, it is important that rhinoplasty surgeons seek to gain a clear understanding of the way a patient's racial, ethnic, and cultural background may influence their perception of beauty.[8–11] Rhinoplasty literature has recently shifted to using the term *non-Caucasian rhinoplasty* rather than *ethnic rhinoplasty,* as this term is more inclusive, avoids previous negative connotations of the term "ethnic," and reflects the shift in demographics of the United States toward larger non-Caucasian and mixed race population.[12,13]

Variations in nasal anthropomorphic observations have been grouped into 3 broad categories: *leptorrhine, platyrrhine,* and *mesorrhine* (**Fig. 1**).[14,15]

The *leptorrhine* nose is described as "tall and thin." This nasal type has a strong bony and cartilaginous framework with a high radix, narrow dorsum, and often having a bony-cartilaginous hump. The nasal tip is often large and well projected. The septal cartilage is well-developed, with greater strength and thickness. The nostrils are narrow and oval-shaped, with a narrower alar base. The nasolabial angles are slightly obtuse, with adequate rotation. The soft tissue envelope is normal to thin. It is associated with patients of Caucasian or European descent.[11,15]

The *platyrrhine* nose is described as "broad and flat," with characteristics opposite of the leptorrhine nose. This nasal type is characterized by small nasal bones with a low radix and flat and wide dorsum. The cartilaginous dorsum is often less supported, flat, and wide. The nasal tip has less projection and rotation due to thin and less robust alar cartilages. The cartilaginous septum also tends to be thinner and smaller compared to leptorrhine noses, leading to limited septal cartilage available for grafting. Platyrrhine noses have a wide alar base, and more rounded alar lobules, producing increased nostril flare and large nostrils. The soft tissue envelope is often thick and sebaceous. It is common in patients of African descent.[14,15]

The *mesorrhine* nose is the intermediate nasal type between leptorrhine and platyrrhine noses. Compared to leptorrhine noses, this nasal type has a normal to low radix

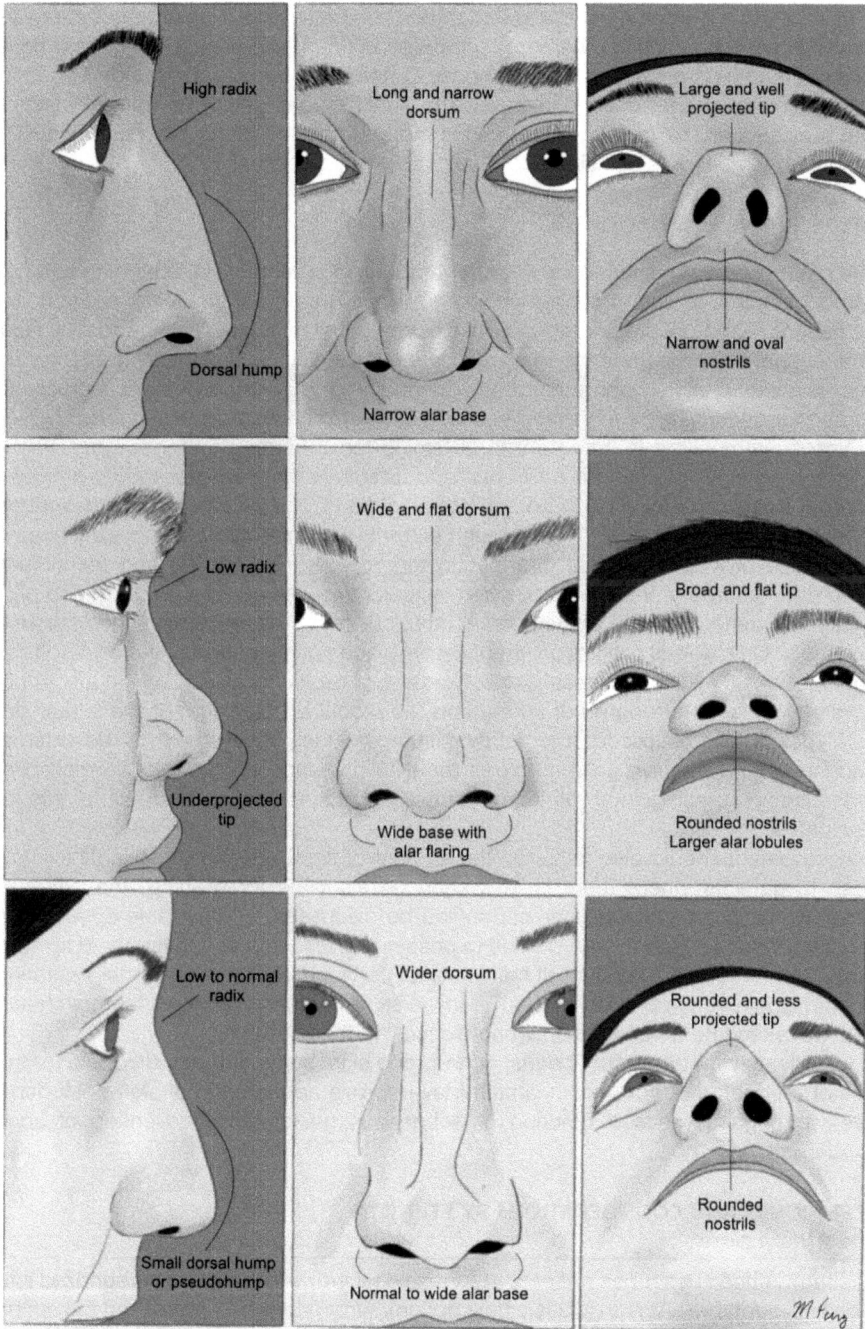

Fig. 1. Examples of leptorrhine (*top row*), platyrrhine (*middle row*), and mesorrhine (*bottom row*) nasal characteristics. Lateral (*left column*), frontal (*middle column*), and base (*right column*) views are shown. Common characteristics for each are labeled. (*Image Courtesy*: Max Feng.)

with widened nasal bridge and a pseudohump or small hump. The length of the nasal bones is normal to short. The septal cartilage is often less robust. The nasal tip is rounded and less projected. The alar base is normal to wide, with rounded nostrils, and a hidden or shortened columella. The soft tissue envelope is normal to thick and sebaceous. The cartilaginous vault is more supported than platyrrhine noses. It is common in patients of Asian and Mestizo/Hispanic descent.[14–16]

PREOPERATIVE EVALUATION

The preoperative consultation is important for gaining greater understanding of a patient's background and ethnicity, which can impact treatment goals and esthetic expectations. Although the primary purpose of functional rhinoplasty is to address nasal obstruction, a deeper understanding of a patient's ethnicity and esthetic ideals can aid in preserving ethnically congruent traits during surgery.[17] Furthermore, it is crucial to screen for underlying psychiatric disease, such as body dysmorphic disorder.[10,11]

Nasofacial analysis is important in obtaining facial harmony after surgery. Facial symmetry, height, and width on frontal and lateral views are assessed. Systematic nasal analysis is performed on frontal, lateral, oblique, and basal views, as described extensively in the literature.[18] A thorough external and internal nasal physical examination can provide important information regarding surgical goals and techniques used during surgery. Visual examination includes assessment of the length and projection of the nose, shape of the nose and tip, columella, osseocartilaginous dorsum, and radix. On external evaluation, emphasis is placed on palpation of the skin-soft tissue envelope (S-STE) to assess skin thickness and elasticity, as well as the amount of fibrofatty tissue. The degree of tip support, tip recoil, and strength of the lateral alar cartilages is also assessed. Internal evaluation includes assessment of the external and internal nasal valve (INV), angle of the INV, presence of dynamic alar collapse, presence of cartilaginous or bony septal deviations, and size of the inferior turbinates.[15,17–19]

Assessment should also focus on the amount of septal cartilage available for harvest. In patients where there is less cartilage available for grafting, the potential need for ear or rib cartilage harvest should be discussed.[15] Platyrrhine noses often require greater structural support due to possessing less robust cartilage and tip support. Furthermore, the amount of native septal cartilage is often limited, necessitating rib cartilage, even in primary cases.[15] However, cultural and religious factors should also be taken into consideration when discussing these options.

In patients with thick, sebaceous, acne-prone skin, some authors advocate for the use of preoperative isotretinoin, which may improve appearance of skin postoperatively through decreased function of sebaceous glands and prevention of acne exacerbations.[20–22]

TECHNIQUES AND CONSIDERATIONS BY ETHNICITY
The African Nose

The term *African* describes patients of African descent, which can be categorized into 3 distinct subtypes: African (classic description), Afro-Caucasian (increased projection and narrower), and Afro-Indian (longest variant with "plunging" tip and dorsal hump).[23,24] These nasal types can be broadly described by the platyrrhine configuration. The classic description of the African nose includes a short nasal length and bony vault with decreased projection, wide base and dorsum, thick and sebaceous skin, flattened and bulbous tip, and wide nostrils.[25] The alar cartilage was previously viewed as small and weak. However, in anatomic studies, the medial crura were found to be of similar size to Caucasian noses. Between the different subtypes, the medial crura were observed to be larger in Afro-Caucasian and Afro-Indian type noses, with African noses having the smallest cartilage size.[26,27] There is a particularly strong desire to maintain ethnic congruency amongst patients of African descent.[28]

Functional rhinoplasty in patients of African background often necessitates an open approach combining transcolumellar and marginal incisions. Keloid formation is rare if meticulous wound edge alignment and eversion is performed.[15,27,29] The thick skin and soft tissue envelope limits the utility of direct palpation. Once the soft tissue envelope is elevated from the bony-cartilaginous framework, direct visualization can aid in intraoperative assessment of areas of anatomic obstruction.[30] Decreased tip projection and a shortened columella are common. While it is common for patients of African descent to have less tip support than their Caucasian counterparts, the rhinoplasty surgeon must determine if this is an underlying cause of the patient's nasal obstruction. If it determined to be a contributing factor, a columellar strut graft or septal extension graft (SEG) can be used to provide additional support.[21]

There is often a paucity of septal cartilage in patients of African descent. A radiological study found 30% less quadrangular cartilage in Black African noses compared to Caucasian noses.[31] Thus, cartilage grafts from auricular or costal cartilage may be needed. Auricular cartilage harvesting should be undertaken with extreme caution, as this region has a high propensity for keloid formation. Preoperative discussion of this possibility should be undertaken with patients if auricular cartilage harvest is being considered.

The Asian Nose

The term *Asian* includes patients of East and Southeast Asian descent. The Asian nose can be broadly described as mesorrhine. It shares similarities with Hispanic patients.[11] The classic description includes a short nasal length, broad, flat dorsum, low radix, wide and under-projected nasal tip, less robust alar cartilages, and wide and horizontally oriented lobules.[25,32] The columella may be retracted. The nostrils are typically horizontally oriented.[32] The literature describes variations between Korean, Chinese, and Japanese noses. Chinese noses fit the classical description, Korean noses sometimes feature a dorsal hump, and Japanese noses are observed to have a narrower, higher dorsum with occasional dorsal convexity.[32–34]

In a cadaveric study of Korean noses, the distance between the medial portion of the lower lateral cartilage (LLC) to the alar rim in the area of the soft tissue triangle was shorter compared to Caucasian noses, potentially increasing the risk of postoperative notching in that area with marginal incisions.[35] The angle of the INV in computed tomography (CT) measurements was 21.6° ± 4.5° in Asian noses, compared to 11.4° ± 2.6° in Caucasian noses. An endoscopic measurement of the INV in Asian noses was 19.3° ± 3.6°, though there was poor correlation between CT and endoscopic measurements.[36] In a study of 57 Asian patients with INV dysfunction undergoing functional rhinoplasty, only 22.8% had dynamic collapse, which could be due to the relatively wider INV and thicker S-STE preventing dynamic collapse.[37] Rhinoplasty surgeons with extensive experience performing Asian rhinoplasty note the relative low observed rate of INV dysfunction in Asian patients.[36] This may limit the effectiveness of spreader grafts in Asian patients.

Tip support is often decreased due to the relatively smaller cartilaginous framework, which is further impacted by contractile forces of the thicker S-STE at the tip. Strong structural support is required to increase projection, reconstruct caudal septal deformities, and augment the tip and dorsum, sometimes necessitating the use of rib cartilage for grafting material.[38] The thickness of the septal cartilage was greatest at the posterior portion near the junction of the perpendicular plate of the ethmoid bone and vomer (1.4 ± 0.3 mm), making that cartilage an ideal choice for load-bearing grafts.[35] The SEG is frequently used to support the alar cartilages.[39] Inclusion of septal bone in the inferior portion of the SEG can increase the rigidity of the graft.[40]

The Indian Nose

The term *Indian* refers to patients of South Asian descent. This region represents a multitude of different ancestries from the Middle East, the Indian subcontinent, and the Caucasus, producing significant variation in the morphologies of the Indian nose. Broadly, the Indian nose can be categorized into a North Indian and South Indian subtype. The North Indian nose shares similar features with the Middle Eastern nose and includes an underrotated, overprojected tip, increased nasal length, presence of a dorsal hump, and a wide base and bony vault. The South Indian nose shares more features with the African nose and includes an overrotated, underprojected, bulbous tip, infratip lobular excess, caudally positioned radix with less dorsal projection, wide alar base and bony vault.[25,41] Among both subtypes, there is greater pigmentation, thicker skin, and less robust cartilages compared to the Caucasian nose.

The open approach is often used for functional rhinoplasty in the North Indian patient. Not only does this allow for better visualization, but the division of tip support ligaments can also facilitate a reduction in tip projection, as this nasal type is frequently overprojected. Due to their relative lack of strength, the upper lateral cartilages (ULCs) and LLCs should be preserved as much as possible. If cephalic trim is performed, alar rim grafts may be needed to prevent external valve collapse or alar notching.[42]

South Indian noses often require additional tip support and projection. This can be achieved using a columellar strut graft or SEG. Spreader or extended spreader grafts can be used to increase the INV angle, augment the dorsum, and derotate the tip. The increase in tip projection often helps decrease alar flaring.[42,43]

The Mestizo/Hispanic Nose

The terms Hispanic, Mestizo, or Latino are used interchangeably to refer to patients from Spanish-speaking countries.[25] However, there is an incredibly large diversity in nasal characteristics in Mestizo populations due to racial contributions from European, African, and American Indian ancestries.[23] Due to the extensive diversity of ancestries, there is not a single predominating feature in these populations.[44]

Broadly, the Mestizo/Hispanic nose resembles mesorrhine characteristics. This ethnic group tends to have a thick S-STE, a low radix, wide dorsum, short nasal bones, less supported middle vault and nasal tip, wide base, short columella, and more flared nostrils. Tip support can be insufficient due to less robust caudal septal cartilage and alar cartilages, along with a smaller nasal spine.[44,45] Similar to Asian noses, the INV is more obtuse in this nasal type. In an endoscopic study of INV angles in Mexican Hispanic noses, the mean INV angle was 24.1 ± 4.8° on the right and 25.07 ± 5.0° on the left.[46] In conjunction with a large external nasal valve due to larger nostrils and base, nasal airflow issues are less common unless a septal deviation is present.[47]

A functional approach to this nasal type focuses on preserving and reinforcing existing support structures, along with sutures and grafts to improve support and definition.[48] An open approach is widely preferred.[44,45,47] There is typically a limited amount of septal cartilage available for harvesting, so grafts must be chosen wisely.[49] Due to the short nasal bones, overaggressive dorsal reduction can disrupt the attachment of the ULCs. Postoperative INV collapse can be prevented with placement of spreader grafts.[45] Spreader grafting can also help support less robust ULCs and correct dorsal septal deviations.[49] Deficient tip support from the short and less sturdy LLCs can be strengthened with an SEG, which can also improve tip projection and rotation. Alternatively, a columellar strut graft can be used to provide support to the tip and medial crura. Alar rim grafting can be utilized to prevent postoperative collapse of the lateral crura.[49] Alternatively lateral crural strut grafts may be used to support the external valve.

The Middle Eastern Nose

The Middle Eastern nose refers to people of Arabic, Turkish, North African, and Persian descent.[50] Classically, this nasal type features thick and sebaceous skin, a bulbous tip with infratip lobular excess, relatively decreased medial crural strength, wide and overprojected bony and middle vaults, significant dorsal hump, more cephalic and overprojected radix, and overprojected tip with underrotated nose.[25,50,51] However, there is wide variation in the classically observed anatomic characteristics.[52] Significant caudal septal deviation and osseocartilaginous vault asymmetry have been observed.[51] There is prominent fibrofatty tissue in the S-STE, particularly in the intercartilaginous areas, which may contribute to weakening of the stability and strength of the cartilaginous framework through infiltrating of the ligamentous attachments.[50,53] Tip strength is also weakened due to the posterocaudal location of the tip complex relative to the high anterior septal angle. More vertically oriented lower lateral crura can increase risk of postoperative tip position loss, or pollybeak deformity, and external valve dysfunction.[50]

Surgery is often approached in an open fashion. The combination of thin medial crura and thick S-STE necessitates frequent use of a columellar strut graft or SEG to establish adequate tip support. The lateral crura are typically thin, wide, and cephalically displaced, leading to external valve collapse. External valve function can be improved with use of lateral crural strut grafts, batten grafts, or alar contour grafts.[36,40]

Dorsal hump reduction is commonly performed in Middle Eastern rhinoplasty.[50,51] The keystone traverses the dorsal hump, which has important structural contributions from the fusion of the paired nasal bones, ULCs, perpendicular plate of the ethmoid bone, and quadrangular cartilage.[54] With en-bloc resection of the dorsal hump, there is a risk of collapse of the ULC attachment to the septum and inverted-V deformity, leading to INV narrowing. Spreader grafts can be placed to stabilize the INV and prevent postoperative nasal obstruction.[50,55]

POSTOPERATIVE CARE

The thicker S-STE in non-Caucasian noses leads to a propensity for increased postoperative edema, which can take up to 12 to 24 months to fully resolve. Prolonged postoperative taping and splinting of the nose, meticulous hemostasis during surgery, application of silicone sheeting, and perioperative steroids can help prevent edema. Applying ice to the periorbital and nasal areas and head of bed elevation to 40° can also decrease swelling postoperatively.[15,19,27] Isotretinoin can also be used in the postoperative setting for patients with thicker S-STE.[20,22]

Hypertrophic scarring and keloid formation is rare in non-Caucasian rhinoplasty.[15,27] This can be mitigated through meticulous columellar incision closure and early suture removal at 6 to 7 days.[56] There is increased risk of excess skin tension at the nasal tip due to the thick, sebaceous skin and soft tissue envelope, particularly when tip projection is increased. A single buried deep suture using 5-0 Monocryl at the apex of the inverted-V incision can facilitate tension-free closure.

Table 1
Classical descriptions of nasal anatomy amongst ethnicities[a]

Characteristic	Ethnicity				
	African American	Asian	Indian	Mestizo/ Hispanic	Middle Eastern
Skin/soft tissue envelope	Thicker	Thicker	Thicker	Thicker	Thicker
Nasal length	Shorter	Shorter	Longer (North) Shorter (South)	Shorter	Longer
Bony vault	Shorter	Shorter, wider	Wider	Shorter, wider	Wider
Middle vault	Wider	Wider	Wider	Wider	Wider
Radix	More caudal and less projected	More caudal and less projected	More projected (North) More caudal and less projected (South)	Variable	More cephalic and more projected
Alar base	Wider	Wider	Wider	Wider	Wider
Tip quality	More bulbous and flatter	More bulbous and wider	Wider (North) More bulbous (South)	More bulbous	More bulbous
Tip projection	Less projected	Less projected	More projected (North) Less projected (South)	Less projected	More projected

[a] Relative to Caucasian nasal anatomy.

SUMMARY

As ethnic and racial diversity increases in the United States, the variety of patients presenting for functional rhinoplasty will increase in tandem. There is a significant amount of nasal anatomic variance amongst ethnicities (**Table 1**), and understanding these differences is crucial in optimizing functional outcomes while simultaneously preserving facial congruence for patients undergoing rhinoplasty.

CLINICS CARE POINTS

- Nasal anatomic morphologies can be broadly divided into 3 types: leptorrhine, mesorrhine, and platyrrhine noses.
- The 5 distinct non-Caucasian nose types in the United States are the African, Asian, Hispanic/Mestizo, Indian, and Middle Eastern.
- A deeper understanding of the anatomic variances amongst these nasal types can guide operative planning to maximize functional outcomes while maintaining ethnic congruence.
- There is often less harvestable septal cartilage in non-Caucasian patients, so the use of ear, rib, or donor cartilage should be considered.
- Tip support often requires augmentation in non-Caucasian patients. The workhorse for establishing strong tip support is the columellar strut graft or septal extension graft.
- Care should be taken to avoid over-resection during dorsal hump reduction. The placement of spreader grafts can help prevent postoperative narrowing of the internal nasal valve.
- Prolonged postoperative edema is a common postoperative complication in patients with thick, sebaceous skin.

REFERENCES

1. Broer PN, Buonocore S, Morillas A, et al. Nasal aesthetics: a cross-cultural analysis. Plast Reconstr Surg 2012;130(6):843e–50e.
2. Zacharopoulos GV, Manios A, De Bree E, et al. Neoclassical facial canons in young adults. J Craniofac Surg 2012;23(6):1693–8.
3. Doddi NM, Eccles R. The role of anthropometric measurements in nasal surgery and research: a systematic review. Clin Otolaryngol Off J ENT-UK Off J Neth Soc Oto-Rhino-Laryngol Cervico-Facial Surg. 2010;35(4):277–83.
4. Davis R. Rhinoplasty and concepts of facial beauty. Facial Plast Surg 2006;22(3): 198–203.
5. Farkas LG, Hreczko TA, Kolar JC, et al. Vertical and horizontal proportions of the face in young adult North American Caucasians: revision of neoclassical canons. Plast Reconstr Surg 1985;75(3):328–38.
6. U.S. Census Bureau. Projected Population by Single Year of Age, Sex, Race, and Hispanic Origin for the United States: 2022 to 2100. 2023. Available at: https://www2.census.gov/programs-surveys/popproj/technical-documentation/file-layouts/2023/np2023_d1.pdf.
7. Kandathil CK, Saltychev M, Patel PN, et al. Natural history of the standardized cosmesis and health nasal outcomes survey after rhinoplasty. Laryngoscope 2021;131(1).
8. Sturm-O'Brien A, Brissett A, Brissett A. Ethnic trends in facial plastic surgery. Facial Plast Surg 2010;26(02):069–74.

9. Brissett AE, Ishii LE, Boahene KDO. Ethnically sensitive rhinoplasty. Otolaryngol Clin North Am 2020;53(2):xiii–xiv.

10. Deeb R. Ethnically sensitive rhinoplasty. Facial Plast Surg FPS 2023;39(5): 527–36.

11. Patel PN, Most SP. Concepts of facial aesthetics when considering ethnic rhinoplasty. Otolaryngol Clin North Am 2020;53(2):195–208.

12. Leong SC, Eccles R. Race and ethnicity in nasal plastic surgery: a need for science. Facial Plast Surg 2010;26(02):063–8.

13. O'Connor K, Brissett AE. The changing face of America. Otolaryngol Clin North Am 2020;53(2):299–308.

14. Kim DW, Hwang HS. Traumatic rhinoplasty in the non-caucasian nose. Facial Plast Surg Clin N Am 2010;18(1):141–51.

15. Cobo R. Ethnic rhinoplasty. Facial Plast Surg FPS 2019;35(4):313–21.

16. Newsome HA, Chi JJ. The use of race-based terminology in the rhinoplasty literature. Curr Opin Otolaryngol Head Neck Surg 2022;30(4):236–40.

17. Porter JP. Non-Caucasian rhinoplasty: preoperative analysis. Facial Plast Surg Clin N Am 2003;11(3):327–33.

18. Rohrich RJ, Ahmad J. Rhinoplasty. Plast Reconstr Surg 2011;128(2):49e–73e.

19. Nolst Trenité GJ. Considerations in ethnic rhinoplasty. Facial Plast Surg FPS 2003; 19(3):239–45.

20. Cobo R, Vitery L. Isotretinoin use in thick-skinned rhinoplasty patients. Facial Plast Surg 2016;32(06):656–61.

21. Patrocinio LG, Patrocinio TG, Patrocinio JA. Approach for rhinoplasty in African descendants. Facial Plast Surg Clin N Am 2021;29(4):575–88.

22. Yahyavi S, Jahandideh H, Izadi M, et al. Analysis of the effects of isotretinoin on rhinoplasty patients. Aesthetic Surg J 2020;40(12):NP657–65.

23. Heiman AJ, Nair L, Kanth A, et al. Defining regional variation in nasal anatomy to guide ethnic rhinoplasty: A systematic review. J Plast Reconstr Aesthetic Surg JPRAS 2022;75(8):2784–95.

24. Ofodile FA, Bokhari FJ, Ellis C. The black American nose. Ann Plast Surg 1993; 31(3):209–18 [discussion 218-219].

25. Villanueva NL, Afrooz PN, Carboy JA, et al. Nasal analysis: considerations for ethnic variation. Plast Reconstr Surg 2019;143(6):1179e–88e.

26. Ofodile FA, James EA. Anatomy of alar cartilages in blacks. Plast Amp Reconstr Surg 1997;100(3):699–703.

27. Rohrich RJ, Muzaffar AR. Rhinoplasty in the African-American Patient. Plast Reconstr Surg 2003;111(3):1322–39.

28. Boahene KDO. Management of the nasal tip, nasal base, and soft tissue envelope in patients of African Descent. Otolaryngol Clin North Am 2020;53(2): 309–17.

29. Boyette JR, Stucker FJ. African American rhinoplasty. Facial Plast Surg Clin N Am 2014;22(3):379–93.

30. Harris MO. Rhinoplasty in the patient of African descent. Facial Plast Surg Clin N Am 2010;18(1):189–99.

31. Pisapia F, Cottone G, Stutterheim J, et al. The quadrangular cartilage in rhinoplasty: a surgically focused CT dimensional analysis of black African and Caucasian Populations. Facial Plast Surg FPS 2024. https://doi.org/10.1055/a-2302-9456.

32. Fang F, Clapham PJ, Chung KC. A systematic review of interethnic variability in facial dimensions. Plast Reconstr Surg 2011;127(2):874–81.

33. Shirakabe Y, Suzuki Y, Lam SM. A systematic approach to rhinoplasty of the Japanese nose: a thirty-year experience. Aesthetic Plast Surg 2003;27(3):221–31.
34. Yoo JY, Kim JN, Lee JY, et al. Anatomical characteristics of the nasal cartilages for successful rhinoplasty in Koreans. Ann Plast Surg 2014;73(1):77–80.
35. Kim CH, Jung DH, Park MN, et al. Surgical anatomy of cartilaginous structures of the Asian nose: clinical implications in rhinoplasty. Laryngoscope 2010;120(5):914–9.
36. Suh MW, Jin HR, Kim JH. Computed tomography versus nasal endoscopy for the measurement of the internal nasal valve angle in Asians. Acta Otolaryngol 2008;128(6):675–9.
37. Jung HJ, Park MW, Shim WS, et al. Functional and esthetic outcomes of functional rhinoplasty for internal nasal valve dysfunction in Asian patients. Braz J Otorhinolaryngol 2024;90(4):101430.
38. Park JH, Mangoba DCS, Mun SJ, et al. Lengthening the short nose in asians: key maneuvers and surgical results. JAMA Facial Plast Surg 2013;15(6):439–47.
39. Kim JH, Song JW, Park SW, et al. Effective septal extension graft for Asian Rhinoplasty. Arch Plast Surg 2014;41(01):3–11.
40. Kim EK, Daniel RK. Operative techniques in Asian rhinoplasty. Aesthetic Surg J 2012;32(8):1018–30.
41. Mehta N, Srivastava RK. The Indian nose: An anthropometric analysis. J Plast Reconstr Aesthetic Surg 2017;70(10):1472–82.
42. Nagarkar P, Pezeshk RA, Rohrich RJ. The Indian Nose. Plast Reconstr Surg 2016;138(5):836e–43e.
43. Patel SM, Daniel RK. Indian American rhinoplasty: an emerging ethnic group. Plast Reconstr Surg 2012;129(3):519e–27e.
44. Cobo R. Management of the mestizo nose. Otolaryngol Clin North Am 2020;53(2):267–82.
45. Patel A, Kridel R. Hispanic-American Rhinoplasty. Facial Plast Surg 2010;26(02):142–53.
46. Jasso-Ramírez E, Sánchez Y, Béjar F, et al. Nasal valve evaluation in the Mexican-Hispanic (mestizo) nose. Int Forum Allergy Rhinol 2018;8(4):547–52.
47. Higuera S, Hatef D, Stal S. Rhinoplasty in the hispanic patient. Semin Plast Surg 2009;23(03):207–14.
48. Cobo R. Structural rhinoplasty in Latin American Patients. Facial Plast Surg 2013;29(03):171–83.
49. Cobo R. Hispanic/Mestizo rhinoplasty. Facial Plast Surg Clin N Am. 2010;18(1):173–88.
50. Rohrich RJ, Ghavami A. Rhinoplasty for middle eastern noses. Plast Reconstr Surg 2009;123(4):1343–54.
51. Daniel RK. Middle eastern rhinoplasty in the United States: part i. primary rhinoplasty. Plast Reconstr Surg 2009;124(5):1630–9.
52. Daniel R. Middle eastern rhinoplasty: anatomy, aesthetics, and surgical planning. Facial Plast Surg 2010;26(02):110–8.
53. Adams WP, Rohrich RJ, Hollier LH, et al. Anatomic basis and clinical implications for nasal tip support in open versus closed rhinoplasty. Plast Reconstr Surg 1999;103(1):255–61 [discussion 262-264].
54. Simon PE, Lam K, Sidle D, et al. The nasal keystone region: an anatomical study. JAMA Facial Plast Surg 2013;15(3):235–7.
55. Afrooz PN, Rohrich RJ. The keystone: consistency in restoring the aesthetic dorsum in rhinoplasty. Plast Reconstr Surg 2018;141(2):355–63.
56. Rohrich RJ, Bolden K. Ethnic rhinoplasty. Clin Plast Surg 2010;37(2):353–70.

Functional and Cosmetic Considerations in Gender-Affirming Feminization Rhinoplasty

Shayan Fakurnejad, MD[a,1], Suresh Mohan, MD[b],
Rahul Seth, MD[c,d,2], Philip Daniel Knott, MD[d,*]

KEYWORDS

- Rhinoplasty • Gender-affirming facial surgery • Gender-affirming rhinoplasty
- Feminization rhinoplasty

KEY POINTS

- Interest in gender-affirming facial surgery continues to rise, and rhinoplasty plays an integral role in feminizing the face.
- Feminization rhinoplasty has unique considerations in regard to facial aesthetics and nasal function.
- The field of gender-affirming facial surgery, including feminization rhinoplasty, is relatively understudied, and future work is required to clarify the role and impact this procedure has on transgender and gender diverse individuals.

INTRODUCTION

Approximately 1 in every 250 individuals in the United States self-identifies as transgender or gender diverse (TGD), and between 5 to 14 in every 1000 adult males and between 2 to 3 in every 1000 adult females report experiencing gender dysphoria.[1,2] Data suggest that the prevalence of individuals identifying as transgender is increasing, and this trend is expected to continue to rise.[1] Discordance between

[a] Department of Otolaryngology–Head & Neck Surgery, University of California, 2233 Post Street, 3rd Floor, San Francisco, CA 94117, USA; [b] Facial Plastic and Reconstructive Surgery, Division of Otolaryngology, Yale School of Medicine, 47 College Street Suite 216A, New Haven, CT 06510, USA; [c] Golden State Plastic Surgery, San Francisco, CA, USA; [d] Division of Facial Plastic and Reconstructive Surgery, Department of Otolaryngology–Head & Neck Surgery, University of California, San Francisco, San Francisco, CA, USA
[1] Present address: 7134 Marlborough Terrace, Berkeley, CA 94705.
[2] Present address: 355 Lennon Lane, Suite 235, Walnut Creek, CA 94598.
* Corresponding author. Division of Facial Plastic and Reconstructive Surgery, Suite 102, 2320 Sutter Street, San Francisco, CA 94117.
E-mail address: p.daniel.knott@ucsf.edu

Otolaryngol Clin N Am 58 (2025) 315–323
https://doi.org/10.1016/j.otc.2024.08.001
oto.theclinics.com

gender identity and facial appearance is strongly associated with gender dysphoria,[3] and multiple studies have highlighted the differences between the male and female face using sophisticated facial analytic techniques, including gender specific facial morphometrics.[4,5] Gender-affirming facial surgery (GFS) has become increasingly popular as it may better align appearance with gender identity, resulting in significant improvement in quality-of-life and reduction in gender dysphoria.[6–8] A component of this increase in popularity may be due to improved coverage from insurance companies in regard to gender-affirming care.[9]

In this article, we discuss functional and cosmetic considerations in gender-affirming rhinoplasty, and in particular feminization rhinoplasty. Septorhinoplasty is performed to enhance both nasal form and function. Gender-affirming septorhinoplasty is of particular interest because nasal form displays considerable gender dimorphism; approximately 30% of the variation in the axial nasal profile is gender-related.[5] Rhinoplasty has been found to be one of the most effective surgeries in feminizing facial appearance.[10]

When considering the impact of gender-affirming rhinoplasty on the nasal valve, feminization rhinoplasty, when compared to masculinization rhinoplasty, is of greater importance. This is because feminization rhinoplasty is centered on reductive techniques, which may potentially impact function, whereas masculinization rhinoplasty commonly involves widening the nose with or without dorsal augmentation, which does not generally impact function. As such, this article will focus on feminization rhinoplasty and the balance of harmonizing one's gender identity and nasal function.

PATIENT SELECTION AND PREOPERATIVE EVALUATION

As with any facial plastic intervention, patient selection is of utmost importance when approaching feminization rhinoplasty. Unique to this patient population is that rhinoplasty is seldom performed in isolation. Significant time must be dedicated to discussing all of the surgical techniques and potential modifications available for facial feminization. Recognizing the historic challenges of access and understanding faced by TGD patients, many institutions have established care pathways with gender-affirming multidisciplinary clinics and patient experience navigators.[11] Many candidates likely have initiated hormonal therapy, as well as received mental health related support and extensive psychotherapy.

Many facial plastic surgeons who specialize in GFS cite a preference for initiation of hormonal therapy with exogenous estrogen approximately 1 to 2 y prior to feminization rhinoplasty, with the goal of thinning the nasal envelope, reduction in facial hair, and decreased sebum production.[12–14] As for prior rhinoplasty, rates of revision rhinoplasty in this patient population appear to be on par with large cisgender studies.[15]

Pre-operatively, TGD patients are more frequently sent for pre-operative computed tomography (CT_ scans), particularly when concomitant frontal cranioplasty is planned, or if computer aided design/manufacture (CAD/CAM) is to be used. As such, CT scans can be reviewed with patients with particular attention to septal deviation and spurring, as well as dorsal contour issues, and this may help improve patient understanding of the goals of surgery.[16] During a consultation, much like during cisgender rhinoplasty, use of pre-operative photography with 3D morphing or simulation software can be helpful when discussing the patient's goals. Patients experiencing gender dysphoria may have a desire for a "hyper-feminine" nose, and it is the surgeon's responsibility to balance these desires with the ultimate goal of creating facial harmony while feminizing the face.

Pre-operative patient reported outcome measures (PROMs), are commonly employed prior to cisgender rhinoplasty, particularly when there are functional reasons for pursuing septorhinoplasty. Commonly reported PROMs such as the NOSE and SCHNOS can be employed; however, there is no nasal airway survey specifically designed for the transgender population, and to our knowledge there are no studies that have presented data regarding the impact of gender-affirming or feminization rhinoplasty on functional PROM data. Gender-Q is in the process of being validated and may offer high-quality data for TGD individuals undergoing gender affirming facial surgery.[17]

Lastly, a welcoming, inclusive environment is of utmost importance. Clinic staff and surgeons should be educated on using inclusive language, and attention should be paid to the patient's preferred pronouns. The language used on social media and practice websites should also be inclusive in nature. Additionally, intake forms should identify the patient's preferred pronouns and name, although legal names should be kept in the electronic medical record for insurance purposes.[13]

DISCUSSION

The discussion of aesthetic and functional features to consider during feminization rhinoplasty can be organized into the osseous upper third, the cartilaginous middle vault, and the lower third.

DORSUM/RADIX

Many surgeons prefer to approach GFS from a top-down approach, including the senior author. When addressing the nasal radix and dorsum, there are unique considerations in this patient population. Access to the radix can be achieved through traditional endonasal or open septorhinoplasty approaches, or can be managed superiorly via a trichophytic or coronal approach performed during concomitant frontal cranioplasty, browlifting, and hairline repositioning procedures. These different approaches provide varying degrees of visualization and perspective and the appropriate approach should be chosen for a given functional/aesthetic goal. Particular to feminization septorhinoplasty, consideration of the radix includes potent potential alteration of the nasofrontal angle. In general, perceived "ideal" male noses have more acute nasofrontal angles,[10,18,19] and this is due in part because of a larger, more pronounced glabella resulting from frontal sinus pneumatization, but also due to a larger, more projected dorsum. This can be seen in **Fig. 1**A, B. As such, when addressing the nasofrontal angle in feminization rhinoplasty, reduction of the dorsum is important, but often is not sufficient in widening and thereby feminizing the nasofrontal angle. Frontal sinus setback or feminizing frontal cranioplasty permits widening of the nasofrontal angle and softening of the appearance of the radix, providing a more feminine aesthetic. Reduction of the orbital roof, inferoposterior rotation of the anterior table, and removal/reduction of the bone high along the lateral nasal sidewall/dorsum during feminizing frontal cranioplasty typically widens the nasofrontal angle by 12 to 15°.[20]

There is sexual dimorphism in the dorsal width as well, with the male nose being generally wider at the dorsum when compared to the female nose.[18] This can be seen in **Fig. 1**. Given this anatomic generality, it is not surprising that osteotomies are commonly utilized during feminization rhinoplasty. Hage and colleagues described this early on, where all of the patients in their series underwent lateral and medial osteotomies to narrow the appearance of the dorsum.[15] In regards to the type of lateral osteotomies performed, the most common described in the literature is the

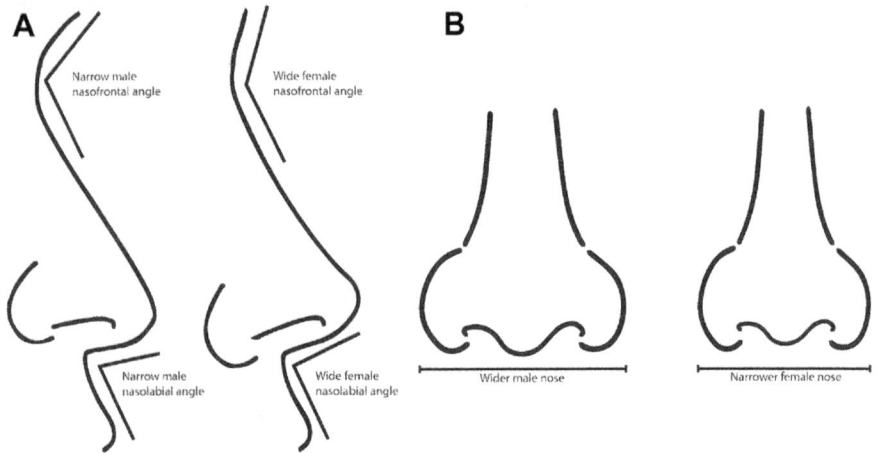

Fig. 1. A representation of gender dimorphism of the nose. (*A*) The nasofrontal and naso-labial angle of the male nose is narrower when compared to the female nose. (*B*) The width of the dorsum and lower third of the male nose is wider when compared to the narrower female nose.

"high-low-high" osteotomy, which is common in cisgender rhinoplasty as well.[21] However, some surgeons describe starting the lateral osteotomies out further laterally in gender-affirming rhinoplasty, to allow for further narrowing of the insertion point of the nasal base at the nasomaxillary junction, which ideally should be roughly two-thirds of the width of the alar base.[13] When doing so, however, there should be great care in the functional impact of this maneuver, as it can result in internal nasal valve narrowing and result in increased rates of obstruction.

When approaching the presence of a dorsal convexity and/or excess dorsal height, structural rhinoplasty is largely favored, as preservation techniques may not adequately narrow and reduce the larger dorsum found in the male nose.[22] However, as dorsal preservation continues to gain traction, it is likely that modifications may be developed for application to feminizing rhinoplasty. Creation of a narrowed upper third with a gentle, feminine dorsal concavity may be obtained with rasps, osteotomes, or powered instruments. It should be noted that the relatively thicker skin at the radix in males may hide some of the dorsal irregularities that may occur with non-preservation techniques. The occasional use of camouflage grafting can be beneficial in improving the aesthetic outcome of the dorsum. Diced or crushed cartilage grafts can help address minor asymmetries. Many patients presenting for feminizing rhinoplasty will focus on the shape of the dorsum on profile view. Again, this is an important area to discuss at the pre-operative visit, and having simulation photographs available in the operating room can assist the surgeon in achieving the patient's desired outcome during surgery.

MIDDLE VAULT

Functional considerations when approaching the radix and dorsum largely revolve around the impact on the mid-vault. Transfemale patients will often favor mid-vault narrowing, and given the relatively thicker bone and skin typically found in male noses, they may eschew maintenance of functionally competent mid-vault support. This may be particularly problematic among patients favoring more aggressive dorsal reduction and dorsal concavity. Given that patients' goals may be more oriented toward appearance than function, surgeons should carefully consider balancing the maintenance of nasal airway patency with appearance-related outcomes.

Maneuvers such as spreader grafting or upper lateral cartilage turn-in flaps, also known as "autospreaders", are commonly employed in functional rhinoplasty to address mid-vault narrowing. These can prevent internal nasal valve collapse, inverted-V deformity, or mid-vault asymmetry, which are potential complications in the setting of more aggressive reductive maneuvers in feminizing rhinoplasty. Often when aggressive osteotomies are performed the use of spreader grafts can mitigate the impact of upper vault narrowing with support of the nasal valve. In the absence of good quality data on post-operative nasal function, in our experience, lateral wall support grafts are employed in 25% to 50% of patients undergoing feminizing rhinoplasty. These include lateral crural strut grafting, spreader grafting, and alar rim grafts. Maintenance of the integrity of the scroll may be particularly important among patients that undergo other nasal valve compromising surgical maneuvers.

TIP/LOWER THIRD

When approaching the lower third and tip of the nose, morphometric analyses have consistently shown that male noses are wider at the nasal base, have a greater linear distance between the insertion of the ala, as well as lateral alar extent, or alar flaring.[23] This is also an area where ethnic differences are particularly apparent.[24,25] As such, this is an area of particular interest for the cosmetic outcomes of feminization rhinoplasty. However, functional rhinoplasty surgeons will commonly counsel patients on the potential of widening the appearance of the nose at these regions, as maneuvers to strengthen the internal and external nasal valves and maintain the alar contour and tip lobule to alar lobule stability will commonly require grafting that impacts the appearance. This is another area where cosmetic and functional considerations are at odds.

To address the sexual dimorphism of lower third nasal width, it is important to distinguish the difference between alar base width and excessive alar flaring. Alar base excision, which has been described extensively in the cisgender literature,[26] can significantly reduce nasal width. If the alar lobule is of appropriate size, diamond-shaped excisions can be performed within the lateral vestibular entrance, with the inferior extent not transgressing the base of the sill. If the lobule needs to be reduced as well, then this can be done via a Weir incision, when the excision extends into the alar facial groove. It should be noted that these incisions can be incorporated into the lip-lift incision, which is commonly performed via a bullhorn incision under the nose, or they can be kept separate. The bullhorn incision can be extended into the nasal sill and a diamond wedge of the sill is removed and the ala can be repositioned medially. The senior author uses an absorbable cinching suture that is passed subdermally through both alar bases, permitting symmetric and even alar base tightening, thereby potentially reducing the incidence of post-operative asymmetries. The various techniques described can be seen in **Fig. 2**A–D.

Another consideration of this area is the nasolabial angle. Much like the nasofrontal angle, morphometric analyses have shown that the "ideal" nasolabial angle for female noses is greater than that for male noses.[10,27] This can be seen in **Fig. 1**. However, much like the nasofrontal angle, this characteristic of the nose is influenced by other interventions, such as lip lifts or lip augmentation, which are commonly performed during gender-affirming facial surgeries. Goals of feminization rhinoplasty, from a cosmetic standpoint, are to maintain or de-project the tip, increase rotation, and decrease the nasal tip width. Lateral crural steal is rarely employed, as additional tip

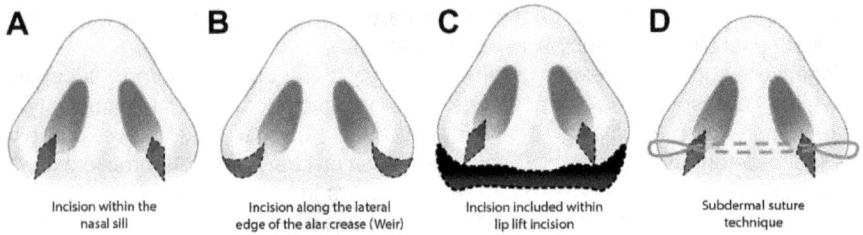

Fig. 2. Different techniques employed to narrow the nasal ala. (*A*) The incisions can be made medially within the nasal sill or (*B*) laterally along the alar crease (Weir incision). (*C*) The alar base incisions can also be incorporated into the lip lift incisions. (*D*) Subdermal suture technique for narrowing the base symmetrically.

projection is not desired in the vast majority of cases. Caudal septal extension grafts, tongue-in-groove tip-plasty, and columellar strut grafting are the techniques of choice in most circumstances by our group. Tip narrowing is accomplished likewise by a variety of maneuvers. Medial cephalic trim can maintain the external nasal valve while narrowing the tip. Intra-domal sutures, with or without domal grafting offers tip narrowing without tip projection. Among patients with particularly thick, sebaceous skin, tip grafting offers the potential for considerable tip width modification.

FUNCTIONAL CONSIDERATIONS

The functional considerations of rhinoplasty in this patient population are often in opposition to the cosmetic goals. Nevertheless, the authors address any functional issues such as septal deviation or spurring, inferior turbinate hypertrophy, internal or external nasal valve narrowing or compromise in the same fashion as with a cisgender rhinoplasty, with the perspective of maintaining the goal of feminization. Septoplasty and inferior turbinate reduction are often highly effective in improving the nasal airway and are done in almost all cases of feminization rhinoplasty. The septum is also often an excellent source of cartilage for the aforementioned grafting techniques. As mentioned previously, in instances when aggressive osteotomies are performed to feminize the nose, the use of spreader grafting or autospreaders can maintain the patency of the middle vault and mitigate the functional impacts of aggressive reduction of the bony vault.

It has been suggested that, amongst transfemales, the rate of obstructive sleep apnea is higher than in cisgendered females.[28] This is likely a result of the fact that the upper airway of males is more prone to obstructive sleep apnea than females. This should be discussed at preoperative visits, as any impact to the nasal airway may have an impact on the patient's sleep.

COMPLICATIONS

Post-operative complications after GFS and in particular gender-affirming rhinoplasty are uncommon. Studies from groups performing high volume of feminization surgery have reported no increased risk of complication when performing feminization rhinoplasty at the same time as GFS, and complications specifically related to rhinoplasty are the minority of complications.[29,30] Epistaxis occurred in 2.5% of patients in a study published by Chou and colleagues[30] Both studies do, however, note 1 patient in each cohort who developed venous thromboembolism, potentially attributed to hormone replacement therapy in the post-operative setting. As mentioned previously, rates of revision rhinoplasty in this patient population appear to be on par with large cisgender studies.[15]

Nevertheless, there are unique considerations when performing feminization rhinoplasty. Many of the aforementioned maneuvers that are commonly employed in feminization rhinoplasty are reductive in nature. When addressing the dorsum, aggressive reduction can result in an open roof deformity, so care must be made to close this with appropriate lateral osteotomies. Narrowing the midvault, reduction of the alar base, and de-projecting the nose and tip can all potentially lead to nasal obstruction, so care must be made to counter these and support the nasal valves. However, further studies are needed to clarify the functional outcomes after feminization rhinoplasty.

SUMMARY

Standardized gender-affirming septorhinoplasty paradigms are underdeveloped. Maneuvers typically performed to enhance form and function during cis-gender septorhinoplasty may or may not be applicable to transgender septorhinoplasty. Given the gender-associated differences in nasal form, varying approaches are used to achieve gender congruity with a general reductive paradigm of upper, middle, and lower third narrowing, dorsal reduction, and tip narrowing.[12,13,31] Common approaches include medial and lateral osteotomies, radix and dorsal takedown, and cartilage grafting for functional support and tip definition. Alar base reduction has also been described in the cis-gender population for addressing alar flaring, vertical excess, as well as alar asymmetry; however, the frequency of utilization of this technique has not been described in the GFS literature.[26,32] Ultimately, there is still considerable work required to further understand the impact of rhinoplasty in this population, particularly as the field continues to expand and evolve.

CLINICS CARE POINTS

- Surgical maneuvers for transgender feminization rhinoplasty may differ from approaches typically used during cis gender feminization rhinoplasty.
- Careful pre-surgical planning is necessary to most faithfully align desired ethnicity, femininity, and nasal airway patency.
- As reductive techniques are almost universally employed in transgender feminization rhinoplasty, meticulous technique and attention is required among individuals at risk for nasal airway compromise.

DISCLOSURES

The authors have nothing to disclose.

REFERENCES

1. Meerwijk EL, Sevelius JM. Transgender population size in the united states: a meta-regression of population-based probability samples. Am J Publ Health 2017;107(2):e1–8.
2. Zucker KJ. Epidemiology of gender dysphoria and transgender identity. Sex Health 2017;14(5):404–11.
3. van de Grift TC, Cohen-Kettenis PT, Steensma TD, et al. Body satisfaction and physical appearance in gender dysphoria. Arch Sex Behav 2016;45(3):575–85.

4. Russel SM, Frank-Ito DO. Gender differences in nasal anatomy and function among caucasians. Facial Plast Surg Aesthet Med 2023;25(2):145–52.

5. Bannister JJ, Juszczak H, Aponte JD, et al. Sex differences in adult facial three-dimensional morphology: application to gender-affirming facial surgery. Facial Plast Surg Aesthet Med 2022;24(S2):S24–30.

6. Ainsworth TA, Spiegel JH. Quality of life of individuals with and without facial feminization surgery or gender reassignment surgery. Qual Life Res 2010;19(7): 1019–24.

7. Morrison SD, Satterwhite T. Lower jaw recontouring in facial gender-affirming surgery. Facial Plast Surg Clin North Am 2019;27(2):233–42.

8. Nolan IT, Kuhner CJ, Dy GW. Demographic and temporal trends in transgender identities and gender confirming surgery. Transl Androl Urol 2019;8(3):184–90.

9. Movement advancement project. Available at: https://www.lgbtmap.org/equality-maps/healthcare_laws_and_policies. Accessed June 4, 2024.

10. Noureai SAR, Randhawa P, Andrews PJ, et al. The role of nasal feminization rhinoplasty in male-to-female gender reassignment. Arch Facial Plast Surg 2007; 9(5):318–20.

11. Salehi P, Divall SA, Crouch JM, et al. Review of current care models for transgender youth and application to the development of a multidisciplinary clinic - the seattle children's hospital experience. Pediatr Endocrinol Rev 2018;15(4): 280–90.

12. Berli JU, Loyo M. Gender-confirming rhinoplasty. Facial Plast Surg Clin North Am 2019;27(2):251–60.

13. Flaherty AJ, Stone AM, Teixeira JC, et al. Feminization rhinoplasty. Facial Plast Surg Clin North Am 2023;31(3):407–17.

14. Hamidi O, Davidge-Pitts CJ. Transfeminine Hormone Therapy. Endocrinol Metab Clin North Am 2019;48(2):341–55.

15. Hage JJ, Vossen M, Becking AG. Rhinoplasty as part of gender-confirming surgery in male transsexuals: basic considerations and clinical experience. Ann Plast Surg 1997;39(3):266–71.

16. Callen AL, Badiee RK, Phelps A, et al. Facial feminization surgery: key ct findings for preoperative planning and postoperative evaluation. AJR Am J Roentgenol 2021;217(3):709–17.

17. Kaur M, Morrison S, Deibert S, et al. D151. The gender-Q: A rigorous, modular, patient-reported outcome measure for gender-affirming care. Plast Reconstr Surg Glob Open 2023;11(4S):132–3.

18. Springer IN, Zernial O, Nölke F, et al. Gender and nasal shape: measures for rhinoplasty. Plast Reconstr Surg 2008;121(2):629–37.

19. Bellinga RJ, Capitán L, Simon D, et al. Technical and clinical considerations for facial feminization surgery with rhinoplasty and related procedures. JAMA Facial Plast Surg 2017;19(3):175–81.

20. David AP, House AE, Targ S, et al. Objective photoanalysis of feminizing frontal cranioplasty outcomes. Craniomaxillofac Trauma Reconstr 2024;17(2):143–5.

21. Azizzadeh B, Reilly MJ. Primary Caucasian Female Rhinoplasty. In: Shiffman MA, Di Giuseppe A, editors. Advanced aesthetic rhinoplasty: art, science, and new clinical techniques. Berlin Heidelberg: Springer; 2013. p. 147–61.

22. Patel PN, Most SP. Overview of dorsal preservation rhinoplasty. Facial Plast Surg Clin North Am 2023;31(1):1–11.

23. Sforza C, Grandi G, De Menezes M, et al. Age- and sex-related changes in the normal human external nose. Forensic Sci Int 2011;204(1–3):205.e1–9.

24. Liu Y, Kau CH, Talbert L, et al. Three-dimensional analysis of facial morphology. J Craniofac Surg 2014;25(5):1890–4.
25. Kau CH, Wang J, Davis M. A cross-sectional study to understand 3d facial differences in a population of african americans and caucasians. Eur J Dent 2019; 13(4):485–96.
26. Cerkes N. Alar Base Reduction: Nuances and Techniques. Clin Plast Surg 2022; 49(1):161–78.
27. Armijo BS, Brown M, Guyuron B. Defining the ideal nasolabial angle. Plast Reconstr Surg 2012;129(3):759–64.
28. Lin CM, Davidson TM, Ancoli-Israel S. Gender differences in obstructive sleep apnea and treatment implications. Sleep Med Rev 2008;12(6):481–96.
29. Gupta N, Wulu J, Spiegel JH. Safety of combined facial plastic procedures affecting multiple planes in a single setting in facial feminization for transgender patients. Aesthetic Plast Surg 2019;43(4):993–9.
30. Chou DW, Tejani N, Kleinberger A, et al. Initial facial feminization surgery experience in a multicenter integrated health care system. Otolaryngol Head Neck Surg 2020;163(4):737–42.
31. Das RK, Sharma RK, Kassis SA, et al. Differences in patient characteristics and spending among individuals undergoing gender-affirming rhinoplasty in the United States from 2016 to 2019. Facial Plast Surg Aesthet Med 2023;25(6): 533–5.
32. Kridel RWH, Starr N. Reducing the alar base while minimizing visible sequalae: a review of three alar base reduction techniques over 35 years. Facial Plast Surg Aesthet Med 2023;25(5):384–90.

Functional and Cosmetic Considerations in Saddle Nose Deformity Repair

Tiffany T. Pham, MD, MS[a], Andrew A. Winkler, MD[b],
Shekhar K. Gadkaree, MD[a],*

KEYWORDS

- Saddle nose deformity • Functional • Cosmetic • Dorsal augmentation
- Nasal reconstruction

KEY POINTS

- The saddle nose deformity can contribute to nasal obstruction by narrowing the nasal cavities, abnormally widening the internal and external nasal valves, and altering airflow dynamics, sinonasal drainage pathways, and olfaction.
- The saddle nose is associated with various cosmetic changes to the nose and disrupts facial esthetic harmony, which can contribute to psychological and emotional distress, decreased quality of life, and social stigma.
- The saddle nose is associated with specific challenges of decreased skin elasticity, scarring, lack of donor graft material, and challenges in esthetic integration.
- Treatments vary from minor cosmetic treatment with dorsal augmentation to severe cases requiring reconstruction of the nasal framework with flaps to fill soft tissue defects.
- Each patient case is unique and can be challenging to treat, requiring high skill and expertise.

INTRODUCTION

The saddle nose deformity represents collapse of the cartilaginous and/or bony nasal support structures resulting in dorsal height loss. The saddle nose derives its name from the scooped appearance of the dorsum on the lateral view, resembling a saddle (**Fig. 1**).[1] From the frontal view, the nasal dorsum appears broad. The saddle nose is associated with loss of tip support and definition, columellar retrusion, flattened nasal

[a] Department of Otolaryngology-Head and Neck Surgery, University of Miami Miller School of Medicine, 1120 Northwest 14th Street, Floor 5, Miami, FL 33136, USA; [b] Department of Otolaryngology-Head and Neck Surgery, University of Colorado School of Medicine, 12631 East 17th Avenue B205, Aurora, CO 80045, USA
* Corresponding author. Department of Otolaryngology-Head and Neck Surgery, University of Miami Miller School of Medicine, 1120 Northwest 14th Street, Floor 5, Miami, FL 33136.
E-mail address: sgadkaree@miami.edu

Otolaryngol Clin N Am 58 (2025) 325–341
https://doi.org/10.1016/j.otc.2024.07.016
0030-6665/25/© 2024 Elsevier Inc. All rights reserved, including those for text and data mining, AI training, and similar technologies.

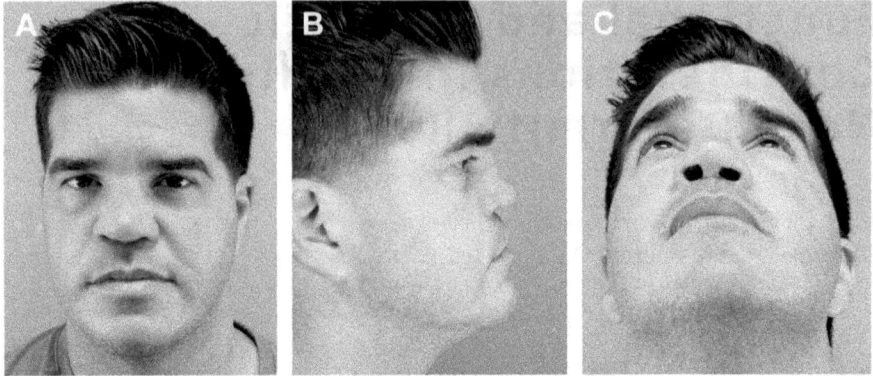

Fig. 1. Male patient with saddle nose deformity from significant nasal trauma. As seen in the (*A*) frontal, (*B*) lateral, and (*C*) base views, there is collapse of the midvault and nasal tip, with flattening of lobules.

lobules, a shortened vertical length, tip over rotation, and recessed maxilla (**Fig. 2**).[1,2] In 1887, John Orlando Rose performed the first rhinoplasty for a "pug nose" deformity. Since that time, there have been many advances in understanding the etiology, challenges, and treatments for the saddle nose deformity, which has been one of the most formidable nasal deformities due to the need to support the nasal structures to improve breathing and esthetics, albeit combating intrinsic challenges such as skin contracture. Herein we discuss functional and cosmetic considerations for saddle nose deformity repair.

DISCUSSION
Etiologies

There are multiple etiologies for the saddle nose, with the most predominant being acquired. Most acquired cases in literature are due to trauma or surgery.[3] Nasal trauma may result in mechanical disruption of the septum, and/or lead to hematoma formation and subsequent cartilage necrosis. Saddle nose from excessive surgical removal of cartilage, dorsal hump reduction, or disruption of surrounding septal attachments can present early on or delayed over months to years. Additionally, a saddle nose can result from a septal perforation, which can be iatrogenic, traumatic, due to either vasoconstriction agents (cocaine or oxymetazoline) or autoimmune disorders such as granulomatosis with polyangiitis (GPA), sarcoidosis, Crohn's disease, or relapsing polychondritis. Prior to the popularity of rhinoplasty, infectious causes were the most frequent cause, including septal abscesses, rarely syphilis, leprosy, leishmaniosis, and tuberculosis.[3–5] Congenital hypoplasia of the nose also contributes to the saddle nose and is seen in syndromes such as Down, Binder, and Williams syndromes.

Classification Systems

The complexity of the saddle nose is reflected in the numerous proposed classification systems. Despite these efforts, there is no consensus regarding the most suitable classification. Tardy and colleagues[6] have described a 3 "M" category classification system: minimal, moderate, and major. Vartanian and Thomas[7] categorized saddling into 4 categories based on the extent of anatomic deficit. Daniel and Brenner[1] introduced a more intricate classification system considering appearance, degree of septal support compromise, and appropriate surgical treatment (**Table 1, Fig. 3**). These

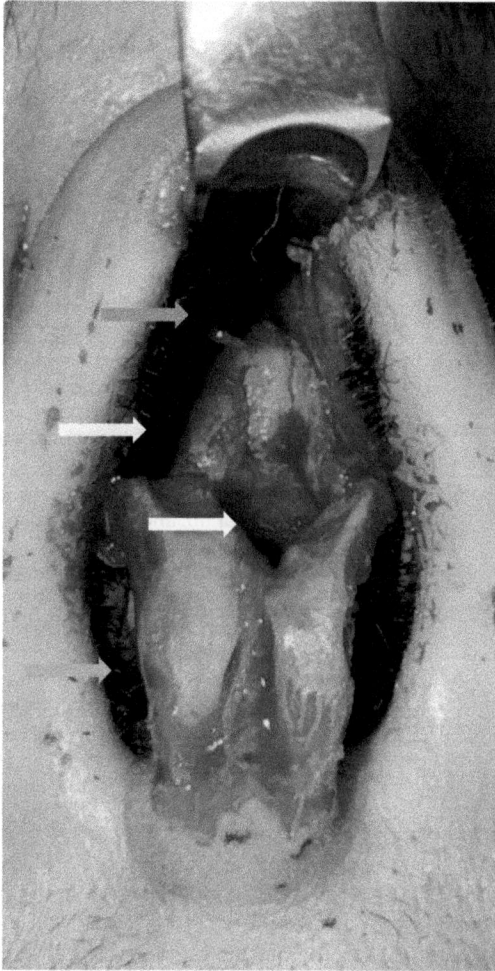

Fig. 2. Intraoperative view of saddle nose deformity. Depicted is a collapsed septum, leading to complete dorsal midvault collapse, and loss of upper lateral cartilage and tip support. Blue arrow: nasal bones, yellow arrow: collapsed upper lateral cartilages, white arrow: collapsed septum, green arrow: lower lateral cartilages.

classification systems can be useful to describe complexity of the saddling and guide treatment approach. However, each patient case and saddle presentation can be quite unique, requiring slightly different surgical plans.

Functional and Cosmetic Considerations

The saddle nose deformity can lead to various functional and cosmetic problems. The collapsed dorsum increases the nasofrontal angle and the nasal dorsum appears widened on frontal view. Nasal airway obstruction is a prominent feature due to septal deformities and decreased septal structural integrity, leading to midvault collapse and diminished nasal airways. Furthermore, the upper lateral cartilages can be weakened and collapsed without septal support. Loss of structural support for the upper lateral cartilages can lead to dynamic internal and external nasal valve narrowing.

Table 1
Summary of Daniel and Brenner classification of saddle nose deformity

Type	Description
Type 0: Pseudosaddle	• Dorsal depression of cartilaginous vault • Absolute depression owing to over resection of cartilaginous vault • A relative depression of the cartilaginous dorsum • Excellent septal support • A standard secondary rhinoplasty is performed
Type 1: Minor-cosmetic concealment	• Weakening of septal support • Excessive supratip depression and columellar retraction • Cosmetic concealment or structural correction is performed
Type 2: Moderate-cartilage vault restoration	• Compromise of septal support • Cartilaginous vault collapse, columellar retraction, and loss of tip support • Combination of extended vault grafts and a columellar strut are performed
Type 3: Major-composite reconstruction	• Total absence of septal support for the cartilaginous vault, columellar, nasal tip, and external valves • Flattening of nasal lobules • A composite reconstruction is performed to re-establish nasal support, followed by esthetic contour
Type 4: Severe-structural reconstruction	• End-stage septal collapse with cartilage vault depression and columellar shortening, compounded by bony vault disruption and severe contracture of nasal lining • Cantilevered dorsal graft with columellar strut is performed
Type 5: Catastrophic-nasal reconstruction	• Progression from reconstructive esthetic rhinoplasty to esthetic reconstruction of nose and adjacent tissue • Requires reconstruction of internal lining of nose or skin coverage, and extensive bone grafting or plating

A collapsed septum can lead to nasal tip deprojection and cephalic rotation. As there is decreased support for the lateral wall, the lobule flattens, "ballooning," or abnormally widening both the internal and external nasal valves, which contributes to turbulent airflow and nasal airway obstruction (**Fig. 4**).[8–10] The airflow is directed downward toward the inferior meatus instead of normal physiology, which directs airflow upward toward the middle meatus and olfactory area.[11] Additionally, midvault collapse may physically block the olfactory area, leading to a decreased sense of smell.

In cases of septal perforation, airflow can be turbulent and cause nasal dryness, crusting, and epistaxis, which further make breathing difficult. Moreover, these structural changes can alter the natural sinonasal drainage pathways, leading to recurrent sinus infections or chronic sinusitis. Inflammatory conditions like GPA and relapsing polychondritis often are associated with cartilage necrosis, septal perforation, sinusitis, and saddle nose.[12] In Holme and colleagues'[13] study of 116 patients with GPA, those with severe osteitis on computed tomography had more bony destruction, including saddle nose deformity.

Furthermore, subsequent columellar retraction and shortening can be seen in severe saddle cases, where the nasolabial angle becomes more acute and the alar columellar complex becomes distorted.[1] Columellar retraction can cause the caudal base to widen. The upper lip can appear elongated and alar hooding can be seen on lateral view. In severe cases, there can be premaxillary recession due to nasal spine and

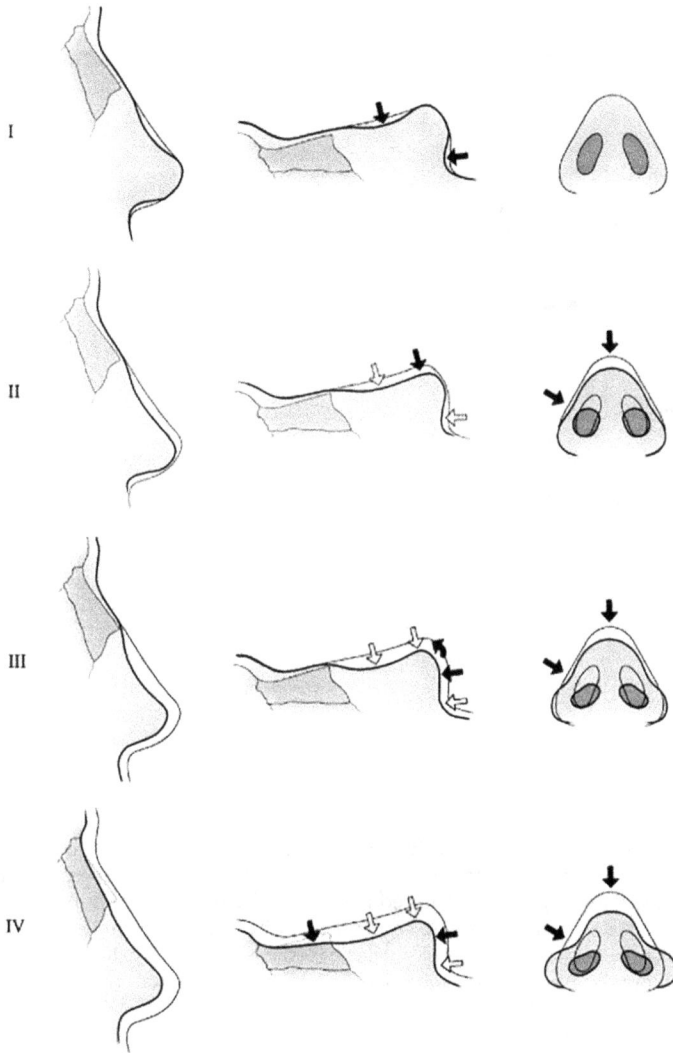

Fig. 3. Daniel and Brenner Classification for Saddle Nose Deformity. Type I has supratip depression and columellar retraction. Type II is more advanced with loss of tip projection and septal support. Type III has total loss of cartilage vault integrity and flattening of the nasal lobule. Type IV shows progression with involvement of the bony vault. (*From* Daniel RK, Brenner KA, Saddle Nose Deformity: A New Classification and Treatment, Facial Plastic Surgery Clinics of North America, 14/4, Pages 301-312, Copyright (2006), with permission.)

caudal septum retrusion. Prolonged skin retraction can complicate repair, both in immediate and long-term postoperative time frames.

Given the aforementioned cosmetic changes associated with the saddle nose, there can be significant alterations to patients' esthetics and facial harmony. Those with nasal deformities may have psychological distress and increased emotional role difficulty, leading to decreased quality of life.[14] Additionally, social stigma and altered perceptions from others can potentially impact social functioning. In their quantitative study, Van Schijndel and colleagues[15] found that observers had longer fixation times

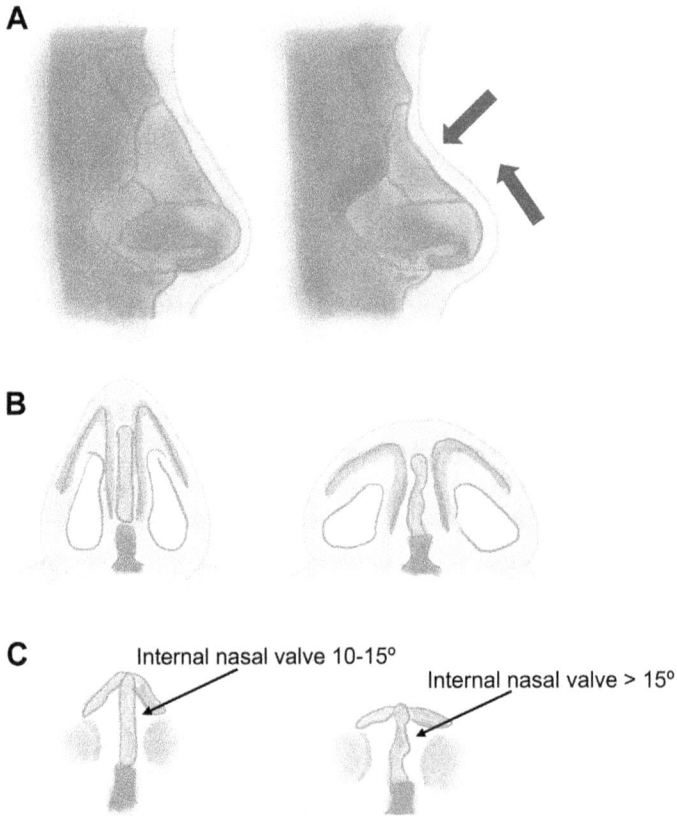

Fig. 4. Abnormal widening of the internal and external nasal valves in saddle nose deformity (*A*) Left: normal nasal anatomy, Right: Saddle nose deformity with collapsed midvault and deprotected and cephalically rotated nasal tip. (*B*) Left: normal nasal tip cross section, Right: Saddle nose deformity nasal tip cross section with septal deformities, deprojected tip, flatted lobules, widened alar and columellar bases, and widened external nasal valves. (*C*) Left: normal internal nasal valve, Right: Saddle nose deformity with widened internal nasal valve.

and more negative personality perceptions of those with nasal deformities. It has been shown that those with nasal deformity have higher social anxiety and avoidance.[14]

Special Challenges

The saddle nose deformity poses many distinctive challenges to surgeons.

Decreased skin elasticity and scarring

First and, perhaps, most importantly, the nasal skin can contract over time with decreased elasticity and tight adherence to underlying tissues.[16] The limited stretch of the skin envelope restricts how much the dorsum and tip can be built up and supported, as it hinders smooth draping of the nasal framework. Some surgeons may ask patients to try to massage or stretch the tissue preoperatively, though the benefit of this is unclear. Retraction of the skin and additionally the mucosa are very limiting in the amount of projection is attainable. These issues lead to surgeons using various local flap techniques to release the tissues, such as V-to-Y advancements of the columella and Z-plasties of the mucosal lining. Patients must be cautioned that excellent immediate postoperative results may be worsened long term by skin retraction.

Lack of autologous graft materials
The greater the saddle deformity, the less septal cartilage that is typically available for donor tissue, and the less adequate conchal cartilage becomes. For example, in a case of prior rhinoplasty wherein the upper lateral cartilages have disarticulated from the keystone, extended spreaders using auricular cartilage are sufficient. In severe retraction, costal cartilage provides adequate strength and volume for nasal reconstruction.

Challenges in esthetic integration
Achieving a "natural look" after reconstruction can be a significant challenge in severe saddle noses. The skin and soft tissue envelope must seamlessly incorporate with the new nasal framework, which can be challenging either if there is significant grafting, contracted skin, thin skin, dorsal irregularities or if there is not a skin texture and color match, particularly with the use of flaps.

Increased risk of complications
There is an increased risk of complications with saddle nose reconstruction, such as poor wound healing, infection, and necrosis, particularly around the nasal tip where skin tension is the greatest.[16,17] These patients are prone to thin skin with decreased vascularity, which can complicate healing. In Hyun and colleagues' study, 22% of patients with saddle nose deformity undergoing rhinoplasty had fair or poor outcomes, with a revision rate of 9%. Additionally, in patients with GPA undergoing rhinoplasty, the complication rate has been shown to be 20%, mostly attributed to infection and resorption of graft material with resorption rates ranging from 0% to 19%.[16,18] Furthermore, immunosuppression of these patients can contribute to poor wound healing.[16]

Addressing these great challenges requires careful planning and execution, demanding meticulous techniques to minimize skin tension and proper graft selection and shaping.

Surgical Treatment

Treatment of saddle nose deformity is aimed at restoring physical appearance and improving or maintaining nasal function. Treatment is highly individualized, depending on the severity of the saddle nose deformity and specific needs for breathing and esthetics. Herein, we review treatment approaches (**Fig. 5**). Multiple techniques can address both the cosmetic and functional concerns, while others address each individually.

Dorsal augmentation
Dorsal augmentation is a mainstay of cosmetic surgical correction of the mild or moderate saddle nose. This technique involves building up or camouflaging the depressed nasal dorsum. A variety of graft materials can be employed for dorsal onlay grafts. First, autologous grafts, including cartilage harvested from the septum, rib, or ear; bone grafts from the septum, turbinate, rib, iliac crest, or calvarium (split); or fascia from temporalis fascia or fascia lata.[19] Autologous materials are preferred due to their biocompatibility and lower risk of rejection. Septal cartilage can be utilized for mild-to-moderate saddle noses, whereas rib cartilage, with its strength, is reserved for severe cases where greater structural support is needed or where there is a lack of septum for grafting. Rib cartilage tends to warp, thus should be allowed time in warm sterile saline

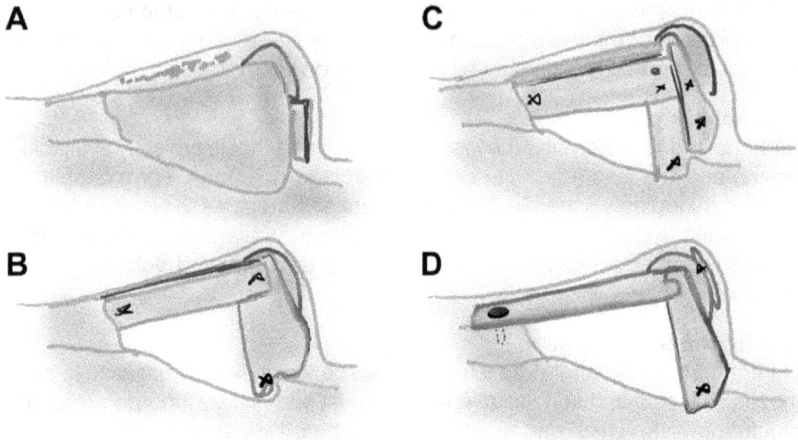

Fig. 5. Different surgical treatments for saddle nose deformity. (*A*) Diced cartilage for dorsal augmentation with cartilage for columellar augmentation. (*B*) L-strut reconstruction with caudal septal extension graft. (*C*) Composite reconstruction with L-strut reconstruction and columellar strut. Alloderm dorsal overlay is shown for dorsal augmentation. (*D*) Reconstruction of nasal framework with cantilever rib cartilage graft, screwed into the nasal bones. Shield graft is shown to project the nasal tip.

(mixed with antibiotic) for it to declare its shape.[20] If a full rib onlay graft is used, the senior author uses an osteocartilaginous rib segment, contoured to recreate the dorsum, with a small amount of bony overlap with remnant nasal bones or frontal bones to allow for osteointegration and securing the onlay graft with transcutaneous Kirschner wires (K-wires). Gadkaree and colleagues[19] also described the use of vomer onlay grafts, which lacks the risk of warping, provides increased structural support, and can allow for bone-to-bone healing.

Allografts can also be utilized as they can be easily available without donor site morbidity. Irradiated cadaveric costal cartilage can be useful; however, a higher rate of resorption and infection is thought to occur, although controversial.[21,22] AlloDerm (Allergan Aesthetics, Birmingham, AL), an acellular human dermal matrix, has also been widely used as a dorsal onlay graft to augment the nasal dorsum, over a stable framework.[23]

Alloplastic grafts, such as silicone, Gore-Tex, and porous high-density polyethylene (MEDPOR, Stryker, Kalamazoo, MI), are synthetic options that can be utilized as a dorsal onlay graft. These materials are relatively easy to shape and insert. However, they have increased risks of infection, migration, and extrusion,[24] and for these reasons, they are almost never used by the senior author. More commonly, cases of saddle nose after removing infected implants or implants that have fistulized through skin have been encountered. Silicone implants remain widely used in dorsal augmentation, especially in Asia. They do not integrate with the adjacent tissue but instead a fibrous capsule surrounds these implants, and they, therefore, are prone to shifting and buckling.[3] Being aware of these materials is important, as one should obtain imaging if an implant is suspected to evaluate the potential defect after removal, and timing of removal of implant, and immediate versus delayed reconstruction must be undertaken.

Diced cartilage can be utilized to fill in small dorsal depressions and smooth dorsal irregularities. Diced cartilage can also be wrapped in temporalis fascia, AlloDerm, or

Surgicel (a resorbable oxidized cellulose mesh; Johnson & Johnson, New Brunswick, NJ).[25] These grafts can be molded intraoperatively to camouflage dorsal irregularities, and subsequently reshaped and molded postoperatively if needed.

Lastly, in a preservation "push up" technique, Toriumi and colleagues[26] has described the subdorsal cantilever graft, which can raise the nasal dorsum by releasing the midvault and caudal nasal bones from the septum (high strip) and can be elevated to accommodate increases in nasal tip projection. He also describes a variation of the subdorsal cantilever graft that can raise the radix with the graft extending through a radix osteotomy site.

Midvault reconstruction

To better address functional aspects, particularly nasal obstruction, spreader grafts or extended spreader grafts can be employed to treat internal nasal valve insufficiency or support the dorsal strut.[27] These can be useful for cases of previous surgery, where the midvault was not adequately supported or may have collapsed. Spreader grafts, however, are limited in their ability to adequately support the lower lateral nasal wall. Grafts to better support the lateral nasal wall include either alar batten grafts or lateral crural strut grafts.[20,28] Furthermore, a butterfly graft can greatly improve the internal nasal valve, and an extended butterfly graft allows correction of both midvault collapse and a deficient bony pyramid.[29]

Reconstruction of the nasal framework

In cases of saddle nose deformity with compromised septal support, extensive reconstruction of the nasal framework is required. Techniques include L-strut reconstruction, columellar strut, or major reconstruction with cantilevered cartilage or bone grafts.

L-strut reconstruction involves shaping a stable "L"-shaped dorsal and caudal strut, providing robust structural septal support. The L-strut graft can be made with 2 extended spreader grafts and a columellar strut. The caudal end of the strut is placed between the medial crura of the lower lateral cartilages and secured to the anterior nasal spine, while the cephalic ends of the extended spreader grafts are attached on both sides to the existing dorsal septum. Where a dorsal onlay costal cartilage graft is used for severe saddle, this itself can articulate with an extended spreader graft to help support and recreate the L-strut. Moreover, cartilage vault restoration can be used to re-establish the dorsal height and tip projection. In this case, the restored cartilage vault profile must be significantly higher than the saddled septum.[1] Additionally, caudal septal extension grafts have been useful in supporting the caudal strut and enhancing tip projection and support.[17]

In cases of end-stage saddle nose deformity with severe septal collapse, often associated with bony vault disruption, drastic contracture of nasal lining, columellar retraction and shortening, nasal tip deprojection and cephalic rotation, and broad nostril; major reconstruction is required. Major reconstruction may involve the use of cantilevered cartilage (**Fig. 6**) harvested from the rib or bone grafts to reconstruct the nasal framework and restore both form and function. These grafts can be secured to the nasal bones using sutures, K-wires, or surgical screws, or they may be left to naturally adhere to the underlying nasal bones in certain cases. Some surgeons, including the senior surgeon, prefer osteocartilaginous costal cartilage with dorsal graft fixed with percutaneous K-wires proximally and sutures distally.[10] The caudal strut is inserted between the crura down to the premaxilla, and secured bilaterally to the nasal spine with suture through a drill hole. An osteotome may be needed to create a slit in the

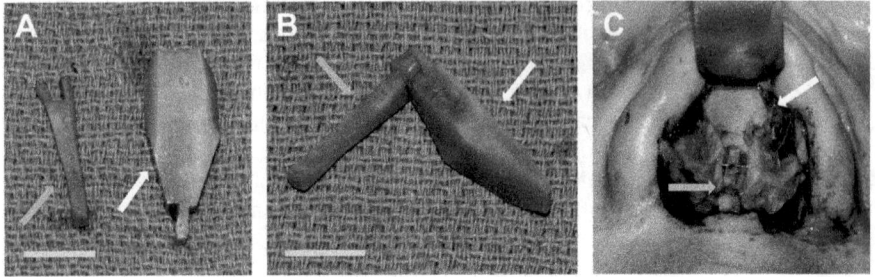

Fig. 6. Cantilever graft. (*A*) Dorsal and caudal components of the cantilever graft unassembled. (*B*) Dorsal and caudal components of the cantilever graft fixed in a tongue and groove fashion. (*C*) Cantilever graft inset in vivo and secured through the lower lateral cartilages. White arrow points to dorsal strut. Green arrow points to caudal strut. Yellow bar represents 1 cm.

bone for the caudal graft to sit in, as periosteum around the nasal spine is often stripped away due to previous surgery or the disease causing the saddle nose deformity.

For type V catastrophic saddle nose deformity, the bony deformity extends further into the skull and thus can be quite challenging to treat. These cases require a degloving approach and extensive bone grafting or plating.

Nasal tip augmentation

Nasal tip augmentation often accompanies the cosmetic correction of the saddle nose deformity to refine the nasal tip's shape and improve projection and decrease rotation. Interdomal and transdomal sutures, tip grafts, such as cap or shield grafts, can augment the nasal tip. A columellar strut can provide support for the medial crura to support the nasal tip. Furthermore, the caudal septal extension graft can provide further tip projection and support. Often, external valve collapse due to retraction is severe. Laterally, batten grafts can reconstruct the support structure of the nasal tripod, and these grafts can extend and help support the tip. A columellar V-Y flap extending the full length of the columella and onto the upper lip may allow for improved tip projection, while a Z-plasty can help free the mucosa.

Columellar augmentation

A columellar strut in between the medial crura can correct retraction. Additionally, premaxillary or additional columellar plumping cartilage grafts can be placed anterior to the columellar strut.[10]

Alar rim augmentation

While batten grafts may be required to fully reconstruct the flattened lateral ala and replace deficient cartilage, alar rim support grafts can be used to treat both the external valve collapse and esthetic contour of the alar rim. Articulated rim grafts have provided excellent correction of alar rim deformities.[30,31] Other options that may be required include conchal cartilage grafts.

Reconstruction of nasal soft tissue

For cases with severe loss of nasal support, lining, and skin coverage seen in type V deformity, reconstructive options include the use of either rotational forehead flaps or microvascular free flaps to restore both the shape and function of the nose (**Fig. 7**).[3]

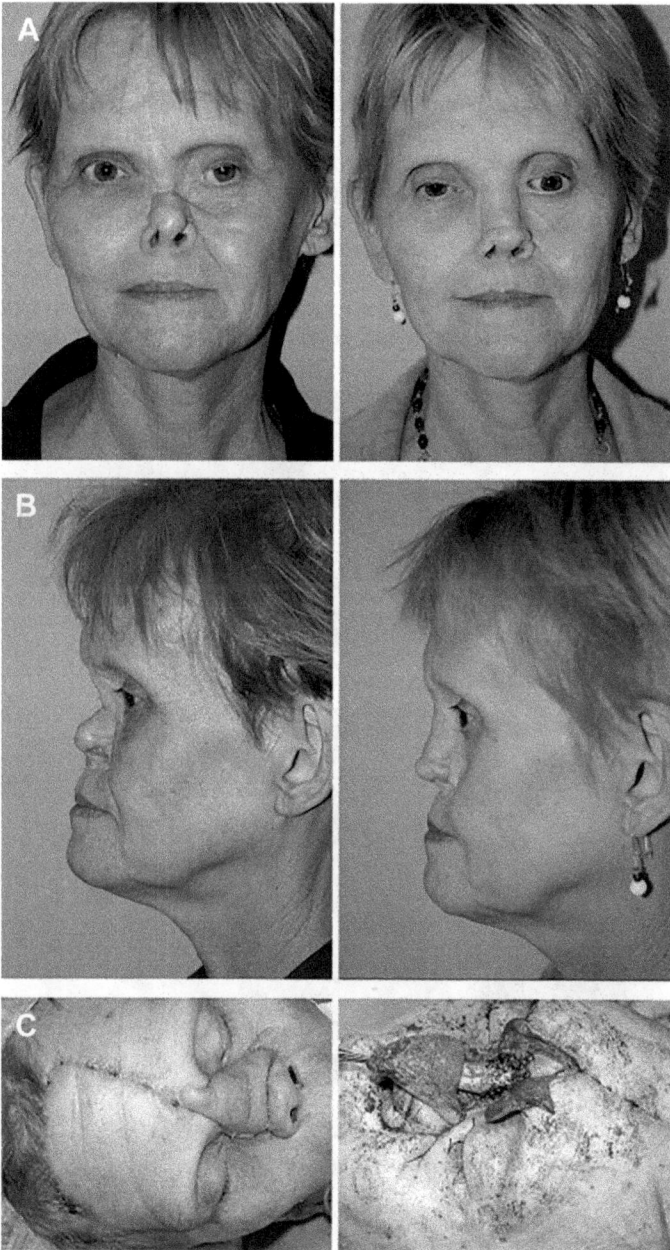

Fig. 7. Reconstruction of type V deformity. (*A*) Preoperative and postoperative frontal views of type V deformity repaired in 2 stages. (*B*) Preoperative and postoperative lateral views. (*C*) First-stage forehead flap to re-establish nasal lining and skin coverage, followed by can-tilevered rib cartilage graft. (*From* Pribitkin EA, Ezzat WH. Classification and Treatment of the Saddle Nose Deformity, The Otolaryngologic Clinics of North America, 42/3, Pages 437-461, Copyright (2009), with permission.

Composite reconstruction

Effective treatment of saddle nose deformity often necessitates a combination of multiple techniques, particularly in severe cases of saddle nose where it is accompanied by a combination of esthetic and functional changes to the nose. In major cases with total absence of septal support for the dorsum, columella, nasal tip, internal and external valves, a composite reconstruction is preferred. In composite reconstruction, the structural support is re-established first and then the desired esthetic contouring is performed.[10,17] In traditional rhinoplasty, nasal tip projection, shape, and rotation are mainly controlled by septal extension grafts or columellar structure. They are part of the load-bearing nasal framework and contribute to most of the tension on the closure. With the composite reconstruction, the contour of the nasal tip and dorsum are controlled mainly by the esthetic layer above the principal load-bearing framework,

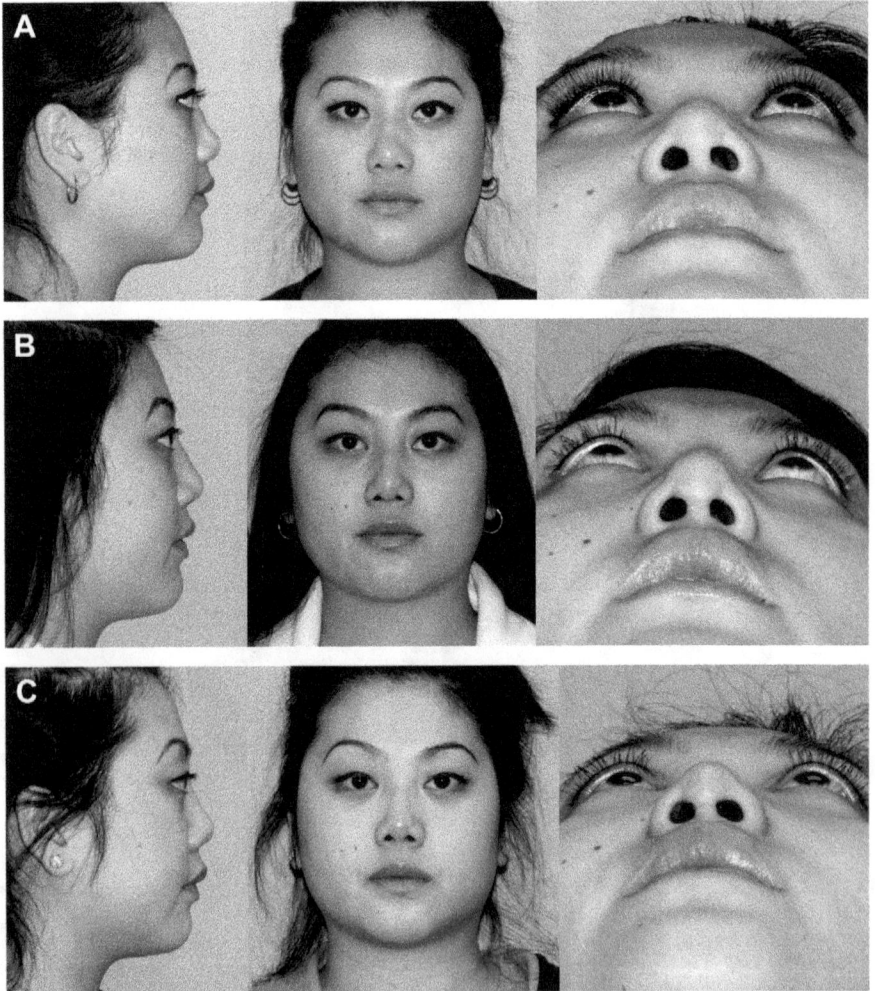

Fig. 8. Case 1. (*A*) Preoperative lateral, frontal, and base views of patient with a saddle nose deformity from a septal perforation. (*B*) One month postoperative views after dorsal augmentation with first, 2 auricular cartilage dorsal onlay grafts followed by a 2 layer temporoparietal fascia/temporalis fascia onlay graft. (*C*) Four months postoperative views.

thus sharing the force on the esthetic layer and potentially minimizing distortion of the esthetic layer.[17]

Nonsurgical Treatment

Injections

For cases of mild saddle nose or for patients that are not good surgical candidates, injection of hyaluronic acid, calcium hydroxyapatite, or adipose-derived products has been a recent innovation to treat cosmetic concerns.[32,33] Ossanna and colleagues[34] describe immediate high patient satisfaction after injection of hyaluronic acid, fat, Dermgraft, and Nanograft, but decreasing satisfaction rate over time. In

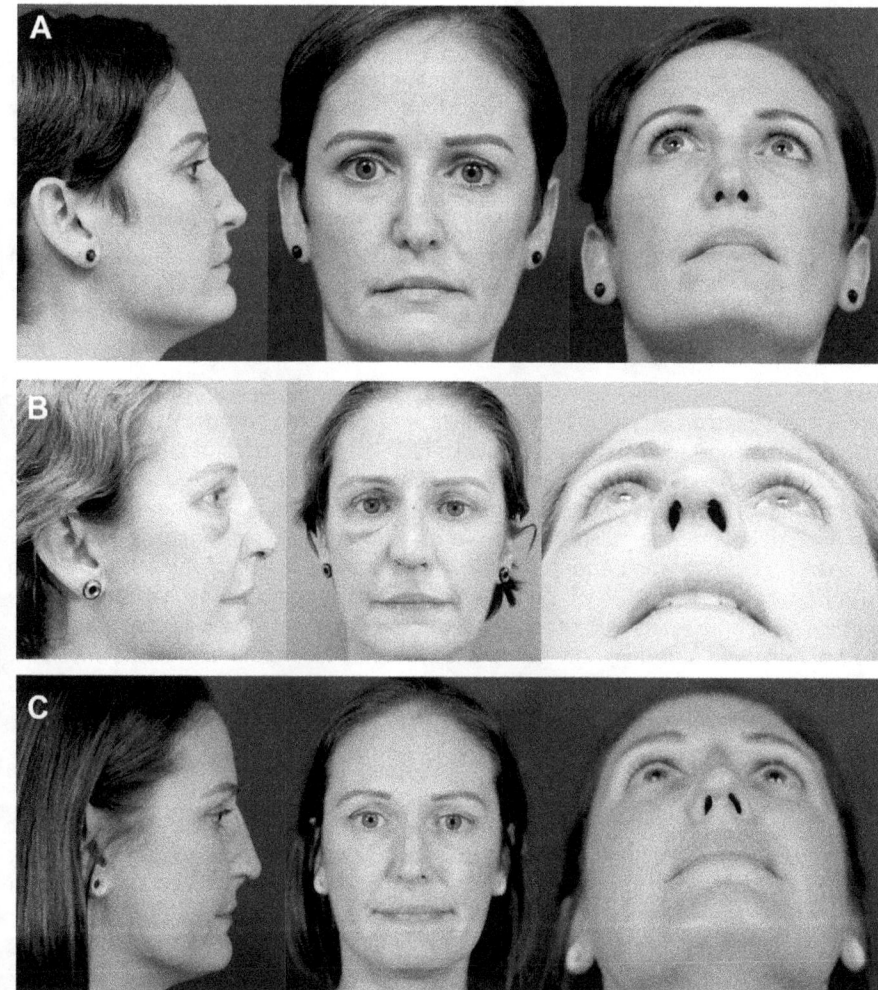

Fig. 9. Case 2. (*A*) Preoperative lateral, frontal, and base views of patient with a saddle nose deformity from a septal perforation. (*B*) Two weeks postoperative views after total reconstruction of the L-strut, dorsal onlay graft, caudal septal extension graft, bilateral articulated alar rim grafts, and a cap graft, using autologous rib cartilage. (*C*) Three months postoperative views.

patients with tight skin envelopes, injecting in the correct plane can be challenging with increased risks of incorrect placement, vascular injury, or injection under high pressure, thus treatment should be avoided or counseling of increased risks should be performed. Although data are limited, it is suggested that patients with GPA can undergo temporizing filler injections during active disease states until they can safely undergo rhinoplasty during remission.[35]

Prosthetics
For cases of severe saddle nose deformity, a nasal prosthesis can be used to achieve excellent cosmetic camouflage.

Case Presentations

Case 1
This is a 20 year old Asian female patient with chronic rhinosinusitis, prior sinus surgery, GPA in remission and maintained on chronic prednisone, who presented with a saddle nose deformity. She denied difficulty breathing. Preoperatively, the nasal dorsum was relatively straight with a collapsed midvault and an inverted V deformity (**Fig. 8**A). Her septum was straight but with diffuse granular change. An open septorhinoplasty with bilateral interior turbinate outfracture was performed. For dorsal augmentation, 2 auricular cartilage dorsal onlay grafts were placed first on the dorsum, followed by a 2 layer temporoparietal fascia/temporalis fascia onlay graft. She is depicted at 1 (**Fig. 8**B) and 4 months (**Fig. 8**C) postoperatively. She had an excellent correction of saddling however with intranasal crusting. At 4 months, she had a flare up of her GPA, and there was a small visible and palpable nodule on the right aspect of the rhinion, likely cartilage but could represent a granuloma.

Case 2
This is a 39 year old Caucasian female patient who presented with complaints of saddle nose deformity and total septal perforation secondary to a history of chronic drug use, now 5 years sober at the time of preoperative evaluation (**Fig. 9**A, B). Her examination demonstrated total septal perforation, loss of turbinates, collapse of the midvault, and a C-shaped deviation of her nasal dorsum. The columella was intact with nasal tip clefting. An open rhinoplasty was performed using autologous rib cartilage for grafting. Grafts included total reconstruction of the L-strut, dorsal onlay graft, caudal septal extension graft, bilateral articulated alar rim grafts, and a cap graft. At 2 weeks postoperatively, she had improved saddling; however, given the contraction of her soft tissue envelope, she developed some deprojection of her nasal tip. **Fig. 9**C depicts her 3 months postoperatively.

SUMMARY

The saddle nose deformity describes midvault collapse and is associated with other cosmetic changes, including nasal tip deprojection and rotation, columellar retraction, and flattening of the nasal lobules. Nasal obstruction is a prominent functional concern for patients with saddle nose deformity. Furthermore, the esthetic features of the saddle nose can be associated with psychological distress and social anxiety. Treating saddle nose deformity requires a comprehensive approach that considers the severity of the deformity, the functional and cosmetic concerns, and the unique challenges of the saddle nose, in particular skin contracture. Surgical options range from minor dorsal augmentations to major reconstructions with composite rib cartilage or bony reconstruction of the nasal framework, followed by esthetic contouring. In the most complex cases, bone grafting and plating, and forehead flaps or free flaps may be required to fill or correct soft tissue deficits. Given the complexity of the saddle nose, a thorough understanding and skilled execution of techniques are essential for achieving optimal functional and cosmetic outcomes in patients with saddle nose deformity.

CLINICS CARE POINTS

- The saddle nose deformity contributes to nasal obstruction via ballooning of the valves eliciting abnormal airflow dynamics and dynamic nasal valve narrowing.
- The saddle nose deformity elicits cosmetic changes, which can contribute to social and emotional distress.
- The saddle nose deformity can be challenging to treat given its decreased skin elasticity, contracture, and scarring.
- Expertise is needed to treat the saddle nose, given its complexity.

DISCLOSURE

The authors have nothing to disclose.

REFERENCES

1. Daniel RK, Brenner KA. Saddle nose deformity: a new classification and treatment. Facial Plast Surg Clin North Am 2006;14(4).
2. Gerow FJ, Stal S, Spira M. The totem pole rib graft reconstruction of the nose. Ann Plast Surg 1983;11(4):273–81.
3. Pribitkin EA, Ezzat WH. Classification and treatment of the saddle nose deformity. Otolaryngol Clin North Am 2009;42(3):437–61.
4. Durand ML. In: Durand ML, Deschler DG, editors. Nasal infections. Cham, Switzerland: Springer International Publishing AG; 2018. https://doi.org/10.1007/978-3-319-74835-1_9.
5. Andrade M, Santos Fernandes V, Boléo-Tomé JP. Saddle nose: Our approach to the problem. Aesthetic Plast Surg 1999;23(6):403–6.
6. Tardy ME, Schwartz M, Parras G. Saddle nose deformity: autogenous graft repair. Facial Plast Surg 1989;6.
7. Vartanian AJ, Thomas JR. Saddle-nose rhinoplasty. Medscape 2022. Available at: https://emedicine.medscape.com/article/840910-overview#a9. [Accessed 2 June 2024].
8. Pirsig W. Physiology of the nasal cartilages and their importance to rhinosurgery. In: Önerci TM, editor. Nasal physiology and pathophysiology of nasal disorders. Berlin, Heidelberg: Springer Berlin Heidelberg; 2013. p. 475–503.
9. Bloching MB. Disorders of the nasal valve area. GMS Curr Top Otorhinolaryngol, Head Neck Surg 2007;6. Available at: http://www.ncbi.nlm.nih.gov/pubmed/22073083%0Ahttp://www.pubmedcentral.nih.gov/articlerender.fcgi?artid=PMC3199841.
10. Daniel RK. Rhinoplasty: Septal saddle nose deformity and composite reconstruction. Plast Reconstr Surg 2007;119(3):1029–43.
11. Meyer R, Berset J-C, Emeri J-F, et al. Residual deformities of the dorsum. In: Secondary rhinoplasty: including reconstruction of the nose. Berlin, Heidelberg: Springer Berlin Heidelberg; 2002. p. 165–87. https://doi.org/10.1007/978-3-642-56267-9_19.

12. Hanci D, Uyar Y, El-Saggan A. Rheumatological diseases of the nose and paranasal sinuses. In: Cingi C, Bayar Muluk N, editors. All around the nose: basic science, diseases and surgical management. Cham: Springer International Publishing; 2020. p. 431–40.

13. Holme SS, Kilian K, Eggesbø HB, et al. Impact of baseline clinical and radiological features on outcome of chronic rhinosinusitis in granulomatosis with polyangiitis. Arthritis Res Ther 2021;23(1):1–11.

14. Kucur C, Kuduban O, Ozturk A, et al. Psychological evaluation of patients seeking rhinoplasty. Eurasian J Med 2016;48(2):102–6.

15. van Schijndel O, Tasman A-J, Litschel R. The nose influences visual and personality perception. Facial Plast Surg 2015;31(5).

16. Unadkat SN, Pendolino AL, Kwame I, et al. Nasal reconstructive surgery for vasculitis affecting the nose: our two-centre international experience. Eur Arch Oto-Rhino-Laryngology. 2020;277(11):3059–66.

17. Song Z, Xu Y, Zhang X, et al. Application of a modified costal cartilaginous framework in Correction of Severe Saddle Nose Deformity. Aesthetic Surg J 2023;43(8):830–9.

18. Ezzat WH, Compton RA, Basa KC, et al. Reconstructive techniques for the saddle nose deformity in granulomatosis with polyangiitis: A systematic review. JAMA Otolaryngol - Head Neck Surg. 2017;143(5):507–12.

19. Gadkaree SK, Weitzman RE, Fuller JC, et al. Review of literature of saddle nose deformity reconstruction and presentation of vomer onlay graft. Laryngoscope Investig Otolaryngol. 2020;5(6):1039–43.

20. Kirgezen T, Yigit O, Bertossi D. Reconstruction of the Saddle Nose Deformity. In: Cingi C, Bayar Muluk N, editors. All Around the Nose: Basic Science, Diseases and Surgical Management. Cham, Switzerland: Springer Nature Switzerland AG; 2020. p. 879–88.

21. Pfaff MJ, Bertrand AA, Lipman KJ, et al. Cadaveric costal cartilage grafts in rhinoplasty and septorhinoplasty: a systematic review and meta-analysis of patient-reported functional outcomes and complications. J Craniofac Surg 2021;32(6):1990–3.

22. Wee JH, Mun SJ, Na WS, et al. Autologous vs irradiated homologous costal cartilage as graft material in rhinoplasty. JAMA Facial Plast Surg 2017;19(3):183–8.

23. Gryskiewicz J. Dorsal augmentation with alloDerm. Semin Plast Surg 2008;22(2):090–103.

24. Ferril GR, Wudel JM, Winkler AA. Management of complications from alloplastic implants in rhinoplasty. Curr Opin Otolaryngol Head Neck Surg 2013;21(4):372–8.

25. Onur Ö. Techniques in cosmetic surgery the turkish delight: a pliable graft for rhinoplasty. Plast Reconstr Surg 2000;105(6):2229–41.

26. Toriumi DM. Subdorsal cantilever graft for elevating the dorsum in ethnic rhinoplasty. Facial Plast Surg \& Aesthetic Med. 2022;24(3):143–59.

27. Teymoortash A, Fasunla JA, Sazgar AA. The value of spreader grafts in rhinoplasty: A critical review. Eur Arch Oto-Rhino-Laryngology 2012;269(5):1411–6.

28. Ballert Stephen SJAP. Functional rhinoplasty: treatment of the dysfunctional nasal sidewall. Facial Plast Surg 2006;22(01):49–54.

29. Vega-Cordova X, Brenner MJ, Putman HC. Extended butterfly graft for functional and cosmetic correction of saddle nose deformity. JAMA Facial Plast Surg 2019;21(6):568–9.

30. Ballin AC, Kim H, Chance E, et al. The articulated alar rim graft: reengineering the conventional alar rim graft for improved contour and support. Facial Plast Surg 2016;32(4):384–97.

31. Lyrio T, Maricevich P, Andrade AA, et al. New concept for articulated alar rim graft positioning. Plast Reconstr surgery Glob open 2024;12(3):e5686.
32. Bertossi D, Lanaro L, Dell'Acqua I, et al. Injectable profiloplasty: Forehead, nose, lips, and chin filler treatment. J Cosmet Dermatol 2019;18(4):976–84.
33. Yu AY. Nose tip elongation and elevation: a novel filler injection technique. Aesthetic Surg J 2022;42(6):660–76.
34. Ossanna R, Ghazanfar Tehrani S, Dallatana A, et al. Innovative non-surgical plastic technique for saddle nose correction: a study on 97 patients. J Clin Med 2024;13(8).
35. Thomas WW, Bucky L, Friedman O. Injectables in the nose: facts and controversies. Facial Plast Surg Clin North Am 2016;24(3):379–89.

Repairing the Nasal Valve in Revision Surgery

Aniruddha C. Parikh, MD[a], Jessyka G. Lighthall, MD[a,b],*

KEYWORDS

- Nasal obstruction • Internal nasal valve • External nasal valve
- Lateral wall insufficiency • Revision rhinoplasty

KEY POINTS

- In patients undergoing revision nasal airway surgery, meticulous preoperative evaluation must be performed to identify specific causes of persistent nasal airway obstruction, which may have been inadequately treated during initial surgery.
- External nasal valve compromise may be due to caudal septum deviation, tip ptosis, over-projection of the nasal tip, tension nose deformity, malpositioned or misshapen lateral crura, or a widened columella, and systematically addressing these abnormalities will help alleviate nasal obstruction.
- Internal nasal valve compromise can be repaired by a variety of techniques such as spreader grafts, spreader flaps, flaring sutures, and the butterfly graft.

INTRODUCTION

Nasal airway obstruction is a frequent complaint in an otolaryngology clinic and is often multifactorial. Anatomic contributors may include a nasal septal deviation, inferior turbinate hypertrophy, and nasal valve compromise (NVC). Septoplasty and inferior turbinate reduction are one of the most common procedures performed by an otolaryngologist. Unfortunately, 25% of patients are dissatisfied with their nasal breathing after this surgery.[1] In many of these patients, persistent NVC may be the etiology of their ongoing nasal airway obstruction. Sixty-seven percent of patients undergoing primary evaluation for nasal airway obstruction and 82% of patients undergoing evaluation for revision surgery have been found to have clinically significant NVC.[2] This suggests that

[a] Department of Otolaryngology-Head and Neck Surgery, Penn State Health Milton S. Hershey Medical Center, Hershey, PA, USA; [b] Division of Facial Plastic and Reconstructive Surgery, Department of Otolaryngology-Head & Neck Surgery, Penn State College of Medicine, Facial Nerve Clinic, Esteem Penn State Health Cosmetic Associates, 500 University Drive H-091, Hershey, PA
* Corresponding author. Division of Facial Plastic and Reconstructive Surgery, Facial Nerve Clinic, Esteem Penn State Health Cosmetic Associates, Department of Otolaryngology-Head & Neck Surgery, Penn State College of Medicine, 500 University Drive H-091, Hershey, PA
E-mail address: jlighthall@pennstatehealth.psu.edu

Otolaryngol Clin N Am 58 (2025) 343–359
https://doi.org/10.1016/j.otc.2024.07.009
oto.theclinics.com

NVC is often not appropriately diagnosed during initial evaluation and highlights the importance of careful preoperative evaluation for patients undergoing primary and revision nasal airway surgery to ensure optimal outcomes. If persistent NVC is identified, treating it should be one of the main focuses during revision rhinoplasty.

Persistent nasal airway obstruction may also be secondary to initial surgery. In patients with history of a septoplasty, it is possible that the septum was overresected, leading to tip ptosis or a saddle nose deformity. The keystone region may have been disrupted during initial surgery and not reconstructed, which may lead to an inverted V deformity and static vestibular stenosis. Additionally, traditional reductive rhinoplasty techniques where the nasal cartilages are weakened or resected are common causes of nasal obstruction after rhinoplasty.[3] These can occur immediately after initial surgery or years later as the aging process leads to cartilage weakening and soft tissue laxity of the lateral nasal wall and subsequent NVC.

While not frequently discussed, the nasal musculature plays a role in either widening or narrowing the nasal airway. Chronic hypertonicity of the nasal constrictors can lead to persistent nasal obstruction, which can be improved with chemodenervation treatment or biofeedback via surface electromyography.[4,5] Nasal obstruction could be related to persistent inflammatory/reactive disease, such as allergic rhinitis, nonallergic rhinitis, chronic rhinosinusitis, or a sinonasal or nasopharyngeal mass. These diagnoses can be ruled out through a thorough history, physical examination with rigid nasal endoscopy, and potentially a computed tomography (CT) scan of the sinuses. In patients who have had aggressive surgical treatment, the diagnosis of empty nose syndrome should be considered. This can be a challenging disorder to treat and surgical therapy should be avoided in most cases as it will not improve patient symptoms.

ANATOMY AND NASAL VALVE PHYSIOLOGY

When discussing nasal valve surgery, it is critical to differentiate between the external nasal valve (ENV) and internal nasal valve (INV). The ENV is the area bounded by the alar rim anterolaterally; the columella, medial crura, and septum medially; and the nasal sill inferiorly (**Fig. 1**). The anatomy of the ENV is closely related to the size, shape,

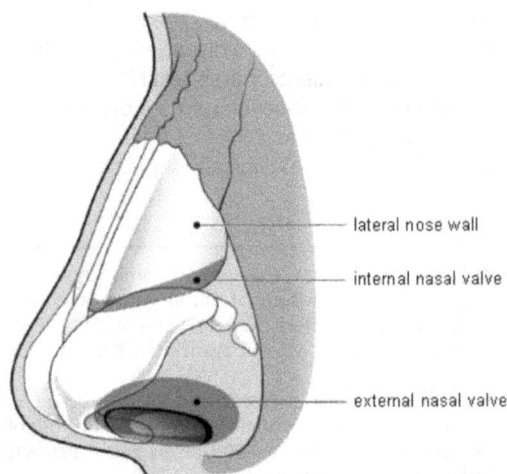

lateral nose wall

internal nasal valve

external nasal valve

Fig. 1. Anatomy of the internal and external nasal valves. (*Reproduced from* Bloching MB. Disorders of the nasal valve area. GMS Curr Top Otorhinolaryngol Head Neck Surg. 2007;6:Doc07.)

orientation, and strength of the lateral crura and the position of the caudal septum.[6] Any significant abnormalities of these structures may lead to external NVC (ENVC), which should be addressed to improve nasal breathing.

The INV is the area formed by the dorsal septum, the caudal edge of the upper lateral cartilage, the head of the inferior turbinate, and the nasal floor (see **Fig. 1**). In the Caucasian nose, the angle between the upper lateral cartilage and nasal septum is typically 10° to 15°.[7] The INV accounts for one-half to two-thirds of total airway resistance, and thus, small changes in the patency of this angle lead to very large changes in nasal airway function.[8,9] Thus, the INV is a critical area to address during primary and revision surgery to ensure patients have optimal functional outcomes.

The physiology of the nasal valve is related to Poiseuille's law and Bernoulli's principle.[10] Poiseuille's law pertains to static compromise and states that flow through a tube is inversely proportional to the radius of the tube to the fourth power, meaning that very slight changes in the patency of the nasal valve can have dramatic effects on the nasal airflow. In contrast, Bernoulli's principle relates to dynamic NVC and states that as the velocity of a fluid increases through a tube, the pressure within that tube decreases.[11] Thus, intraluminal pressure within the nasal cavity will decrease during inspiration, and if this pressure gradient can overcome the strength and resiliency of the lateral nasal wall, then it will collapse on inspiration and lead to nasal obstruction.[10]

PREOPERATIVE EVALUATION

When evaluating a patient with persistent nasal obstruction after previous nasal airway surgery, it is critical to obtain a detailed history and physical examination. Details regarding the onset of symptoms, prior history of trauma, fluctuation of symptoms, previous surgical history, and the use of nasal sprays or oral allergy medications should be obtained. A comprehensive nasal analysis should be performed with special attention paid to the caudal septum and nasal valves, which when unaddressed at initial surgery, may cause persistent nasal obstruction. It should be noted if there is lateral nasal wall collapse when the patient breathes normally and upon more forceful inhalation. The lateral nasal walls should be palpated to determine if there is an underlying structural deficiency. The location of the tip should be noted and if the tip is severely ptotic, it can be gently raised to a position that is achievable through surgery to note if there is an improvement in nasal obstruction. On the base view, the shape of the nostrils, the location of the caudal septum, the width of the columella, and the presence of dynamic collapse should be observed.

Next, a speculum should be inserted into the vestibule and gently opened in order to evaluate the patency of the INV. Care should be taken to not advance the speculum too far and obstruct or artificially widen the INV and potentially miss internal NVC (INVC). Finally, the speculum can be advanced fully to evaluate the nasal septum and inferior turbinate. The amount of residual native cartilage remaining should be determined by palpating the septum with a cotton-tipped applicator to identify if cartilage will need to be harvested from other sites.

A Cottle maneuver, where the cheeks are distracted laterally, can improve nasal obstruction symptoms. However, it typically leads to an over improvement that is not achievable surgically and is classically not considered a reliable method to evaluate the nasal valve. However, one should perform a modified Cottle maneuver, where the back end of a cotton-tipped applicator or a small ear curette is placed within the nasal airway along the INV or ENV to support or slightly widen the nasal valve (**Fig. 2A–C**). If the patient's nasal airway obstruction improves, this may indicate NVC that can be

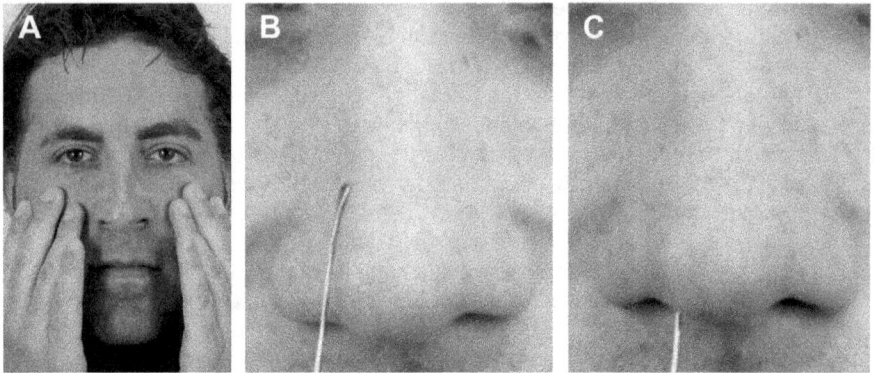

Fig. 2. (*A*) The Cottle maneuver involves laterally distracting the cheeks, which improves nasal valve compromise. This typically leads to an overcorrection and is not a reliable method to evaluate the nasal valve. (*B, C*) The modified Cottle maneuver involves supporting the nasal sidewall and can be an effective method to evaluate for nasal valve compromise. (*Reproduced from* plasticsurgerykey.com with permission.)

improved through surgery. Care must be taken to increase the width of the nasal valve only slightly to what is surgically feasible, as maximal widening will improve nasal air flow in nearly all patients and may not be reproducible in surgery. Finally, a rigid nasal endoscopy may be considered to evaluate the middle meatus, sphenoethmoidal recess, and nasopharynx to rule out other causes of nasal obstruction including chronic rhinosinusitis, concha bullosa, or sinonasal and nasopharyngeal masses. If there is concern for these pathologies, a CT scan of the sinuses should be obtained.

SURGICAL MANAGEMENT
External Nasal Valve

NVC related to the ENV can contribute significantly to nasal airway obstruction and repairing the ENV has the capacity to double nasal airflow compared to preoperative values.[12] ENVC can have a variety of etiologies such as caudal septal deviation, tip ptosis, overprojection of the nasal tip, tension nose deformity, malpositioned or misshapen lateral crura, or a widened columella. Many of these deformities may not have been addressed during primary nasal airway surgery, especially if only a septoplasty was performed initially. These pathologies have varying treatments, and it is important to determine the exact cause of a patient's ENVC in order to select appropriate surgical techniques.

A caudal septal deviation is a common cause of persistent nasal obstruction after primary nasal airway surgery. There are a variety of techniques to address the caudal septum, and these should be tailored to the individual patient. Frequently, the septum may have excess length in the anterior-posterior dimension leading to a deviation of the septum as it inserts onto the maxillary crest. This can typically be treated with a swinging door technique where the excessively long portion of the septum along the maxillary crest is removed so that the septum can be repositioned to the midline and secured to the anterior nasal spine (**Fig. 3**).[13] The septum can also have excess length in the cranio-caudal dimension leading to a deviation of the caudal septum. In these cases, a small amount of caudal septum can be resected to allow the cartilage to sit straight.[14] Additionally, cartilage scoring techniques have been described, which may have variable efficacy. Cartilage scoring can be combined with placement of cartilage or bony

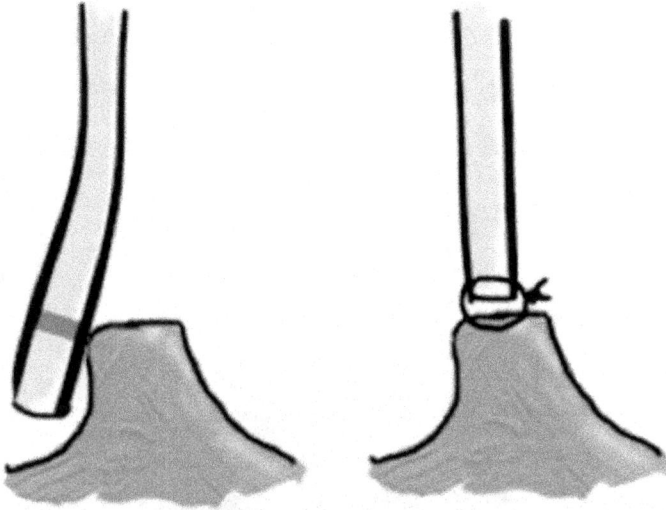

Fig. 3. A swinging door technique is performed where the excessively long septum is trimmed so that it sits on the maxillary crest in a midline position. (*Reproduced from* Delaney SW. Evolution of the Septoplasty: Maximizing Functional and Aesthetic Outcomes in Nasal Surgery. M J Otol. 2018.1(1): 004.)

splinting grafts or a caudal septal extension graft in order to stabilize the caudal septum in a midline position.[15] If there is excess length in the cranio-caudal dimension, an L-strut division with or without batten graft placement can lead to resolution of a caudal septal deviation.[16] Oftentimes, the caudal septal deviation is so severe that cartilage sparing techniques will not be effective. In these cases, the caudal septum should be removed and reconstructed with a caudal septal replacement graft or an anterior septal reconstruction (**Fig. 4**). While these techniques are more aggressive, they can produce reliable results with improvement in the position of the septum.[17]

The position of the nasal tip can have a profound effect on the patency of the ENV. When the tip is ptotic, increasing rotation to a more normal position may improve nasal airway obstruction. This can be performed through a variety of techniques including a columellar strut graft, caudal septal extension or replacement graft, or securing the medial crura to the caudal septum in a tongue-in-groove manner (**Fig. 5A–D**).[18] When the tip is overprojected or there is a prominent tension nose deformity, the nostrils can be overly narrowed and the medial crura may be shortened. By deprojecting the tip, the nostrils can be widened into a more normal orientation and the medial crural footplates can sit closer to the base of the columella.[19] If the columella continues to be widened, a variety of techniques have been described to narrow it by removing the soft tissue between the medial crura and then suturing the footplates to each other.[20]

Alar batten grafts can be utilized to improve dynamic collapse of both the INV and ENV. This technique involves a strip of cartilage that spans over the nasal sidewall to the bony pyriform aperture, which allows for stabilization of the nasal sidewall during inspiration (**Fig. 6**). Preoperatively identifying the region of greatest collapse is critical as this dictates the exact location the graft should be placed. The major drawback of alar batten grafts is that they can lead to lateral nasal wall fullness and visibility.[21,22]

The shape and position of the lateral crura play an important role in the patency and strength of the ENV. They ideally have a slightly convex or flat shape. If the convexity is

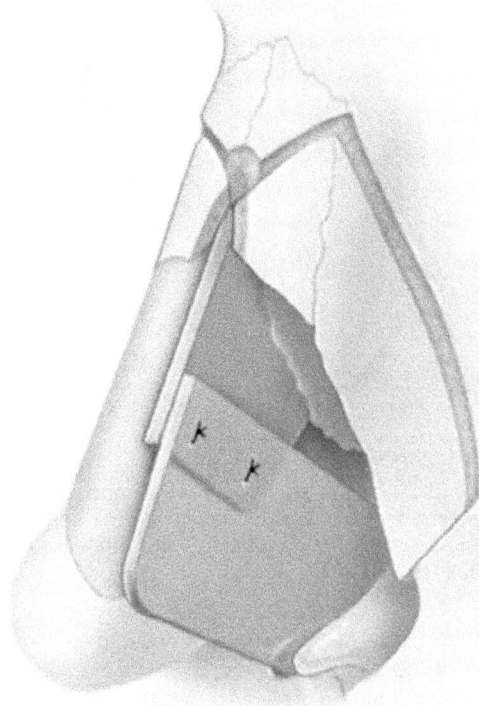

Fig. 4. An anterior septal reconstruction should be performed when there is a severe caudal septal deviation. This technique involves removing the offending caudal strut and then securing the neo-strut to the native dorsal strut. (*Reproduced from* Patel PN, Kandathil CK, Most SP. Outcomes of Combined Anterior Septal Reconstruction and Dorsal Hump Reduction. Laryngoscope. 2020 Dec;130(12):E803-E810 with permission.)

excessive, this can lead to curvature of the lateral aspect of the lateral crura into the nasal vestibule, narrowing the ENV. This can be treated by either trimming the recurved portion of the lateral crus or by supporting it with a lateral crural strut graft.[23] If the lateral crura are concave, this can obstruct the ENV and can be treated by performing a barrel roll or flip–flop maneuver, where the lateral crura are divided, rotated 180°, and sutured to the native residual crus to create a more ideal shape.[24] When the lateral crus is excessively wide, lateral crural hinge or turn-in flaps, where the cephalic edge is elevated off the underlying vestibular skin and folded over itself, can be an effective method to strengthen the lateral crus while also benefiting from the cosmetic improvement of a cephalic trim.[25,26] A review of various lateral crural techniques showed that lateral crural strut grafts alone improved lateral wall insufficiency scores compared to other standalone techniques, such as cephalic overlay or turn in flaps.[27] When the lateral crura have been resected due to previous reductive rhinoplasty, they must be fully reconstructed with cartilage graft that is secured laterally in a soft tissue pocket at the pyriform aperture.[28,29]

When evaluating the lateral crura, it is important to evaluate the long axis, which follows the length of the lateral crura from the dome to its distal aspect, and the short axis, which runs from the caudal to the cephalic aspect of the lateral crus.[23,30] Ideally, the

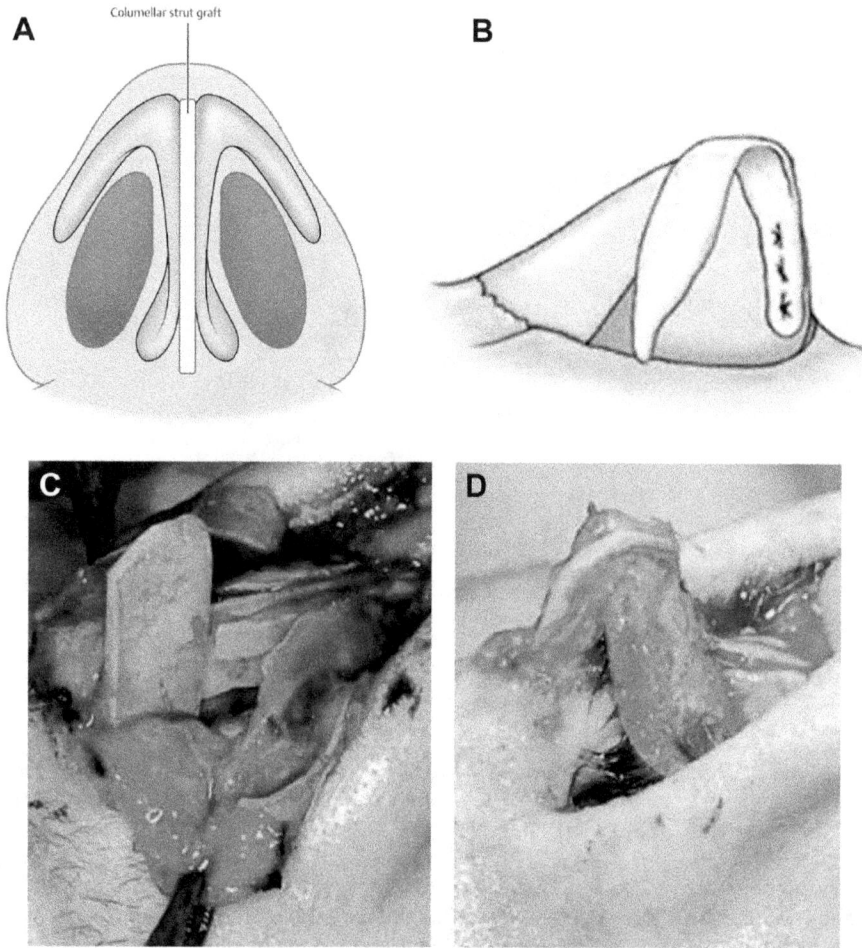

Fig. 5. (A) variety of techniques have been described to reposition the nasal tip. (A) Columellar strut graft. (B) Suturing the media crura to septum in a tongue-in-groove manner. (C, D) Caudal septal extension graft. (Pavri, S. and Steinbacher, D.M. (2019). Rhinoplasty: Control of Tip, Ala, and Tripod Complex. In Aesthetic Orthognathic Surgery and Rhinoplasty, D. Steinbacher (Ed.). https://doi.org/10.1002/9781119187127.ch15 (B–D).)

long axis should be positioned toward the lateral canthus and is considered cephalically malpositioned when it is oriented toward the medial canthus (**Fig. 7**).[30] This can be treated by dissecting the lateral crura free from the nasal vestibular skin, reorienting them into a more favorable position, and supporting them with lateral crural strut grafts (**Fig. 8**).[6] In comparison, sagittal malpositioning is an issue with the orientation of the short axis where the lateral crura are nearly parallel to the septum rather than being perpendicular at nearly a 90° angle to the septum. This deformity can be corrected by a variety of techniques including releasing the scroll and performing a conservative cephalic trim, placing domal sutures on the cephalic aspect of the dome to reorient the position of the lateral crura, potentially excising a wedge of cartilage from the cephalic edge of the lateral crura to reorient the lateral crus, and placing alar suspension sutures.[6,31]

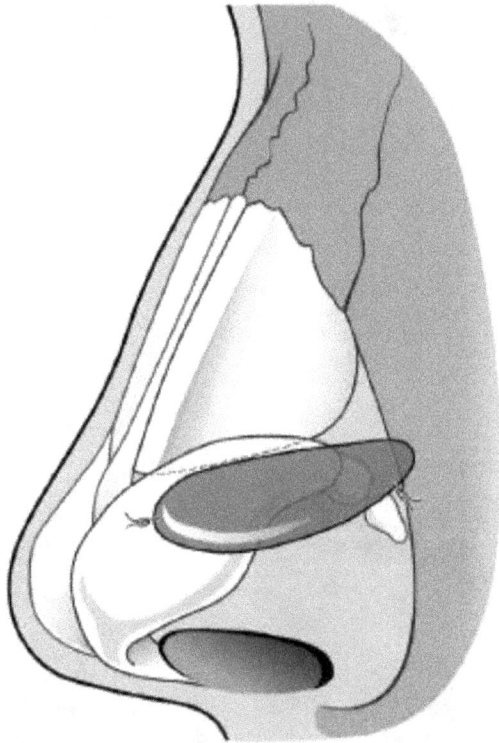

Fig. 6. An alar batten graft can be placed to stabilize the lateral nasal wall and prevent dynamic nasal valve collapse. (*Reproduced from* Bloching MB. Disorders of the nasal valve area. GMS Curr Top Otorhinolaryngol Head Neck Surg. 2007;6:Doc07.)

An effective adjunctive technique are alar rim grafts, which are slips of cartilage placed within the soft tissue of the rim and are used to reinforce the alar margin, elongate and widen the nostril, and prevent the displacement of the alar rim (**Fig. 9**). Although effective, this technique alone is unlikely to completely improve the ENV.[32]

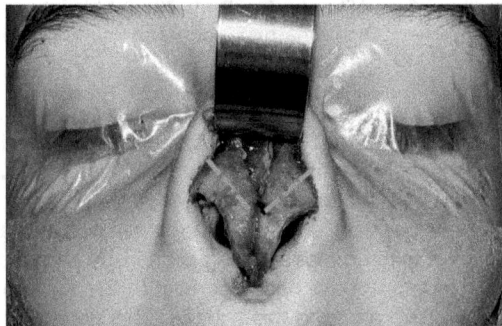

Fig. 7. An example of cephalically malpositioned lateral crura. The green dashed lines represent the long axis of the lateral crura, which when oriented in the direction of the medial canthus are said to be cephalically malpositioned. The blue dashed line represents the short axis of the lateral crura, which when more parallel, rather than nearly perpendicular, to the septum are said to be sagittally malpositioned. (*Photo courtesy* of Dr Mark Mims.)

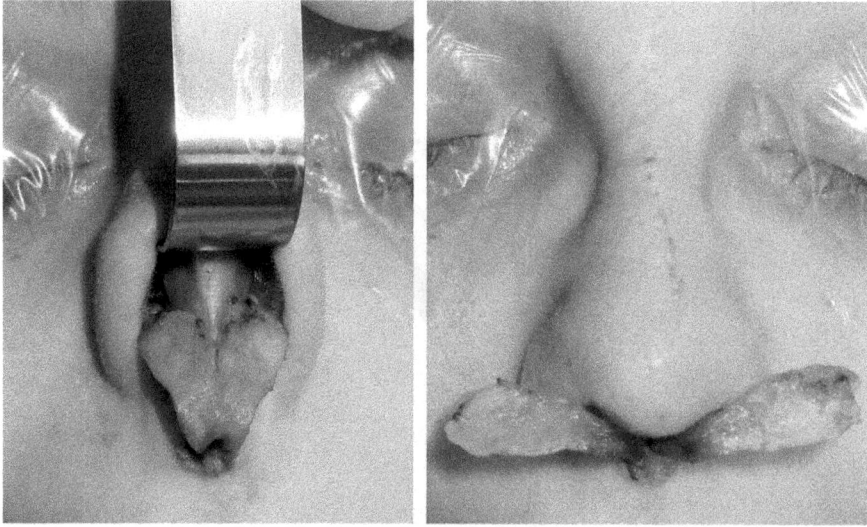

Fig. 8. Severe cephalic malpositioning which was corrected by completely dissecting the lateral crura free from the underlying vestibular skin so they can be reoriented into a more favorable position. (*Photo courtesy* of Dr Jessyka Lighthall.)

A variety of techniques also exist to suspend the nasal valve by suture fixation to the inferior orbital rim or maxilla (**Fig. 10**). This may be approached through a transconjunctival incision, a malar incision, or an incision at the nasal sidewall–cheek junction. While effective, this technique requires another incision and may have associated complications and, therefore, is not generally considered a fist-line technique for nasal valve reconstruction.[33,34] Finally, a study by Stoddard and colleagues[35] found that patients with denser vibrissae had greater nasal obstruction by subjective and objective measurements, and this improved after the vibrissae were trimmed.

In summary, there are a variety of etiologies of nasal valve dysfunction. If the ENV is narrowed in a patient undergoing revision nasal airway surgery, the exact cause of the obstruction must be determined preoperatively so that appropriate techniques can be utilized to reconstruct the nasal valve. The orientation and shape of the lateral crura are often overlooked and play an important role in ENV function, and reorienting the lateral crura in a more favorable position and using lateral crural strut grafts to stabilize the lateral crura are powerful techniques to treat ENV pathology.

Internal Nasal Valve

INVC is one of the most common causes of persistent nasal airway obstruction after primary nasal airway surgery. A variety of techniques have been described to treat INVC in primary and revision rhinoplasty.

Spreader grafts and flaps are a common way to reconstruct the INV. These were initially described by Sheen and gained popularity due to the esthetic and functional improvements noted after placement.[36] This technique involves placing strips of cartilage within submucosal pockets between the upper lateral cartilages and the dorsal septum either unilaterally or bilaterally (**Fig. 11**). Spreader grafts are a valuable technique after dorsal hump reduction, correcting a crooked nose or saddle nose deformity, and when treating a narrow middle vault.[37] Extended spreader grafts can be utilized either unilaterally or bilaterally in order to stabilize the caudal strut during anterior septal

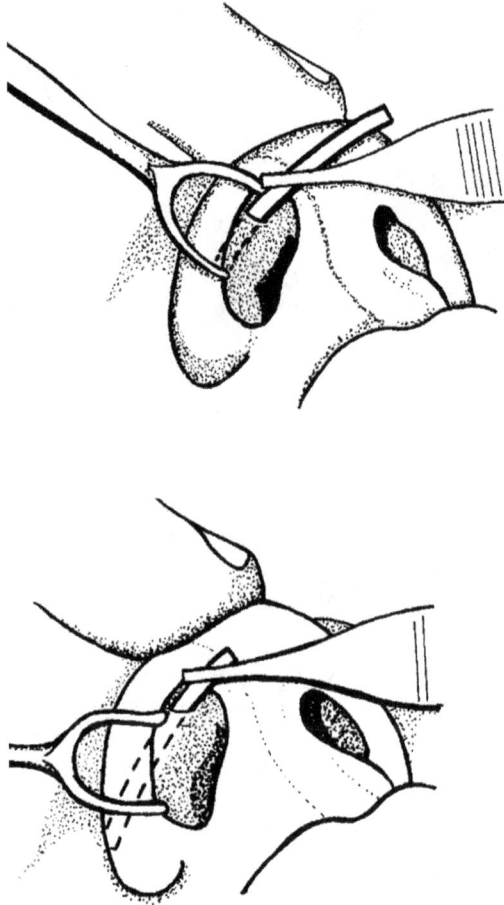

Fig. 9. An alar rim graft can be placed to reinforce the alar margin, elongate and widen the nostril, and prevent displacement of the alar rim. (*Reproduced from* Troell RJ, Powell NB, Riley RW, Li KK. Evaluation of a new procedure for nasal alar rim and valve collapse: nasal alar rim reconstruction. Otolaryngol Head Neck Surg. 2000 Feb;122(2):204-11 with permission.)

reconstruction and extracorporeal septoplasty, and it has been suggested that there are no functional or cosmetic differences between traditional versus extended spreader grafts.[37–39] Spreader flaps, also known as autospreader grafts, are a technique where the medial edges of the upper lateral cartilages are folded onto themselves after dorsal hump reduction to provide a spreader graft effect without the need of additional cartilage.[40] A recent systematic review and metanalysis showed no significant difference in outcomes or complications between spreader grafts versus flaps, and this is a technique that may be considered during revision surgery if a dorsal hump is present.[41]

Additionally, spreader grafts can be placed via an endonasal approach, and a more recent article described the placement of endonasal spreader grafts with a barbed suture, which may make securing the grafts less challenging.[42–44] A recent article has described endonasal spreader graft placement in dorsal preservation rhinoplasty to improve the integrity of the INV without disrupting the dorsum.[45] A retrospective review of 50 patients who underwent open versus endonasal spreader graft placement

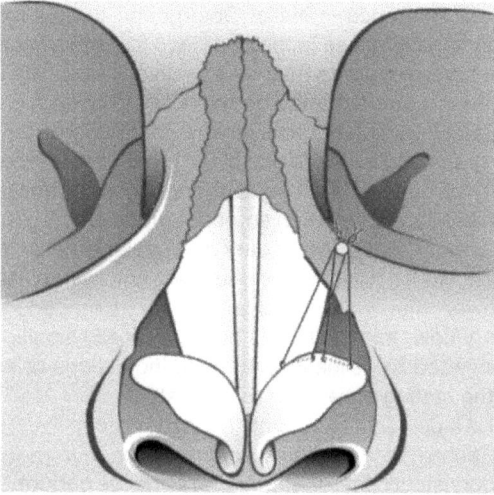

Fig. 10. Suspension sutures can be used to improve nasal valve insufficiency by securing a suture from the lateral nasal wall to the inferior orbital rim or maxilla. While these can be effective, they are generally not considered first-line techniques. (*Reproduced from* Bloching MB. Disorders of the nasal valve area. GMS Curr Top Otorhinolaryngol Head Neck Surg. 2007;6:Doc07.)

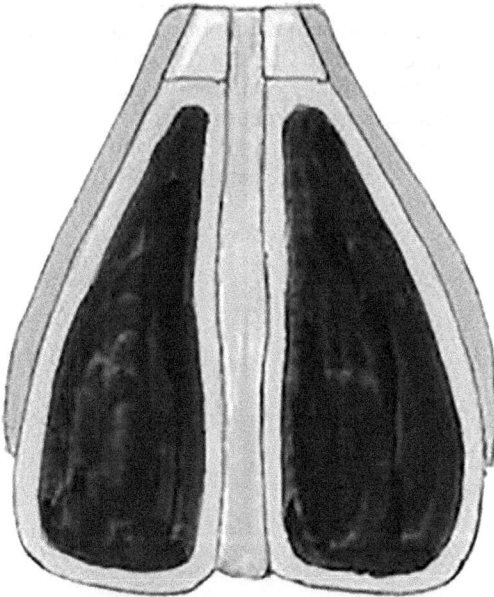

Fig. 11. Spreader grafts are strips of cartilage that are placed between the nasal dorsum and upper lateral cartilages. They are a commonly utilized technique to widen the internal nasal valve. (*Reproduced from* Howard BE, Madison Clark J. Evolution of the butterfly graft technique: 15-year review of 500 cases with expanding indications. Laryngoscope. 2019 Apr;129(S1):S1-S10 with permission.)

showed there was no difference in Nasal Obstruction Symptoms Evaluation score improvement, suggesting that these techniques lead to equivalent functional results.[46] Although endonasal spreader grafts may be effective, in the setting of revision nasal airway surgery, an open approach may be more comprehensive unless INVC is the only identifiable cause of persistent nasal airway obstruction.

Overall, spreader grafts and flaps are one of the most common techniques utilized in structural rhinoplasty to support the midvault and increase the patency of the INV. While there are definite indications when spreader grafts should be utilized, some surgeons believe they are not always necessary and have decreased their usage of this technique.[47] A study of 72 patients who underwent rhinoplasty with or without spreader grafts showed that while spreader grafts did procedure a slightly greater peak nasal inspiratory flow, this result was not statistically significant.[48] In summary, further studies are needed to delineate the exact indications of spreader grafts and flaps, especially in the setting of revision rhinoplasty.

The butterfly graft is a powerful technique that can improve INVC in primary and revision surgeries. This technique was initially described for patients who underwent revision rhinoplasty for persistent nasal obstruction and can be performed through either an open or a closed approach.[49] A single surgeon series of 500 cases showed 87% of patients had complete improvement in their nasal obstruction symptoms, 10% had partial improvement, and 4% had no improvement. Additionally, 53% had improved nasal appearance, 32% had a similar appearance, and 15% had worsened appearance.[50] The technique involves harvesting the concha cavum, which is then thinned anteriorly taking care to leave the posterior perichondrium intact. An open or a closed rhinoplasty approach is performed, and the dorsum is reduced to create space for the graft. The graft is then sutured to the caudal edges of the upper lateral cartilage on each side with the posterior perichondrium facing superficially (**Fig. 12**). The tensioning from the remaining posterior perichondrium and subsequent scar tissue contracture lead to elevation and widening of the INV. Cadaveric studies with computational fluid dynamics have shown that the butterfly graft can reduce nasal airflow resistance by 20% to 51%, whereas spreader grafts reduce resistance by 2% to 21%.[51] A subsequent study showed that the butterfly graft improved nasal airway resistance by

Fig. 12. The butterfly graft is a powerful technique where an auricular cartilage graft is sutured to the caudal aspect of the upper lateral cartilages to widen the internal nasal valve. (*Reproduced from* Howard BE, Madison Clark J. Evolution of the butterfly graft technique: 15-year review of 500 cases with expanding indications. Laryngoscope. 2019 Apr;129(S1):S1-S10 with permission.)

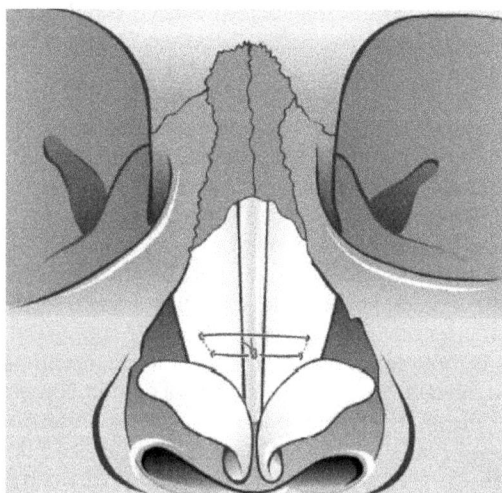

Fig. 13. A flaring suture can be placed along the lateral aspect of the upper lateral cartilage. When tied down, this technique will widen the internal nasal valve. (*Reproduced from* Bloching MB. Disorders of the nasal valve area. GMS Curr Top Otorhinolaryngol Head Neck Surg. 2007;6:Doc07.)

24.9%, whereas spreader grafts and bioabsorbable nasal implants reduced nasal airway resistance by 2.6% and 6.7%, respectively.[52] When an extensive saddle nose deformity is present, an extended butterfly graft can be effective in improving the nasal valve stenosis while also providing camouflage of the saddle nose deformity.[53]

Although extremely effective, some surgeons hesitate to utilize the butterfly graft routinely due to concerns for increased width and supratip fullness.[54] However, a recent survey administered to nonmedical observers who rated either preoperative or postoperative photos of 22 patients who underwent either butterfly graft or spreader graft placement showed no significant difference in ratings of preoperative and postoperative photos in the butterfly graft group and no significant difference in the postoperative photos of the butterfly graft compared to the spreader graft group.[55] Additionally, a recent cadaver study has shown that the butterfly graft can be thinned significantly until only a sliver of cartilage remains attached to the posterior perichondrium but still create enough force to displace the INV.[56] Thus, these results suggest that the majority of cosmetic concerns of the butterfly graft can be mitigated by thinning the graft sufficiently. Overall, the butterfly graft is a powerful technique to treat the INV and should be considered in the revision rhinoplasty patient.

Another technique that has been described to improve NVC is flaring sutures. This is where a horizontal mattress suture is placed along the lateral aspects of the upper lateral cartilages. When the suture is tied down, the lateral aspect of the upper lateral cartilages will flare outwards leading to improvement in NVC (**Fig. 13**). This technique can be performed via either an open or a closed approach.[57,58] As was previously discussed in the ENV section, alar batten grafts can also be used to treat dynamic INVC by placing the graft over the scroll region to provide support during inspiration.[59]

SUMMARY

There are a variety of causes of persistent nasal airway obstruction after primary nasal airway surgery including NVC, previous reductive rhinoplasty leading to structural compromise of the nose, abnormal tone of the nasal constrictors, inferior turbinate hypertrophy, chronic rhinosinusitis, or sinonasal masses. During initial evaluation, a careful examination should be performed to identify these causes so they can be treated appropriately.

ENVC may be secondary to caudal septal deviation, tip ptosis, overprojection of the nasal tip, tension nose deformity, malpositioned or misshapen lateral crura, or a widened columella. During revision surgery, these deformities should be addressed in a systematic manner. Of note, cephalic or sagittal malpositioning of the lateral crura are frequently missed causes of ENVC and can be treated by reorienting the lateral crura in a more favorable position. Finally, a variety of techniques have been described to strengthen the lateral crura; however, the lateral crural strut graft should be considered in the revision rhinoplasty patients as studies have suggested it is more powerful than other methods without requiring other techniques to strengthen the lateral crura.

INVC is one of the most common causes of nasal obstruction. In the setting of revision surgery, it is possible that some of the more common techniques to repair the INV, such as spreader grafts, may have already been utilized. If the INV continues to be narrowed, then more aggressive techniques, such as the butterfly graft, should be considered. Some surgeons have concerns about supratip fullness after butterfly graft placement. However, more recent studies have suggested that these cosmetic concerns are not significant and the graft can be thinned significantly, thus mitigating some of the risks of supratip fullness.

CLINICS CARE POINTS

- Careful preoperative evaluation must be performed on patients undergoing revision nasal airway surgery to identify specific causes of persistent nasal obstruction.
- ENVC and INVC are common causes of persistent nasal airway obstruction.
- Lateral crural strut grafts and lateral crural repositioning are powerful techniques to treat ENVC.
- Although spreader grafts are frequently utilized to treat INVC, the butterfly graft has been shown to be more powerful and should be considered in the revision rhinoplasty patients.
- Updated butterfly graft techniques allow the graft to be camouflaged more effectively, mitigating many of the concerns of postoperative supratip fullness.

DISCLOSURE

The authors have no commercial or financial conflicts of interest and were provided no funding for this article.

REFERENCES

1. Fearington FW, Awadallah AS, Hamilton GS, et al. Long-term outcomes of septoplasty with or without turbinoplasty: a systematic review. Laryngoscope 2024; 134(6):2525–37.
2. Clark DW, Del Signore AG, Raithatha R, et al. Nasal airway obstruction: prevalence and anatomic contributors. Ear Nose Throat J 2018;97(6):173–6.
3. Grymer LF. Reduction rhinoplasty and nasal patency: change in the cross-sectional area of the nose evaluated by acoustic rhinometry. Laryngoscope 1995;105(4 Pt 1): 429–31.

4. Vaiman M, Shlamkovich N, Kessler A, et al. Biofeedback training of nasal muscles using internal and external surface electromyography of the nose. Am J Otolaryngol 2005;26(5):302–7.
5. Aksoy F, Veyseller B, Yıldırım YS, et al. Role of nasal muscles in nasal valve collapse. Otolaryngology-Head Neck Surg (Tokyo) 2010;142(3):365–9.
6. Hamilton G. Form and function of the nasal tip: reorienting and reshaping the lateral crus. Facial Plast Surg 2016;32(01):049–58.
7. Barrett DM, Casanueva FJ, Cook TA. Management of the nasal valve. Facial Plast Surg Clin North Am 2016;24(3):219–34.
8. Wustrow TP, Kastenbauer E. Surgery of the internal nasal valve. Facial Plast Surg 1995;11(3):213–27.
9. Bloching MB. Disorders of the nasal valve area. GMS Curr Top Otorhinolaryngol, Head Neck Surg 2007;6:Doc07.
10. Howard BK, Rohrich RJ. Understanding the nasal airway: principles and practice. Plast Reconstr Surg 2002;109(3):1128–46, quiz 1145-1146.
11. O'Neill G, Tolley NS. Theoretical considerations of nasal airflow mechanics and surgical implications. Clin Otolaryngol Allied Sci 1988;13(4):273–7.
12. Constantian MB, Clardy RB. The relative importance of septal and nasal valvular surgery in correcting airway obstruction in primary and secondary rhinoplasty. Plast Reconstr Surg 1996;98(1):38–54 ; discussion 55-8.
13. Heppt W, Gubisch W. Septal surgery in rhinoplasty. Facial Plast Surg 2011;27(02):167–78.
14. Most SP, Rudy SF. Septoplasty. Facial Plast Surg Clin North Am. 2017;25(2):161–9.
15. Wee JH, Lee JE, Cho SW, et al. Septal batten graft to correct cartilaginous deformities in endonasal septoplasty. Arch Otolaryngol Head Neck Surg 2012;138(5):457.
16. Jang YJ, Yeo NK, Wang JH. Cutting and suture technique of the caudal septal cartilage for the management of caudal septal deviation. Arch Otolaryngol Head Neck Surg 2009;135(12):1256.
17. Haack J, Papel ID. Caudal septal deviation. Otolaryngol Clin North Am 2009;42(3):427–36.
18. Toriumi DM. New concepts in nasal tip contouring. Arch Facial Plast Surg 2006;8(3):136–85.
19. Johnson CM, Godin MS. The tension nose: open structure rhinoplasty approach. Plast Reconstr Surg 1995;95(1):43–51.
20. Lawson W, Reino AJ. Reduction columelloplasty. a new method in the management of the nasal base. Arch Otolaryngol Head Neck Surg 1995;121(10):1086–8.
21. Toriumi DM, Josen J, Weinberger M, et al. Use of alar batten grafts for correction of nasal valve collapse. Arch Otolaryngol Head Neck Surg 1997;123(8):802–8.
22. Chua DY, Park SS. Alar batten grafts. JAMA Facial Plast Surg 2014;16(5):377–8.
23. Hamilton GS. The external nasal valve. Facial Plast Surg Clin North Am 2017;25(2):179–94.
24. Boccieri A, Marianetti TM. Barrel roll technique for the correction of long and concave lateral crura. Arch Facial Plast Surg 2010;12(6):415–21.
25. Janis JE, Trussler A, Ghavami A, et al. Lower lateral crural turnover flap in open rhinoplasty. Plast Reconstr Surg 2009;123(6):1830–41.
26. Barham HP, Knisely A, Christensen J, et al. Costal cartilage lateral crural strut graft vs cephalic crural turn-in for correction of external valve dysfunction. JAMA Facial Plast Surg 2015;17(5):340–5.

27. Abdelwahab M, Patel P, Kandathil CK, et al. Effect of lateral crural procedures on nasal wall stability and tip aesthetics in rhinoplasty. Laryngoscope 2021;131(6): E1830–7.

28. Ishida LC, Ishida J, Henrique Ishida L, et al. Total reconstruction of the alar cartilages with a partially split septal cartilage graft. Ann Plast Surg 2000;45(5):481–4.

29. Balikci H, Yenigun A, Dogan R, et al. Total lower lateral cartilage reconstruction in multiple revision rhinoplasty patients. Aesthetic Plast Surg 2024. https://doi.org/10.1007/s00266-024-04087-x.

30. Constantian MB. The Boxy Nasal Tip, the Ball Tip, and Alar Cartilage Malposition: Variations on a Theme???A Study in 200 Consecutive Primary and Secondary Rhinoplasty Patients. Plast Reconstr Surg 2005;116(1):268–81.

31. Hamilton GS. Correction of sagittally malpositioned lateral crura. Ear Nose Throat J 2009;88(6):961–2.

32. Guyuron B, Bigdeli Y, Sajjadian A. Dynamics of the alar rim graft. Plast Reconstr Surg 2015;135(4):981–6.

33. Paniello RC. Nasal valve suspension: an effective treatment for nasal valve collapse. Arch Otolaryngol Head Neck Surg 1996;122(12):1342–6.

34. White J, Hamilton G. Mitek suspension of the lateral nasal wall. Facial Plast Surg 2016;32(01):070–5.

35. Stoddard DG, Pallanch JF, Hamilton GS. The effect of vibrissae on subjective and objective measures of nasal obstruction. Am J Rhinol Allergy 2015;29(5):373–7.

36. Sheen JH. Spreader graft: a method of reconstructing the roof of the middle nasal vault following rhinoplasty. Plast Reconstr Surg 1984;73(2):230–9.

37. Kim L, Papel I. Spreader grafts in functional rhinoplasty. Facial Plast Surg 2016; 32(01):029–35.

38. Chen YY, Kim SA, Jang YJ. Centering a deviated nose by caudal septal extension graft and unilaterally extended spreader grafts. Ann Otol Rhinol Laryngol 2020; 129(5):448–55.

39. Weitzman RE, Gadkaree SK, Justicz NS, et al. Patient-perceived nasal appearance after septorhinoplasty with spreader versus extended spreader graft. Laryngoscope 2021;131(4):765–72.

40. Gruber RP, Perkins SW. Humpectomy and spreader flaps. Clin Plast Surg 2010; 37(2):285–91.

41. Buba CM, Patel PN, Saltychev M, et al. The safety and efficacy of spreader grafts and autospreaders in rhinoplasty: a systematic review and meta-analysis. Aesthetic Plast Surg 2022;46(4):1741–59.

42. Pontius AT, Williams EF. Endonasal placement of spreader grafts in rhinoplasty. Ear Nose Throat J 2005;84(3):135–6.

43. Bradford BD, Asher SA, Ardeshirpour F. Endonasal (Closed) rhinoplasty technique. JAMA Facial Plast Surg 2016;18(5):395–6.

44. Yoo DB, Jen A. Endonasal placement of spreader grafts: experience in 41 consecutive patients. Arch Facial Plast Surg 2012;14(5):318–22.

45. Go BC, Frost AS, Friedman O. The use of endonasal spreader grafts in preservation rhinoplasty. Plast Reconstr Surg 2023;151(3):398e–401e.

46. Talmadge J, High R, Heckman WW. Comparative outcomes in functional rhinoplasty with open vs endonasal spreader graft placement. Ann Plast Surg 2018; 80(5):468–71.

47. Gerecci D, Perkins SW. The use of spreader grafts or spreader flaps—or not—in hump reduction rhinoplasty. Facial Plast Surg 2019;35(05):467–75.

48. Xavier R, Azeredo-Lopes S, Papoila A. Spreader grafts: functional or just aesthetical? Rhinol J 2015;53(4):332–9.

49. Clark JM, Cook TA. The "butterfly" graft in functional secondary rhinoplasty. Laryngoscope 2002;112(11):1917–25.
50. Howard BE, Madison Clark J. Evolution of the butterfly graft technique: 15-year review of 500 cases with expanding indications. Laryngoscope 2019;129(S1):S1–10.
51. Brandon BM, Austin GK, Fleischman G, et al. Comparison of airflow between spreader grafts and butterfly grafts using computational flow dynamics in a cadaveric model. JAMA Facial Plast Surg 2018;20(3):215–21.
52. Brandon BM, Stepp WH, Basu S, et al. Nasal airflow changes with bioabsorbable implant, butterfly, and spreader grafts. Laryngoscope 2020;130(12):E817–23.
53. Vega-Cordova X, Brenner MJ, Putman HC. Extended butterfly graft for functional and cosmetic correction of saddle nose deformity. JAMA Facial Plast Surg 2019; 21(6):568–9.
54. Chaiet SR, Marcus BC. Nasal tip volume analysis after butterfly graft. Ann Plast Surg 2014;72(1):9–12.
55. Mims MM, Shockley WW, Clark JM. Casual observers' perception on the aesthetics of the butterfly graft. Laryngoscope 2023;133(10):2578–83.
56. Brownlee BP, Hassoun A, Parikh A, et al. Cadaveric assessment of the butterfly graft in rhinoplasty. Laryngoscope 2024;134(4):1638–41.
57. Park SS. The flaring suture to augment the repair of the dysfunctional nasal valve. Plast Reconstr Surg 1998;101(4):1120–2.
58. Rasic I, Pegan A, Kosec A, et al. Use of intranasal flaring suture for dysfunctional nasal valve repair. JAMA Facial Plast Surg 2015;17(6):462–3.
59. Bewick JC, Buchanan MA, Frosh AC. Internal nasal valve incompetence is effectively treated using batten graft functional rhinoplasty. Int J Otolaryngol. 2013; 2013:1–5.

Rhinoplasty for Patients with Cleft Lip-Palate
Functional and Aesthetic Concerns

Tsung-yen Hsieh, MD[a], Isabelle Gengler, MD[a],
Travis T. Tollefson, MD, MPH[b,*]

KEYWORDS

- Cleft lip • Cleft palate • Cleft rhinoplasty • Nasal deformities • Surgical techniques
- Nasal valves • Septal deviation

KEY POINTS

- Understanding the unique anatomic challenges in patients with cleft lip and palate, such as septal deviation, asymmetry of the cartilaginous frame work, and bony and soft tissue deformities is essential for successful surgical planning in cleft rhinoplasty.
- Techniques such as thorough septoplasty, structural grafting, management of the soft tissues, and the use of advanced suturing methods are crucial for achieving desired aesthetic and functional outcomes.
- Primary rhinoplasty can be performed during initial lip repair, intermediate rhinoplasty before skeletal maturity, and definitive rhinoplasty after skeletal maturity, balancing growth concerns, and deformity severity.

INTRODUCTION

Many patients with cleft lip and cleft palate have anatomic features that affect the form and function of their nose. The shape and function of the nose is affected by the deficient bony maxilla, dentoalveolar arch/teeth, and lip soft tissues, impacting them both structurally and aesthetically. This article will define the characteristic nasal deformities found in patients with cleft lip and palate and describe the associated surgical techniques and considerations in cleft rhinoplasty with focus on the nasal valves in both unilateral and bilateral cleft lip nasal deformities. Overall, concepts will include

[a] Facial Plastic and Reconstructive Surgery, Department of Otolaryngology - Head and Neck Surgery, University of Cincinnati College of Medicine, Cincinnati, OH, USA; [b] Facial Plastic and Reconstructive Surgery, Department of Otolaryngology - Head and Neck Surgery, University of California Davis Medical Center, University of California Davis, 2521 Stockton Boulevard, Suite 7200, Sacramento, CA 95817, USA
* Corresponding author.
E-mail address: tttollefson@gmail.com

Otolaryngol Clin N Am 58 (2025) 361–377
https://doi.org/10.1016/j.otc.2024.07.017
0030-6665/25/© 2024 Elsevier Inc. All rights are reserved, including those for text and data mining, AI training, and similar technologies.
oto.theclinics.com

correction of septal deflections, structural cartilage grafting, suture techniques, and nostril soft tissue rearrangements.

BACKGROUND

Cleft lip and/or palate is the most common congenital orofacial anomaly, as 6000 to 8000 children are born with it every year in the United States (1 in 700 births). According to the National Institute of Dental and Craniofacial Research, cleft lip and cleft palate affect 1 in 1600 births, with isolated cleft lip defects in 1 in 2800 births, and 1 in 1700 births with cleft palate only.[1] The etiology of orofacial clefts is complex and multifactorial including genetic, syndromic, environmental, and toxic factors.[2–5] The classically described nasal, oral, and pharyngeal deformities can first impact optimal swallowing and nutrition.[6]

Once these early concerns are addressed, the cleft nasal deformity that persists is one of the hardest technical challenges for the surgeon. The complex nasal architecture that results from either unilateral or bilateral cleft lip deformity can be made even more challenging in older children, considering postsurgical changes, scarring, and modified facial growth.[7]

ANATOMIC CONSIDERATIONS OF THE CLEFT LIP NASAL DEFORMITY

Due to the complexity of the nasal anatomy and patient-specific deformities that are observed in patients with cleft lip and palate, classifications and nomenclatures have been described[8] to guide the novice surgeon in evaluating the cleft nose. This article proposes a description of the nasal anatomy in both unilateral and bilateral cleft lip, and divides the evaluation of the nose into 3 anatomic parts: the nasal tip and columella, the nasal septum, and the nasal valve. Having a thorough understanding of each patient's unique cleft nasal anatomy is critical for surgical planning and patient's specific nasal reconstruction.

Unilateral Cleft Lip and Nasal Deformity

Patients with unilateral cleft lip have several nasal characteristics derived from local embryologic development and muscle attachments that will not be reviewed in this article. On the cleft side, the skeletal deficiency of the maxilla leads to dysmorphic nasal ala with a shorter medial crus and elongated lateral crus, which contribute to nasal tip asymmetry and posterior displacement of the tip. The length and volume of both lower lateral cartilage is comparable to patients without cleft deformity, but the lack of muscle attachments and the resulting vector forces result in cartilage deformity. The nostril appears flattened on the cleft side, and the caudal septum and nasal spine further displaced toward the non-cleft side.[9,10] These deformities are summarized in **Box 1** and can be seen in **Fig. 1**.

Bilateral Cleft Lip and Nasal Deformity

Patients with bilateral cleft lip and palate usually present with an overall more symmetric nasal deformity with some similarities to unilateral cleft patients, but also with critical anatomy differences that impact rhinoplasty surgery. Due to medial and inferior maxillary deficiency, both alar bases are positioned more laterally and posteriorly, contributing to an overall wider and flatter nose. In cases of complete bilateral cleft, the prolabial tissue extends from the nasal septum and is significantly affected during surgical correction of the nasal deformity. The lower lateral cartilage has a shorter medial crura and a longer lateral crura, which further widens the alar bases. Due to the severity of the nasal under-projection, the definition of the tip is poor, the height

---

Box 1

Clinical characteristics of unilateral cleft nasal deformity

Asymmetric tip, usually posteriorly deviated to the cleft side

Posterior cartilaginous and bony septum deviated to the cleft side

Caudal septum deviated to the non-cleft side

Flattening of the nostril on the cleft side

Shorter medial crura and lengthened lateral crura (LLC length is intact)

Alar base is displaced laterally, inferiorly, and posteriorly

Maxillary deficiency on the cleft side

Anterior nasal spine is displaced to the non-cleft side

---

of the nose is decreased, and the remnant columellar skin becomes a limiting factor in reconstructive surgery. The orbicularis oris muscle is absent in the prolabial region and the premaxilla is protruding, which contributes to the short, and sometimes non-existent, columella. Patients with bilateral cleft experience bilateral nasal obstruction secondary to bilateral nasal valve static collapse against the reconstructed nasal floor, while the septum usually remains midline. The external nasal valve is narrow on both sides due to the severe flattening of the nose, and the internal nasal valve is obstructed by the plica vestibularis, from the redundant lower lateral cartilage.[11] These deformities are summarized in **Box 2** and can be seen in **Fig. 2**.

EVALUATION OF THE NASAL TIP AND COLUMELLA

When evaluating the nasal deformity of patients with cleft lip and palate, the surgeon should first consider overall tip support and tip deformity. The major support of the nasal tip is the strength and shape of the medial crura and their relationship with the distal nasal septum, as well as the attachment of the lower lateral cartilage to the caudal aspect of the upper lateral cartilage. The significant asymmetry of the lower lateral cartilages and the soft tissue of the nasal base will create a significant nasal deformity. Assessing the strength of the nasal tip, its symmetry, the length of the medial crura, and the amount of available soft tissue at the columella are important clinical findings to start surgical planning. In case of bilateral cleft, tip support is

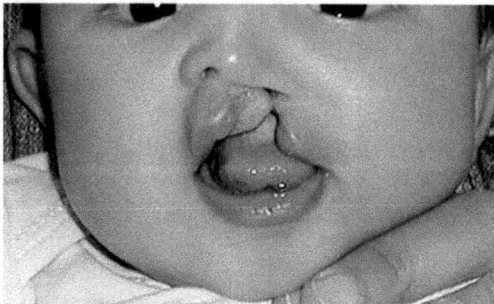

Fig. 1. Infant with unilateral cleft lip and palate demonstrating features of unilateral cleft lip nasal deformity.

Box 2
Clinical characteristics of bilateral cleft nasal deformity

Nasal tip is broad, flat, with poor definition, and grossly asymmetric

Tip is underprojected and posterolaterally displaced domes

Dysmorphic lower lateral cartilages bilaterally

Medial crura is shorter and lateral crura is longer

Short columella with lack of soft tissue

Wider alar base and flattening of both nostrils

Bilaterally absent or deficient nasal floor

---

very deficient, and reconstruction will depend on the amount of columellar skin, the length of both medial crura, the height of the premaxilla, and the possible associated septal deformity.[12] A step-by-step guide to analyze nasal deformity prior to surgery is described in **Table 1**.

EVALUATION OF THE NASAL SEPTUM DEFORMITY

A deviated septum will invariably impact nasal symmetry in the mid vault and contribute to chronic nasal obstruction. Careful treatment of septal deviation is critical to improve overall cosmetic appearance without negative impact on nasal growth. Patients with unilateral cleft lip and palate display a posterior cartilaginous and bony septum deviated toward the cleft side while the caudal septum is deviated to the non-cleft side (**Fig. 3**). Often, the caudal septum is also displaced from its maxillary crest attachment. The strength and thickness of the nasal septum should also be considered, especially in bilateral cleft cases. Finally, the height of the caudal septum in relationship with the premaxilla will also impact the type of surgical reconstruction considered and the grafts required.

ASSESSMENT OF THE NASAL VALVES

The lateral nasal valve is composed of the nasal septum, the position and strength of the lateral crura (LLC), and the relationship of the lateral crura and septum with the

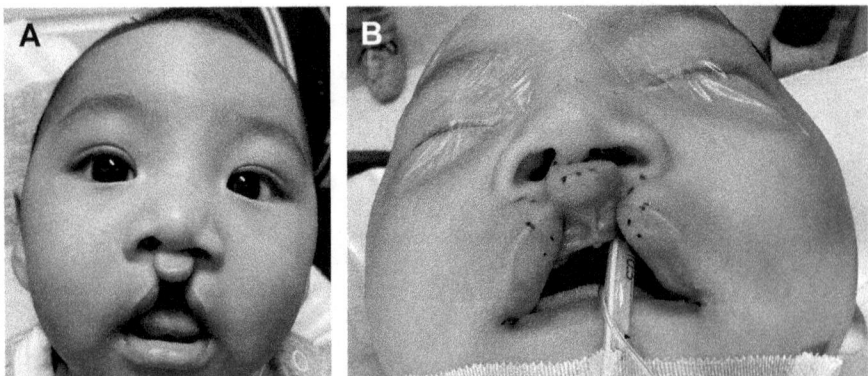

Fig. 2. Patient with bilateral cleft lip and palate demonstrating features of bilateral cleft lip nasal deformity. (*A*) Frontal view. (*B*) Base view.

Table 1
Step-by-step preoperative nasal deformity analysis

Nasal tip and columella	Tip projection, rotation, and support
	Dome asymmetry
	Length and deformity of the columella
	Amount of residual prelabial tissue
	Amount of columellar scar tissue from prior lip surgery
Septum	Length and deformity of the caudal septum
	Posterior bony spur and deviation
	Attachment to the maxillary crest
	Saddle nose deformity
Nasal valve and LLC	Length and position of medial and lateral crura
	Lateral crura dynamic collapse
	Alar base widening
	INV static narrowing
	Inferior turbinate hypertrophy

nostril sill[13] The elongated and weak lateral crura on the cleft side nose in a unilateral cleft lip deformity tends to collapse against the caudal septum, and is sometimes directly in contact with the nostril sill. Specific nomenclatures have been proposed to evaluate the severity of the dynamic collapse of the lateral nasal valve. Maximum nasal inspiration can help grade the severity of the nasal collapse as a percentage of airway obstruction,[14] as well as assess the strength of the crura. In patients with bilateral cleft, the length of the medial crura is a more relevant component of the preoperative assessment.

The internal nasal valve is composed of the nasal septum, the caudal border of the upper lateral cartilage, the head of the inferior turbinate, and the redundant tissue that surrounds these structures.[15] The internal nasal valve can display both static and dynamic collapse in patients with cleft lip and palate, which will affect breathing function, but also olfaction by narrowing the olfactory cleft, and nasal aesthetics due to a narrow mid vault. The internal nasal valve angle is considered normal between 10 and 15°.[16] It

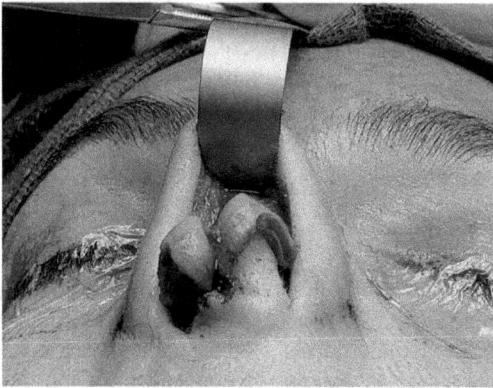

Fig. 3. Intraoperative demonstration of cartilaginous deformities and asymmetry in a patient with unilateral cleft lip. The figure demonstrates severe caudal septal deflection to the non-cleft side with significant differences of the lower lateral alar cartilages in shape, position, and symmetry.

is the narrowest area in the nose, which makes it critical to assess prior to rhinoplasty. The direct and indirect Cottle maneuver can define the extent of the internal nasal valve narrowing. The surgeon can also differentiate between anatomic obstruction versus mucosal swelling by introducing oxymetazoline in the patient's nose.

TIMING AND SEQUENCE OF SURGICAL OPTIONS

Surgeons have differing opinions regarding optimal time to address the nose. If not addressed during primary cleft lip repair, intermediate rhinoplasty may be performed during palatoplasty or later time. Definitive cleft rhinoplasty is often performed in the late teenage years after "skeletal maturity." Advocates for delayed surgery cite weak anecdotal evidence that early surgery may affect facial growth. Factors that may influence timing of surgeries include concern for growth and development, severity of deformity, psychosocial considerations, functional concerns, and surgeon preference. The authors' approach has been to wait until maturity prior to definitive surgery unless there is significant deformity that requires earlier intervention.

Presurgical Management Prior to Primary Cleft Lip Repair and Rhinoplasty

Presurgical infant orthopedics (PISO) have been utilized for the manipulation of the premaxilla since the sixteenth century for patients with cleft lip and palate.[17] The techniques have improved significantly since then. The nasoalveolar molding (NAM) appliances combine an orthodontic device on the premaxilla and lateral alveolar segments with nasal stents. The concept of molding is theorized increase serum maternal estrogen increases elasticity of cartilage via estrogen-mediated release of proteoglycans and hyaluronic acid.[18,19]

Primary objectives of NAM are the following (1) bring maxillary segments closer, (2) retract the premaxilla posteriorly to approximate the maxillary segments in bilateral cleft, and (3) expand the nasal mucosal lining and soft tissues as well as mold the lower lateral cartilages to be more symmetric.[20,21]

It is worth noting that the use of PSIO is debated due to limited long-term outcomes, lack of clear objective outcome measures, and differences in techniques.[22] Therefore, the decision to utilize NAM should consider socioeconomic impact on the parents, parental compliance and cleft severity.[17,23]

Primary Rhinoplasty

Primary cleft rhinoplasty is performed at the time of the cleft lip repair. The objective of the primary cleft rhinoplasty is to achieve early symmetry before deformities become more pronounced with growth. This may reduce the severity of future deformity, thus decreasing the need for multiple revision surgeries.[24] Special care to avoid excessive dissection can prevent excessive scarring, devascularization or inadvertent stenosis of the external nasal valves.

Intermediate Rhinoplasty

Intermediate cleft rhinoplasty is defined as rhinoplasty performed after primary lip repair but before definitive (mature) rhinoplasty at near full skeletal and facial development. Evidence for intermediate rhinoplasty is limited, with the literature focusing on primary and definitive rhinoplasty. A nuanced approach is important for intermediate rhinoplasty as the patients may present with a variety of deformities, scarring, and functional issues. Most cleft surgeons consider the lip and nose as a single unit. Therefore, presurgical NAM and maneuvers performed during primary lip repair can have considerable implications on nasal outcomes. Thus, in the setting of the intermediate stage, small revision techniques are typically applied rather than large reconstructive surgeries.

Orthognathic Surgery and Alveolar Bone Grafting

There is typically maxillary skeletal deficiency and need for establishing a bony foundation for these cases. A multidisciplinary approach with orthodontic preparation and alveolar bone grafting where needed typically happens in the first decade of life. Surgically treatable dentofacial malocclusion (orthognathic surgery), alveolar bone grafting, closure of alveolar clefts/fistulae, and dental preparation should be completed prior to the definitive rhinoplasty to establish the maxillary bony foundation.[25,26]

Definitive (Mature) Cleft Rhinoplasty

Definitive rhinoplasty is performed once nasal and midface growth is completed, usually at ages 14 to 16 in females and ages 16 to 18 in males. The goals of definitive rhinoplasty are to create symmetry and definition of the nose, correct nasal obstruction, repair nasal scarring/stenosis. A customized approach is crucial in the success of definitive cleft rhinoplasty as there are a variety of nasal deformities that include the type and severity of the original lip and nasal defect, changes in nasal growth over time, and sequelae of prior primary and/or intermediate cleft rhinoplasties.[27]

SURGICAL TECHNIQUES
Primary Cleft Rhinoplasty

Unilateral cleft lip primary rhinoplasty
Primary cleft rhinoplasty in unilateral cleft nasal deformity aims to reconstruct the nasal tip symmetry and decrease excess alar hooding on the cleft side. Dissection begins with elevation of the lower lateral cartilages (LLCs) from the soft tissue envelope through the columellar portion of the lip incision (**Fig. 4**). Next, the cleft side LLC is mobilized to a more cephalad and medial position. This can be accomplished through the Skoog technique where an intracartilaginous or marginal rhinoplasty is made to

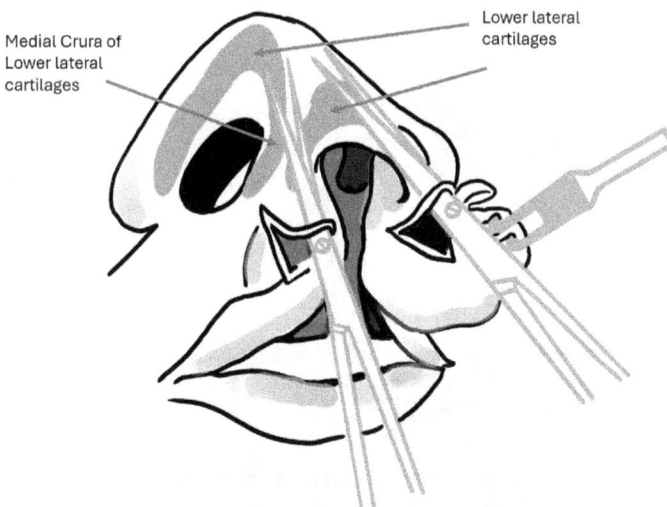

Fig. 4. Demonstration of primary cleft rhinoplasty approach utilizing the lip incisions for access to dissect between the lower lateral cartilages and the soft tissue envelope.

access and secure the cleft side lower lateral cartilages to the upper lateral cartilages (ULCs) and septum to achieve a more symmetric position of the cleft side external nasal valve. Another approach to repositioning the cleft side LLC is to utilize triangular fixation sutures (**Fig. 5**). Transnasal sutures out to the alar crease and back into the nasal vestibule while holding the cleft side LLC cephalad and medially can achieve similar goals of creating symmetry of the external nasal valves.

To address excessive hooding on the cleft side, elliptical excision of the soft tissue hooding or transposition flap utilizing a rim incision (Tajima reverse U) can remove and reposition the soft tissues to decrease hooding of the cleft side nose and repair the external nasal valve on the cleft side (**Fig. 6**).

Lastly, alar base cinching suture can be utilized to place the cleft side alar base in a more symmetry position to the cleft alar base. Often this is done in conjunction with the nasal sill repair as part of the cleft lip repair (**Fig. 7**).

Bilateral cleft lip primary rhinoplasty

In bilateral cleft nasal deformity, primary rhinoplasty is typically performed to reduce alar flare, reposition the LLC, reconstruct the nasal sills, project the nasal tip and lengthen the columella.[28–30] These objectives can be accomplished through bilateral partial marginal incisions to expose the nasal tip fat pad. Excess fibrofatty tissue between the LLCs is removed. Bilateral lateral crural steal (LCS) techniques are then performed and the LLCs sutured together in the midline in a more projected position of the nasal tip. Nostril hooding can be addressed similarly to the unilateral primary cleft rhinoplasty using elliptical excision or the Tajima reverse U rim incision[31] and soft tissue transposition to expand the external nasal valves. Alar base cinching sutures are often utilized as well to facilitate nasal sill positioning. A traditional approach is to add soft tissue and skin from the lip to the columella using a V-Y columellar lengthening.

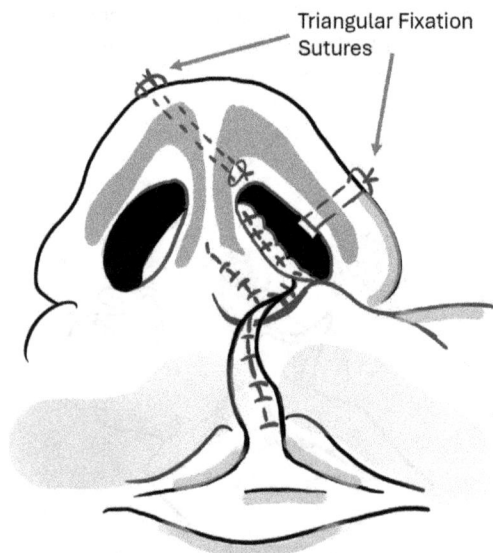

Triangular Fixation Sutures

Fig. 5. Illustration of triangular fixation sutures, which are full thickness mattress sutures that can help position the lower lateral cartilages. Note that symmetric positioning of these sutures can be placed to provide the desired effect on the lower lateral cartilages to create symmetry.

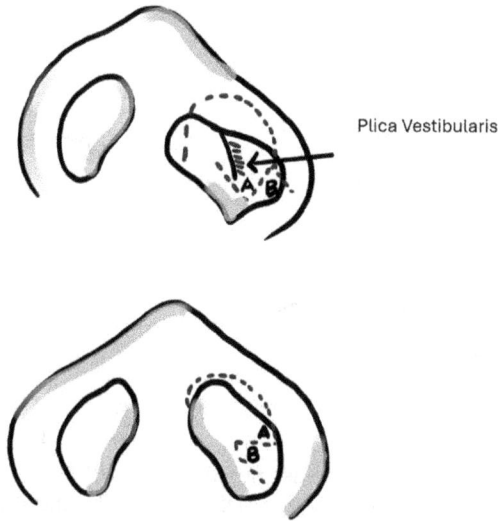

Fig. 6. Tajima reverse-U incision with Z-plasty modification. The lateral wall Z-plasty introduces internal lining to the cleft side vestibule by transposing flap (A) and flap (B).

With the concepts of Mulliken and others, many (including the authors) prefer to go by the philosophy that the "columella is in the nose"[28] and lengthen the columella by transferring soft tissue triangle of the nostril skin into the columella along with LCS of the lower lateral cartilages. This is performed instead of incisions on the lip that recruit soft tissues from the former prolabium/lip (**Fig. 8**)

In primary cleft rhinoplasty, nasal conformers are often utilized to support the nostrils for up to 6 weeks. Nasal conformers should be placed without blanching of the nasal tip skin to avoid pressure necrosis.[32] The evidence of nasal conformer's effectiveness is heterogeneous as shown in a recent systematic review published in 2023 by Nguyen and colleagues, which suggests that stenting is safe and can assist in

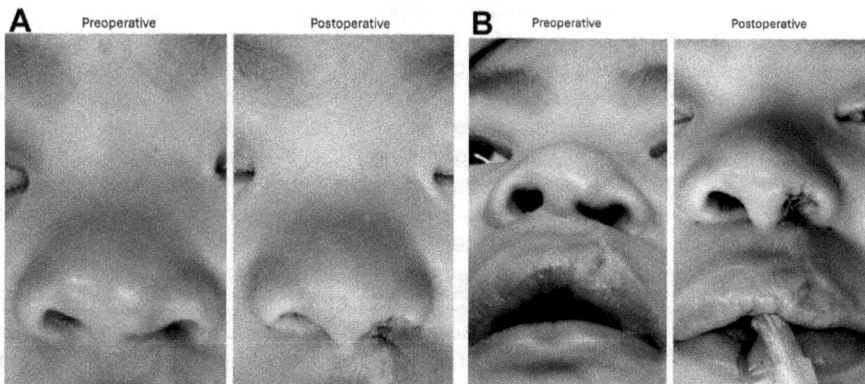

Fig. 7. Preoperative and postoperative photos demonstrating primary rhinoplasty, utilizing various techniques including triangular fixation sutures, Tajima reverse U incision with skin excision and transposition flaps, and alar cinching suture, with improvement in positioning, symmetry, and nasal airway. (*A*) frontal view. (*B*) base view.

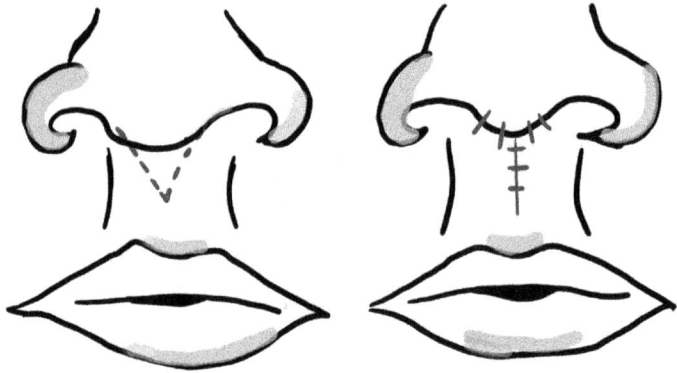

Fig. 8. V-Y advancement flap schematic demonstrating lengthening of the columella by recruiting tissue from the upper lip.

preserving the nasal shape and decrease nostril stenosis.[33] The length of time for stent placement is based on the receptiveness of patient, family, and surgeon with little evidence to suggest a clear answer.

DEFINITIVE (MATURE) CLEFT RHINOPLASTY
Surgical Approach

Utilization of endonasal versus external approach to definitive cleft rhinoplasty is determined by surgeon preference and the extent of reconstruction. In definitive cleft rhinoplasty, there are many factors to consider including the nasal septum, nasal tip, alar rim, alar base, columellar, nasal sill, as well as potential need for revisions of the previous cleft lip repair. These cases can be particularly challenging due to both the extent of the initial deformity as well as scar formation/deformities secondary to prior sutures.

Techniques for Correction of Nasal Deformities with Focus on Nasal Valves

Internal nasal valves
The reconstruction of the internal nasal valve will involve correction of the nasal septum, the ULCs, the scroll area and the inferior turbinates. Beginning with the nasal septum, exposure and detachment of all the mucosal, ligamentous, scar, cartilaginous connections causing septal deviation is crucial. A septoplasty is performed to correct the septal deviation that may affect nasal breathing, but also to harvest septal cartilage for later grafting. Spreader grafts and extended spreader grafts can provide further support to the dorsal septum. These grafts are placed between the dorsal nasal septum and ULCs (**Fig. 9**). These grafts can provide support to the nasal dorsum. Asymmetric spreader grafts can also be positioned to correct and straighten dorsal nasal septal deviations. Lastly, spreader, extended spreader and/or autospreader flaps can enlarge the cross-sectional area of the internal nasal valve to improve nasal airway.[34–36] Other maneuvers to expand/support the internal nasal valves such as suspension sutures, nasal implant placement, or radiofrequency treatments can also be utilized.[37–42] In patients with turbinate hypertrophy, turbinate reduction and out-fracture can be performed concomitantly.

External nasal valve
Techniques to repair the external nasal valve in cleft rhinoplasty can be challenging secondary to the existing cleft nasal and lip deformities as well as scar formation

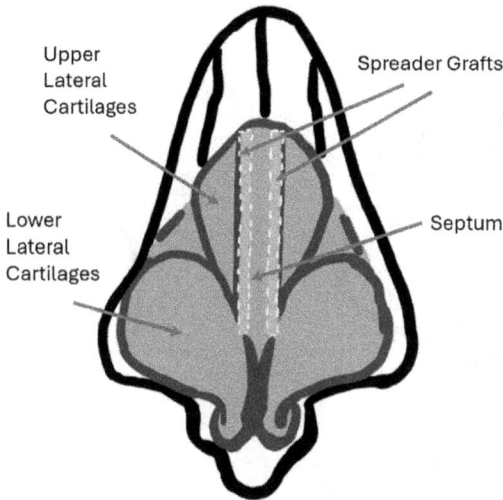

Fig. 9. Spreader graft placement for dorsal septal support and expansion of internal nasal valves.

from previous surgeries. The caudal septum/columella, the nasal ala, and nasal sill all need to be corrected.

To adequately expose the caudal nasal septum, the ligaments connecting the medial crura are often divided. If the caudal septum is severely deviated to the non-cleft side from unimpeded pull of the orbicularis oris and deficient maxilla, it needs to be separated from the nasal spine, mobilized, and repositioned to the midline by securing the caudal septum to the periosteum of the midline maxilla. If necessary, an anterior, inferior wedge of cartilage can be resected from the caudal septum to assist with the septal repositioning (**Fig. 10**). Caudal extension grafting is often utilized to provide more septal support,[43] as well as to provide positioning for the nasal tip. These can be fixated in an end-to-end or end-to-side manner to the existing caudal nasal septum. These grafts can be harvested from septal cartilage, or costal cartilage. While auricular cartilage may also be used, the curvature and decreased strength in the cartilage may be less ideal for large structural grafts.

The nasal tip can then be addressed to establish symmetry, definition and projection. Once the caudal septum is straightened and supported, tongue in groove (TIG) technique can be performed to suspend and position the nasal domes and define the nasal tip position.[44] In unilateral cleft nasal deformity, the cleft side nasal tip is under-projected with hooding of the ala. The TIG technique can be performed asymmetrically by suspending the cleft side alar cartilage further than the noncleft side to the midline structure (caudal septum, columellar strut, or caudal septal extension graft), thereby correcting the cleft LLC flattening and improve symmetry as well as to improve the cleft side external nasal valve. In bilateral cleft nasal deformity, this similar technique can be utilized to project the nasal tip and provide better support to the external nasal valves.

The alar rims all need to be addressed to improve external nasal valve function in cleft rhinoplasty. In unilateral cleft nasal deformity, alar malpositioning results in flattening of the cleft lateral crus of the LLC with inferior and posterior displacement of the cartilage. The resulting concave deformity can create nasal valve collapse. LCS technique,[45] which advances the lateral crura into the medial crura can decrease

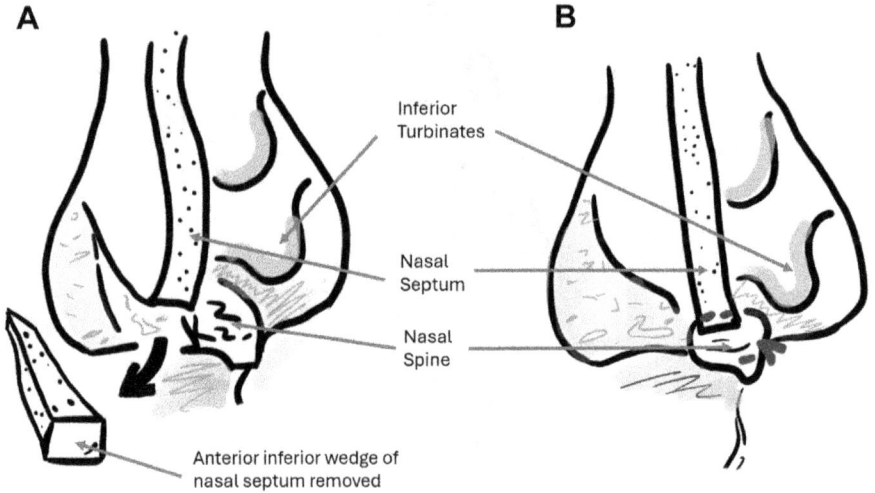

Fig. 10. Caudal septal repositioning. (*A*) deflection of the caudal septum toward the non-cleft side. An anterior inferior wedge of curve caudal septum resected to allow repositioning of the septum to the midline. (*B*) Caudal Septum is sutured to the periosteum of the nasal spine in a more midline position.

the malpositioning in the lateral crus of the LLC in cleft nasal deformities and provide more symmetry as well as less flattening of the lateral crus. In this technique, the vestibular skin is separated from the undersurface of the alar cartilage. If there is significant restriction of the mucosa, a Z-plasty may be performed to help release mucosa. Once the lateral crura is mobilized without restriction from the vestibular skin, the lateral crus is then advanced medially in a curvilinear fashion onto the medial crus and fixed in its new position using mattress sutures (**Fig. 11**). Interdomal sutures and TIG techniques can be performed after to recreate the nasal tip complex and support the external nasal valves. If additional ala support is needed, traditional rhinoplasty techniques can be employed including lateral crural strut grafts (placed between the alar cartilage and vestibular skin down to the pyriform aperture), alar batten grafts (placed over the alar cartilages to the pyriform aperture), alar rim/articulated rim grafts (nonanatomic graft placed within the soft tissues of the alar rim), alar turn in flaps (the cephalic portion of the LLC is transposed on a pedicle and placed under the remaining LLC) (**Fig. 12**). These techniques provide a more laterally positioned alar rim with improved support to the LLC, thereby improving the functional of the external nasal valve.[46]

In severely concave deformities of the LLC, a flip-flop technique can be utilized. The lateral crura of the LLC is dissected completely off of the underlying vestibular skin. The lateral crura is then completely excised, turned over, and sutured back to the medial crura and the vestibular lining, creating a more convex shape of the ala.[47]

Similar to primary cleft rhinoplasty, webbing, significant soft tissue hooding, stenotic scar can be addressed with utilization of rotational flaps, transposition flaps, elliptical soft tissue excision, or Tajima reverse U technique. If there is significant soft tissue contracture, skin grafting or composite grafting may be required.

There is often poor support of the nasal bases on the cleft side secondary to skeletal deficiency. In addition, previous malpositioning of the alar facial junction or the insertion of the alar base can become more exaggerated with growth. These deformities

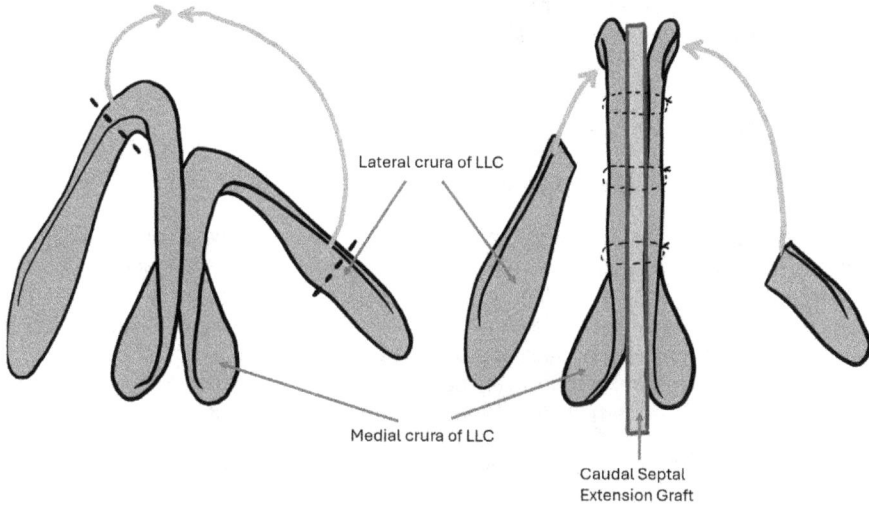

Fig. 11. Lateral Crural Steal Technique—The lateral crura area advanced onto the medial crura, resulting in an increase in the length of the medial crura at the expense of the lateral crura. The medial crura are secured onto the caudal septal extension graft (or native septum/columellar strut) in a mattress fashion to provide symmetry and support.

need to be addressed to achieve better symmetry. Poor skeletal support of the ala base can be addressed with premaxillary cartilage or bone grafting on the cleft-side maxilla and pyriform aperture. This can be placed through a sublabial or nasal sill incision, yet a water-tight closure and sound technique are required for adequate bone graft take.

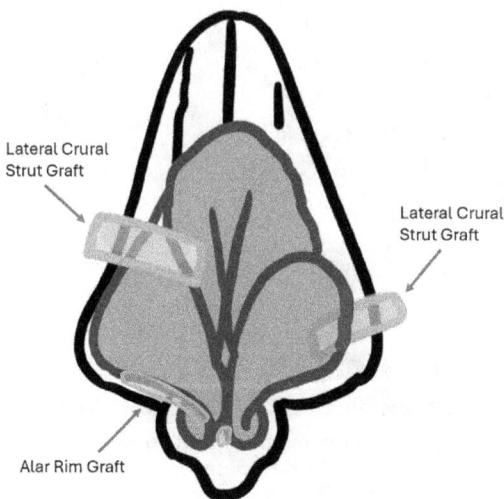

Fig. 12. Structural grafts to external nasal valve support including alar batten graft (placed over the LLC), lateral crural strut graft (placed under the LLC), and alar rim graft (placed along the alar rim).

While there are classic descriptions for unilateral and bilateral cleft lip nasal deformity, the nasal findings can have significant variability along a spectrum of severity. In addition, both congenital and iatrogenic (post-surgical) changes to the nasal architecture make each case unique. Thus, a patient-centered approach to cleft septorhinoplasty is essential (**Fig. 13**).

COMPLICATIONS AND MANAGEMENT

Complications of cleft nasal surgery can be secondary to infections, suture abscess, scarring, residual or recalcitrant septal deviation, recurrent nostril hooding, nasal asymmetry, nasal stenosis resulting in nasal obstruction. Measures to decrease risk of potential complications include (1) meticulous soft tissue dissection and conservation, (2) thoughtful design of incisions to avoid constriction, (3) structural cartilage grafting to provide nasal support, (4) careful presurgical assessment of maxillary bone, dentition, lip scarring and volume, soft tissue thickness, (5) antibiotic

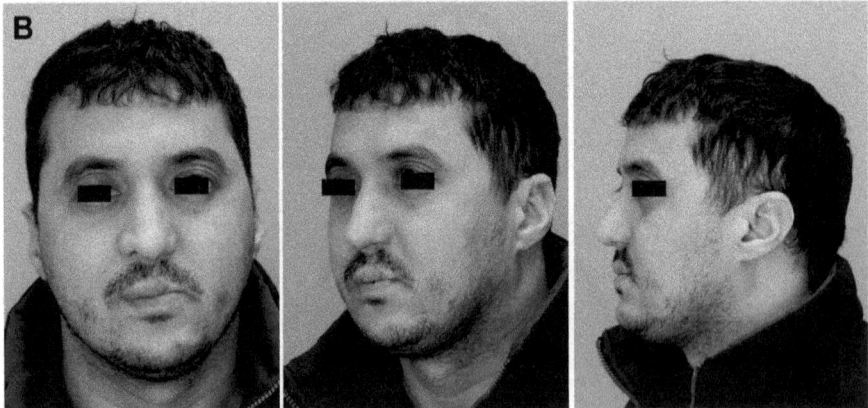

Fig. 13. Example case of a patient with unilateral cleft lip and palate who underwent definitive cleft rhinoplasty. In this patient, the cleft nasal deformity was corrected with extensive septoplasty, bilateral extended spreader grafts, caudal extension graft, bilateral lateral crural strut grafts, tip graft and premaxillary cartilage grafting. Autologous septal and costal cartilage was utilized for the structural grafting. (A) Preoperative in frontal, oblique, profile views. (B) Postoperative in similar views.

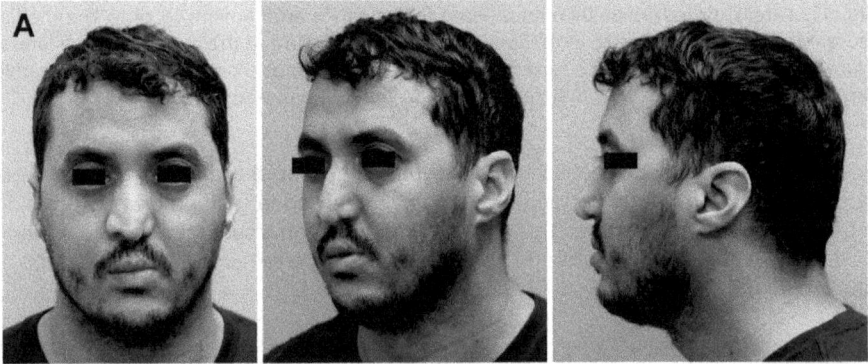

stewardship. As described by rhinoplasty clinical practice guidelines,[48] perioperative antibiotics are utilized for the first 24 hours after surgery unless risk factors are present, such as revision case, significant cartilage grafting or patient immunosuppression.

SUMMARY

Patients with cleft lip nasal deformity need a thorough examination to accurately diagnose and treat the contributions of the nasal valve to nasal airway obstruction. The aim of cleft rhinoplasty is to improve patient quality of life through improving symmetry, proportion of tip projection, and nasal airway function. Reconstruction requires treating the underlying abnormal anatomy with cartilage grafting and suture techniques, but carefully executed alar rim soft tissue adjustments for the alar hooding. The nasal valve treatment will require an assessment of soft tissue symmetry and asymmetric grafts are common making this one of the most challenging rhinoplasty surgeries to plan, execute and manage.

CLINICS CARE POINTS

- When considering the patient complaints regarding nasal obstruction in a typical rhinoplasty practice, many patients have multifactorial nasal complaints. The rhinoplasty surgeon must accurately question the patient about their expectations to best meet their needs, especially when the complexity of rhinoplasty for cleft lip nasal deformities is considered.
- Our approach is to talk with the parents and patients early in their adolescent cleft care cycle. Consultations include gathering patient reported outcome measures including SCHNOS, NOSE, and Cleft-Q, which are helpful for pre and postoperative assessment.
- Effective management of cleft lip and palate patients requires a multidisciplinary approach involving orthodontists, speech therapists, and surgeons, along with long-term follow-up to address evolving anatomic and functional issues.

DISCLOSURE

The authors have nothing to disclose.

REFERENCES

1. Cleft lip & palate | national institute of dental and craniofacial research. (n. d). Available at: https://www.nidcr.nih.gov/health-info/cleft-lip-palate. Accessed June 1, 2024.
2. Leskov A, Nawrocka M, Latkowska M, et al. Can contamination of the environment by dioxins cause craniofacial clefts? Hum Exp Toxicol 2019;38(9):1014–23.
3. Babai A, Irving M. Orofacial clefts: Genetics of cleft lip and palate. Genes 2023; 14(8):1603.
4. Silva K, Messias T, Soares S. Investigation of Flaviviruses emerging in Brazile as etiology factor in nonsyndromic orofacial cleft. J Craniofac Surg 2023;34(3): 987–90.
5. Nasreddine G, El Hajj J, Ghassib-Sabbagh M. Orofacial clefts embryology, classification, epidemiology and genetics. Mutat Res Rev 2021;787:108373.
6. Tahmasebifard N, Briley P, Elis C, et al. Early nutrition among infants admitted to the NICU with cleft lip and palate. Cleft Palate Craniofac J 2023;60(3):299–305.
7. Cuzalina A, Tolomeo P. Challenging rhinoplasty for the cleft lip and palate patient. Oral Maxillofac Surg Clin North Am 2021;33(1):143–59.

8. Naran S, Kirschner R, Schuster L, et al. Simonart's band: its effect on cleft classification and recommendations for standardized nomenclature. Cleft Palate Craniofac J 2017;54(6):726–33.
9. Xue A, Buchanan E, Hollier L. Update in unilateral cleft lip surgery. Plast Reconstr Surg 2021;148(2):262–74.
10. Raymon T, Sitzman T, Allori A, et al. Measuring the unilateral cleft lip nasal deformity: lateral deviation of subnasale is a clinical and morphologic index of unrepaired severity. Cleft Palate Craniofac J 2023;1545–69.
11. Tollefson TT, Shaye D, Durbin-Johnson B, et al. Cleft lip-cleft palate in Zimbabwe: Estimating the distribution of the surgical burden of disease using geographic information systems. Laryngoscope 2015;125(Suppl 1):S1–14.
12. Garri J, O'Leary K, Gabbay J, et al. Improved nasal tip projection in the treatment of bilateral cleft nasal deformity. J Craniofac Surg 2005;16(5):834–9.
13. Surowitz J, Lee M, Most SP, et al. Anterior septal reconstruction for treatment of severe caudal septal deviation: clinical severity and outcomes. Otolaryngol Head Neck Surg 2015;153(1):27–33.
14. Kandathil C, Spataro E, Most SP, et al. Repair of the lateral nasal wall in nasal airway obstruction. Facial Plast Surg 2018;20(4):307–13.
15. Olds C, Sykes J. Cleft rhinoplasty. Clin Plast Surg 2021;49(1):123–36.
16. Englhard A, Wiedmann M, Ledderose G, et al. In vivo imaging of the internal nasal valve during different conditions using optical coherence tomography. Laryngoscope 2018;128(3):105–10.
17. Tollefson TT, Senders CW, Sykes JM. Changing perspectives in cleft lip and palate: from acrylic to allele. Arch Facial Plast Surg 2008;10(6):395–400.
18. Singh G, Moxham B, Langley M, et al. Changes in the composition of glycosaminoglycans during normal palatogenesis in the rat. Arch Oral Biol 1994;39:401–7.
19. Matsuo K, Hirose T. Preoperative nonsurgical overcorrection of cleft lip nasal deformity. Br J Plast Surg 1991;44:5–11.
20. Grayson B, Cutting C, Wood R. Preoperative columella lengthening in bilateral cleft lip and palate. Plast Reconstr Surg 1993;92:1422–3.
21. Grayson B, Cutting C. Presurgical nasoalveolar orthopedic molding in primary correction of the nose, lip, and alveolus of infants born with unilateral and bilateral clefts. Cleft Palate Craniofac J 2001;35:193–8.
22. Abbott MM, Meara JG. Nasoalveolar molding in cleft care: is it efficacious? Plast Reconstr Surg 2012 Sep;130(3):659–66.
23. Aminpour S, Tollefson TT. Recent advances in presurgical molding in cleft lip and palate. Curr Opin Otolaryngol Head Neck Surg 2008;16(4):339–46.
24. Bennum R, Perandones C, Sepliasrsky V, et al. Nonsurgical correction of nasal deformity in unilateral complete cleft lip: a 6-year follow-up. Plast Reconstr Surg 1999;104:616–30.
25. Posnick JC, Thompson B. Modification of the maxillary Le fort I osteotomy in cleft-orthognathic surgery: the bilateral cleft lip and palate deformity. J Oral Maxillofac Surg 1993;51(1):2–11.
26. Converse JM. Corrective surgery of the nasal tip. Laryngoscope 1957;67(1):16–65.
27. Angelos P, Wang T. Revision of the cleft lip nose. Facial Plast Surg 2012;28(4):447–53.
28. Mulliken JB. Primary repair of bilateral cleft lip and nasal deformity. Plast Reconstr Surg 2001;108:181–94.
29. Mulliken JB. Repair of bilateral complete cleft lip and nasal deformity: state of the art. Cleft Palate Craniofac J 2000;37:342–7.

30. Chen PKT, Noordhoff MS. Bilateral cleft lip and nose repair. In: Losee JE, Kirschner RE, editors. Comprehensive cleft care. New York: McGraw-Hill; 2009. p. 331–342.6.
31. Tajima S, Maruyama M. Reverse-U incision for secondary repair of cleft lip nose. Plast Reconstr Surg 1977;60(2):256–326.
32. Yeow VKL, Chen PKT, Chen YR, et al. The use of nasal splints in the primary management of unilateral cleft nasal deformity. Plast Reconstr Surg 1999;103:1347–54.
33. Nguyen DC, Myint JA, Lin AY. The role of postoperative nasal stents in cleft rhinoplasty: A systematic review. Cleft Palate Craniofac J 2023 Jul;28. 10556656231190703. Online ahead of print.
34. Most SP. Trends in functional rhinoplasty. Arch Facial Plast Surg 2008 Nov 3; 10(6):410–3.
35. Cutting C. Cleft lip nasal reconstruction. In: Rees TD, LaTrenta GS, editors. Aesthetic plastic surgery. Philadelphia: Saunders; 1994. p. 497–532.
36. Guryuron B. MOC-PS(SM) CME article: late cleft lip nasal deformity. Plast Reconstr Surg 2008;121(4, Suppl):1–11.
37. Brandon BM, Stepp WH, Basu S, et al. Nasal Airflow Changes With Bioabsorbable Implant, Butterfly, and Spreader Grafts. Laryngoscope 2020;130:E817–23.
38. Clark JM, Cook TA. The 'butterfly' graft in functional secondary rhinoplasty. Laryngoscope 2002;112:1917–25.
39. Gunter JP, Friedman RM. Lateral crural strut graft: technique and clinical applications in rhinoplasty. Plast Reconstr Surg 1997;99:943–52, discussion 953-945.
40. Miller PJ, Dayan SH. The bow-tie mattress suture for the correction of nasal cartilage convexities and concavities. Arch Facial Plast Surg 2010;12:354–6.
41. Stolovitzky P, Sidle DM, Ow RA, et al. A prospective study for treatment of nasal valve collapse due to lateral wall insufficiency: Outcomes using a bioabsorbable implant. Laryngoscope 2018;128:2483–9.
42. Toriumi DM, Josen J, Weinberger M, et al. Use of alar batten grafts for correction of nasal valve collapse. Arch Otolaryngol Head Neck Surg 1997;123:802–8.
43. Hsieh TY, Dedhia R, Tollefson TT. Cleft rhinoplasty: strategies for the multiply operated nose. Facial Plast Surg 2018;34(3):290–7.
44. Kridel RW, Scott BA, Foda HM. The tongue-in-groove technique in septorhinoplasty. A 10-year experience. Arch Facial Plast Surg 1999;1(4):246–56.
45. Foda HM, Kridel RW. Lateral crural steal and lateral crural overlay: an objective evaluation. Arch Otolaryngol Head Neck Surg 1999;125(12):1365–70.
46. Murakami CS, Barrera JE, Most SP. Preserving structural integrity of the alar cartilage in aesthetic rhinoplasty using a cephalic turn-in flap. Arch Facial Plast Surg 2009;11(2):126–8.
47. Ballert JA, Park SS. Functional rhinoplasty: treatment of the dysfunctional nasal sidewall. Facial Plast Surg 2006;22(1):49–54.
48. Ishii LE, Tollefson TT, Basura GJ, et al. Clinical practice guideline: improving nasal form and function after rhinoplasty. Otolaryngol Head Neck Surg 2017; 156(2_suppl):S1–30.

Management of the Nasal Valve in Facial Paralysis

Ciersten A. Burks, MD[a],*, Sofia Lyford-Pike, MD[b,c]

KEYWORDS

- Facial paralysis • Nasal valve compromise • Nasal obstruction • Static suspension

KEY POINTS

- Nasal obstruction is a common, yet often overlooked, symptom associated with flaccid facial paralysis.
- In flaccid facial paralysis, inferomedial displacement of the alar base and lateral nasal sidewall insufficiency contribute to nasal valve compromise.
- Nasal obstruction is corrected in patients with facial paralysis through static suspension of the external nasal valve in a superolateral vector.

INTRODUCTION

Facial paralysis poses significant challenges for patients, affecting not only form, but function. Patients with facial paralysis can present with flaccid paralysis—asymmetry and lack of purposeful movement due to denervation of the facial mimetic muscles— or synkinesis, dysfunction from aberrant reinnervation post-paralysis. In flaccid facial paralysis, there is a loss of tone, increased laxity, and increased asymmetry on the affected side of the face. In the post-paralytic synkinetic face, there is aberrant rein- nervation of the facial mimetic muscles, leading to simultaneous involuntary muscle movement when voluntary facial movement is performed. Patients therefore have the return of movement with the morbidity of synkinesis, hyper-contracture, and limited muscle excursion.

Evaluation of the face in zones is beneficial for assessing the functional conse- quences of facial paralysis.[1] Global facial symmetry, expression, corneal protection, palpebral fissure width, oral competence, and tight platysmal banding are all impor- tant factors to consider. One region that is frequently overlooked is the nasal valve or overall function of the nasal airway.[2,3] Nasal valve compromise, characterized by

[a] Facial Plastic & Reconstructive Surgery, Department of Otolaryngology–Head and Neck Sur- gery, Massachusetts Eye and Ear/Harvard Medical School, Boston, MA, USA; [b] Facial Plastic & Reconstructive Surgery, Department of Otolaryngology–Head and Neck Surgery, University of Minnesota, Minneapolis, MN, USA; [c] Hilger Face Center, 5050 France Avenue South Suite 150, Edina, MN 55410, USA
* Corresponding author. Massachusetts Eye and Ear, 243 Charles Street, Boston, MA 02114.
E-mail address: cburks.ohns@gmail.com

Otolaryngol Clin N Am 58 (2025) 379–386
https://doi.org/10.1016/j.otc.2024.07.018   oto.theclinics.com

static or dynamic collapse or narrowing of the internal and/or external nasal valve, is a common sequelae of facial paralysis. In patients with flaccid paralysis, the lack of muscle tone in the nasal sidewall musculature on the affected side, weight of the cheek and pull from the musculature on the contralateral side (if unilateral disease), and inferomedial displacement of the alar base contribute to nasal valve compromise.[2,4,5] In patients with post-paralytic synkinesis, the lack of coordinated muscle support similarly contributes to nasal valve compromise. Nasal obstruction related to underlying nasal bony and cartilaginous structural deformities may also contribute to nasal valve compromise—frequently addressed by standard cartilage grafting and suture techniques utilized in functional septorhinoplasty. History and physical examination are therefore key in diagnosing and determining strategies to address nasal valve compromise in patients with facial paralysis. This review aims to provide an overview of the etiology and management strategies for nasal valve dysfunction in patients with facial paralysis, encompassing both noninvasive and surgical options.

FOCUSED REVIEW OF ANATOMY AND PHYSIOLOGY

The nasal valve, comprising the internal and external nasal valves, plays a crucial role in regulating airflow and maintaining nasal patency. The anatomic and physiologic details of the internal and external nasal valve are discussed in detail elsewhere (see "Anatomy and Physiology of the Nasal Valves" by Brian Wong in this issue).

Of particular anatomic importance in its relation to patients with flaccid facial paralysis is the nasal musculature. The nasal ala and sidewall are supported significantly by muscle activity acting to stent open those respective regions[5] (**Fig. 1**). The dilator naris muscle and the alar portion of the nasalis muscle insert on the alar and accessory

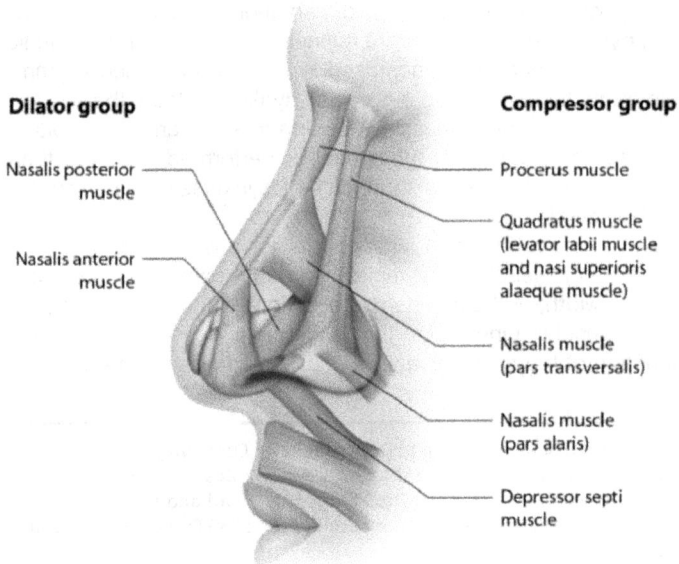

Dilator group

Nasalis posterior muscle

Nasalis anterior muscle

Compressor group

Procerus muscle

Quadratus muscle (levator labii muscle and nasi superioris alaeque muscle)

Nasalis muscle (pars transversalis)

Nasalis muscle (pars alaris)

Depressor septi muscle

Fig. 1. Nasal superficial musculoaponeurotic system. Musculature comprises 2 functional groups: compressor and dilator. (*From* Holger G, et al. "Rhinology in Rhinoplasty." Facial Plastic and Reconstructive Surgery, 4th ed., Thieme, New York, New York, 2016, pp. 1216–1263.)

cartilages respectively, acting to open, strengthen, and provide lateral stability to the lateral nasal sidewall and ala.[5] Additionally, the transverse portion of the nasalis provides stability to the nasal sidewall and valve without direct insertion on the alar cartilages but with action on the overlying soft tissue and skin of the nose.[5]

Evaluation of nasal obstruction in patients with facial paralysis, including assessment for mucosal and structural causes, is unchanged from patients without facial paralysis—a detailed review of preoperative assessment is discussed elsewhere (see James Eng and Jon Robitschek's article, "Preoperative Assessment of the Nasal Valve," in this issue). Cottle and modified cottle maneuvers are fundamental and diagnostic in the evaluation of nasal obstruction. In patients with facial paralysis, lack of tone and function of the nasal musculature contributes to nasal valve compromise and lateral wall insufficiency. Additionally, due to lack of tone in the midface musculature, the alar base is inferomedially displaced on the paretic side (**Fig. 2**).[3] Incomplete muscular support and lack of full muscular excursion contribute to the etiology of nasal obstruction in patients with flaccid facial paralysis and post-paralytic synkinesis, therefore should be a focus of consideration when treating these patients.

NONINVASIVE TREATMENT OPTIONS

It is important to consider all options available to address nasal obstruction in patients with facial paralysis, including noninvasive options. Noninvasive options may be recommended in patients who are poor surgical candidates or those with minimal symptomatology. For patients who demonstrate a mucosal component contributing to nasal obstruction, such as patients with underlying allergic or nonallergic rhinitis,

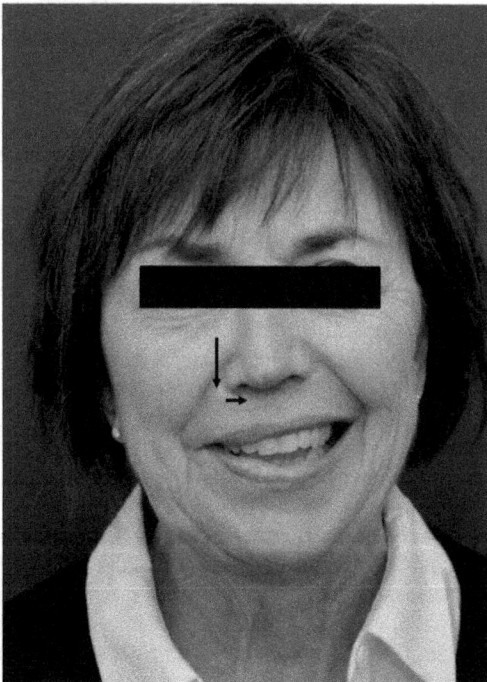

Fig. 2. Patient with right facial paralysis and associated inferomedial displacement of the right alar base (as indicated by the *black arrows*). Patient photo consent obtained.

intranasal steroid spray should be trialed. Ipratropium is often trialed for vasomotor rhinitis. Noninvasive options for patients with structural issues contributing to nasal obstruction include nasal dilators. External nasal dilators, such as the Breathe Right nasal strip (GlaxoSmithKline, Brentford, Middlesex, UK), result in increased nasal valve cross-sectional area, reduced nasal airway resistance, and increased stability of the lateral sidewall.[6] Internal nasal dilators are also effective options for improving the patency of the nasal airway, although use is often limited to nighttime due to unacceptable social appearance with the devices in place and/or discomfort.[7,8] Additionally, one of the primary noninvasive treatment options for nasal valve compromise is the Latera implant (Stryker, Plymouth, Minnesota, USA). This absorbable implant provides structural support to the lateral nasal wall, preventing collapse and improving nasal airflow and can be placed under local anesthesia in an outpatient setting.[9] This option is best indicated for patients who are not surgical candidates and/or have adequate nasal valve aperture at rest but demonstrate dynamic collapse upon inspiration. These noninvasive options often incompletely address significant nasal obstruction or that which has an impact on quality of life.

SURGICAL TREATMENT OPTIONS

Surgical management of nasal valve compromise in patients with facial paralysis often involves reconstructive procedures aimed at restoring nasal support and stability. Standard functional rhinoplasty grafting and suture techniques are common methods to address external nasal valve compromise and lateral wall insufficiency. Alar batten grafts are curvilinear grafts, usually harvested from septal or auricular conchal cartilage, and are placed in a precise pocket at the site of maximal lateral wall insufficiency—which in patients with facial paralysis is caudal to the cephalic edge of the lower lateral crura extending out to the bony pyriform aperture. Lateral crural strut grafts, commonly crafted from septal or auricular conchal cartilage, are placed and sutured deep to the lower lateral crura after freeing the cartilage from the underlying vestibular lining and also extend out to the bony pyriform aperture. Alar batten grafts and lateral crural strut grafts are used to bolster the weakened lateral nasal wall and prevent collapse. Butterfly grafts, for which auricular conchal cartilage is most frequently used, classically span from the caudal border of the nasal bones to the caudal border of the scroll region with lateral extensions along the upper lateral cartilages. However, new modifications have been described (which include decreased length and width of the graft) for improved aesthetic result with similar functional benefit.[10] Butterfly grafts are used to stent open the upper and lower lateral cartilages thus decreasing dynamic movement of the lateral nasal sidewall. Spreader grafts, which are placed in a submucoperichondrial pocket between the upper lateral cartilage and dorsal septum, are the workhorse graft used to increase the aperture of the internal nasal valve.[11] Flaring sutures, or a horizontal mattress from one lower lateral crura to the other spanning the dorsum, can also be used to augment repair of the dysfunctional nasal valve.

The aforementioned techniques, however, do not address the etiology of nasal obstruction that is specific to patients with flaccid facial paralysis.[2] In many patients, there is often nasal valve dysfunction at rest and with dynamic inspiration due to the inferomedial displacement of the alar base and lack of tone of the affected nasal musculature. Thus, non-nasal, but facial approaches are required and most successful.

Suspension of the nasal valve was first described by Paniello[12] in 1996, which redirected the upper lateral crura in a superolateral vector via suture suspension to the inferior orbital rim via transconjunctival incision. This technique was later simplified by Friedman and colleagues[13] in 2004 which described nasal valve suspension to the orbital rim utilizing a bone anchor system with 90% of patients in the study reporting significant improvement in nasal airway breathing. Of note, there were no patients with facial paralysis included in the study by Friedman and colleagues.[13] Other studies, however, have demonstrated significant subjective improvement in nasal airway breathing when nasal suspension techniques have been used in patients with facial paralysis.[4,14,15]

Nasal valve suspension using fascia lata was first introduced by Rose[16] in 2005. After harvest of the fascia lata via serial transverse incisions in the mid and distal lateral thigh, it was secured to the nasal valve and the zygomatic arch in a superolateral vector.[16] Static suspension of the nasal valve in patients with partial or complete facial paralysis demonstrated 80% to 100% subjective improvement in nasal airway breathing.[16] This technique was further modified and postoperative outcomes evaluated by Lindsay and colleagues.[2,3] Fascia lata suspension of the nasal alar accessory cartilages through an incision in the alar crease with fixation to the temporalis fascia was performed.[2,3] All patients reported improvement in their nasal obstruction and demonstrated statistically significant improvement in postoperative Nasal Obstruction Symptom Evaluation scores.[2] Pou and colleagues[17] describe a similar technique of

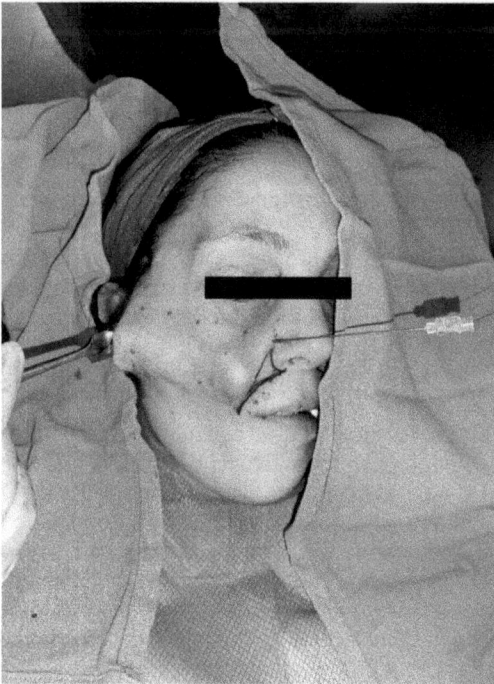

Fig. 3. Intraoperative photo of a patient with right facial paralysis undergoing fascia lata suspension of the nasal valve. A spinal needle is in place at the junction of the lateral nasal wall and nasal ala. This is placed percutaneously and a 4-0 PDS suture (double armed) is passed through the barrel of the needle. The first arm of the suture is passed through the nasal valve. Once all nasal valve sutures have been passed, the second arm of the suture is then passed through the anterior edge of the ribbon of fascia lata. The sutures are then tied down in buried fashion. The posterolateral edge of the fascia lata is then secured to the periosteum of the zygomatic arch, immediately anterior to the root of the helix. Patient photo consent obtained.

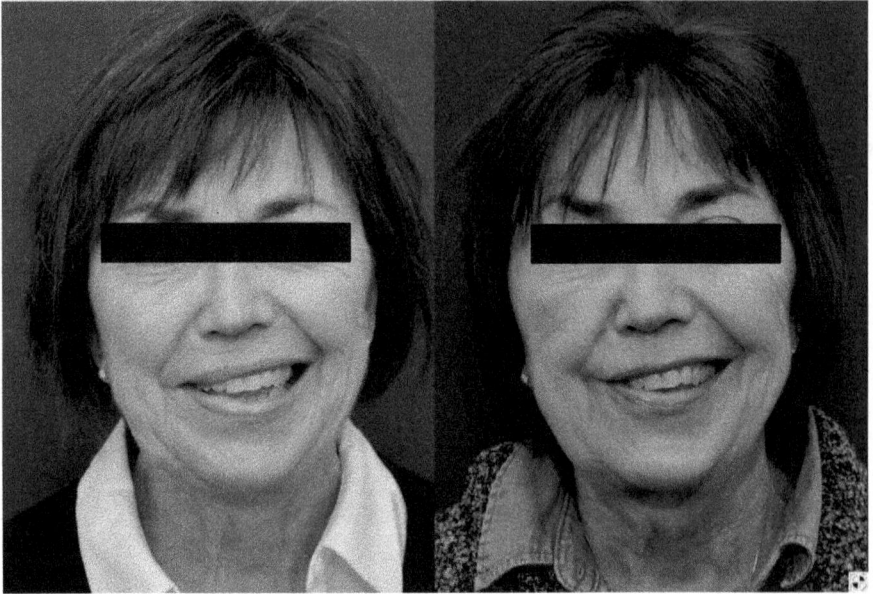

Fig. 4. Preoperative and postoperative photos of a patient with right facial paralysis following fascia lata static suspension of the right external nasal valve. Patient photo consent obtained.

fascia lata suspension; however, a marginal incision is used rather than an incision in the alar crease.

The senior author utilizes a similar technique for static suspension of the nasal valve. The procedure is performed under general anesthesia. The distance from the nasal ala to the helical root is measured. An appropriate length of fascia lata is then harvested from the lateral thigh via two 2 cm horizontal incisions and is then passed off to be placed in saline for later use. Following closure of the incisions, a compression dressing is placed for 1 week.

Attention is then turned to the face where a standard facelift incision is made. In a sub-superficial musculoaponeurotic system (sub-SMAS) plane with care taken to protect the facial nerve branches deep, the dissection (performed without paralytic on board) is carried to the lateral nasal wall and alar cartilage. Subsequently, a ribbon of fascia is designed and used to suspend the lateral nasal wall superolaterally. In a buried fashion with the assistance of passing double-armed sutures through a percutaneous spinal needle, four 4.0 polydioxanone (PDS) sutures are used to secure the fascia lata to the lateral nasal wall (**Fig. 3**). The fascia is then tacked to the periosteum of the zygomatic arch with 4.0 prolene mattress sutures, allowing for superolateral suspension of the nasal valve. The suspension of the nasal valve is typically slightly overcorrected to account for natural relaxation overtime. Once incisions are closed, a compressive dressing is placed for 24 hours. The patient is seen at 1 week postoperatively for suture removal (**Fig. 4**).

COMPLICATIONS

The use of autogenous fascia lata for suspension of the nasal valve is a relatively safe procedure with limited complications. Comparatively, the use of alloplastic materials to suspend the nasal valve, such as expanded polytetrafluoroethylene, is fraught with increased infection rates and concerns related to stretch.[18,19] Complications related to fascia lata harvest include poor wound healing, seroma, infection, hematoma, and pain with walking in the initial perioperative period. In the senior author's experience, these complications are rare, occurring in less than 1% of patients, which is similar to that which has been previously reported.[17]

SUMMARY

Nasal valve compromise in patients with facial paralysis represents an often overlooked clinical challenge. A tailored approach to the evaluation of facial function is required for optimal patient management. While noninvasive interventions may provide symptomatic relief in mild cases and are suitable in patients who are not surgical candidates, surgical intervention to address the etiology of nasal obstruction in the setting of facial paralysis is recommended. Fascia lata suspension of the nasal valve is a safe, effective, and straightforward technique that can be simultaneously combined with various other static or dynamic reanimation procedures.

CLINICS CARE POINTS

- Nasal valve compromise and subsequent nasal obstruction is a common yet overlooked symptom in patients with facial paralysis.

- In facial paralysis, nasal valve compromise is due to lack of tone of the nasal musculature on the affected side and inferomedial displacement of the alar base.

- To address the etiology of nasal valve compromise in patients with facial paralysis, fascia lata static suspension in a superolateral vector with slight overcorrection is recommended.

- Fascia lata static suspension of the nasal valve has demonstrated statistically significant improvement in patient-reported quality-of-life metrics.

DISCLOSURES

The authors have nothing to disclose. No funding.

REFERENCES

1. Hadlock TA, Greenfield LJ, Wernick-Robinson M, et al. Multimodality approach to management of the paralyzed face. Laryngoscope 2006;116(8):1385–9.
2. Lindsay RW, Bhama P, Hohman M, et al. Prospective evaluation of quality-of-life improvement after correction of the alar base in the flaccidly paralyzed face. JAMA Facial Plast Surg 2015;17(2):108–12.
3. Lindsay RW, Smitson C, Edwards C, et al. Correction of the nasal base in the flaccidly paralyzed face: an orphaned problem in facial paralysis. Plast Reconstr Surg 2010;126(4):185e–6e.
4. Soler ZM, Rosenthal E, Wax MK. Immediate nasal valve reconstruction after facial nerve resection. Arch Facial Plast Surg 2008;10(5):312–5.
5. Bruintjes TD, van Olphen AF, Hillen B, et al. A functional anatomic study of the relationship of the nasal cartilages and muscles to the nasal valve area. Laryngoscope 1998;108(7):1025–32.
6. Dinardi RR dAC, Ibiapina Cda C. External nasal dilators: definition, background, and current uses. Int J Gen Med 2014;7:491–504.

7. 2011;25(4):249-251. RBStnafmiaiM-ANCveBRsAJRA.
8. Hellings PW NTGlonbapsbtedAR-.
9. San Nicolo M, Stelter K, Sadick H, et al. A 2-year follow-up study of an absorbable implant to treat nasal valve collapse. Facial Plast Surg 2018;34(5):545–50.
10. Loyo M, Gerecci D, Mace JC, et al. Modifications to the butterfly graft used to treat nasal obstruction and assessment of visibility. JAMA Facial Plast Surg 2016;18(6):436–40.
11. Sheen JH. Spreader graft: a method of reconstructing the roof of the middle nasal vault following rhinoplasty. Plast Reconstr Surg 1984;73(2):230–9.
12. Paniello RC. Nasal valve suspension. An effective treatment for nasal valve collapse. Arch Otolaryngol Head Neck Surg 1996;122(12):1342–6.
13. Friedman M, Ibrahim H, Lee G, et al. A simplified technique for airway correction at the nasal valve area. Otolaryngol Head Neck Surg 2004;131(4):519–24.
14. Nuara MJ, Mobley SR. Nasal valve suspension revisited. Laryngoscope 2007; 117(12):2100–6.
15. Alex JC, Nguyen DB. Multivectored suture suspension: a minimally invasive technique for reanimation of the paralyzed face. Arch Facial Plast Surg 2004;6(3): 197–201.
16. Rose EH. Autogenous fascia lata grafts: clinical applications in reanimation of the totally or partially paralyzed face. Plast Reconstr Surg 2005;116(1):20–32 [discussion 33-25].
17. Pou JD, Patel KG, Oyer SL. Treating nasal valve collapse in facial paralysis: what i do differently. Facial Plast Surg Clin North Am 2021;29(3):439–45.
18. Constantinides M, Galli SK, Miller PJ. Complications of static facial suspensions with expanded polytetrafluoroethylene (ePTFE). Laryngoscope 2001;111(12): 2114–21.
19. Alam D. Rehabilitation of long-standing facial nerve paralysis with percutaneous suture-based slings. Arch Facial Plast Surg 2007;9(3):205–9.

Nasal Valve Considerations in Mohs Reconstruction

Daniel Suarez, MD[a], Hailey Juszczak, MD[a], Sydney C. Butts, MD[b],*

KEYWORDS

- Mohs reconstruction • Nasal lining • Alar subunit • Secondary intention healing
- Cartilage graft • Nasal valve insufficiency

KEY POINTS

- Mohs defects associated with the highest risk of nasal valve compromise involve the alar and sidewall subunits.
- Restoration of nasal lining in full thickness defects is essential to the prevention of scar tissue formation and nasal valve narrowing.
- Cartilage grafting is often needed in both small and large Mohs defects to prevent nasal valve collapse.

INTRODUCTION

The nose is the most frequently involved head and neck site affected by non-melanoma skin cancer.[1–3] Mohs micrographic surgery (MMS) offers high rates of cancer clearance while conserving normal tissue central to limiting impacts on nasal form and function.[4,5] Even when MMS is employed, skin, cartilage, supporting ligaments, nasal muscles, or the nasal lining that support the nasal airway may be excised, weakening the external or internal nasal valves—the major regulators of nasal airflow. The subunits of the nose described by Burget and Menick define its unique external contours and distinct regions shaped by the underlying cartilaginous or bony framework (**Fig. 1**A, B).[6,7] The subunits that primarily support and correspond to the location of the nasal valves include the ala and lateral sidewalls. These have been deemed high-risk zones given the potential impact of surgery of these subunits on airway function.[8] In several reports of nasal reconstruction after MMS, the ala is the most frequent location of skin cancer with 35% to 41% of cases in reports requiring reconstruction of the alar subunit.[3,9,10] As such, nasal obstruction is a significant potential risk that may develop after excision of nasal skin cancers.

[a] Department of Otolaryngology, SUNY Downstate Health Sciences University, Brooklyn, NY, USA; [b] Facial Plastic and Reconstructive Surgery, SUNY Downstate Health Sciences University, 450 Clarkson Avenue, Brooklyn, NY 11201, USA
* Corresponding author.
E-mail address: sydney.butts@downstate.edu

Otolaryngol Clin N Am 58 (2025) 387–398
https://doi.org/10.1016/j.otc.2024.08.013
0030-6665/25/© 2024 Elsevier Inc. All rights are reserved, including those for text and data mining, AI training, and similar technologies.

A   B

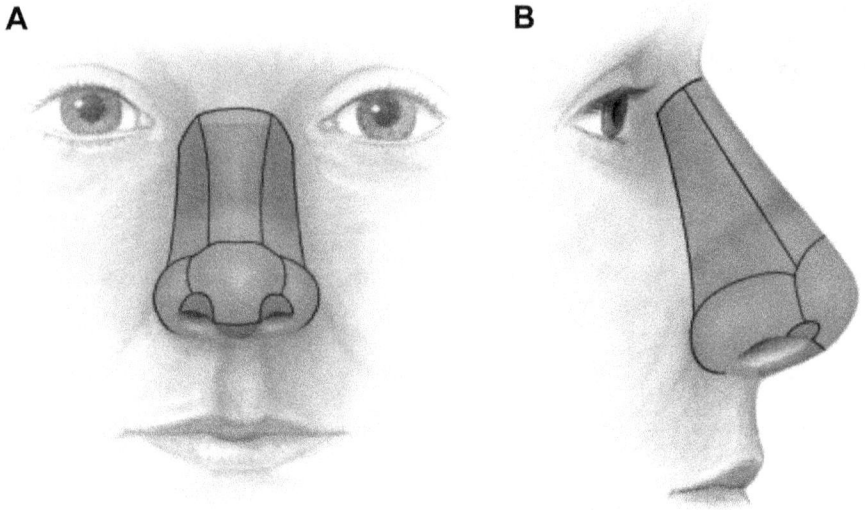

Fig. 1. (*A, B*) Aesthetic subunits of the nose. Blue areas represent thin-skinned regions and red represent thicker-skinned regions. Three central subunits include the columella, tip, and dorsum. The paired subunits include the soft tissue facets, alar, and sidewall subunits. (*Reprinted with permission from* Baker SR. Reconstruction of the Nose. In: Baker SR, editor. Local Flaps in Facial Reconstruction. 3 ed. Philadelphia, PA: Elsevier Saunders; 2014. p. 415–80.)

Given the frequency of skin cancers involving subunits of the nose that support the nasal valves, there has been increasing attention to the prevention and correction of nasal valve compromise as a complication of MMS and reconstruction of resulting nasal defects (**Table 1**).[8–14] Maintenance of airway patency is a key element of the final treatment goals and more frequently reported among outcomes of reconstructive procedures (see **Table 1**).

The objective of this article is to explore the ways in which nasal valve patency is at risk in patients undergoing reconstruction of Mohs surgical defects. We will review measures the reconstructive surgeon can take to prevent and treat nasal valve compromise. Ideally, the valve area is restored at the initial reconstructive setting, but patients may also present after initial repair with airway obstruction when valve compromise has developed secondarily. Approaches to reconstruction will be reviewed in the context of evidence-based recommendations supported by outcomes data.

Nasal Valve Anatomy

Nasal airflow is controlled at the internal and external nasal valves. The internal nasal valve is the area of greatest resistance to airflow along the nasal airway and is bound by the septum medially, the upper lateral cartilage laterally (creating an angle that ideally measures 10–15°), the head of inferior turbinate, and the nasal floor.[15] The external nasal valve is located at the entrance of the nasal airway surrounding the nasal vestibule and bound by the caudal septum and the medial crura of the lower lateral cartilages medially and the alar sidewall laterally (**Fig. 2**).[16] Most describes the concept of lateral wall insufficiency (LWI), referring to dynamic collapse in which nasal obstruction is exacerbated by airflow according to the Bernoulli effect, during which increases in air speed result in the development of negative pressure, collapsing the lateral nasal

Table 1
Case series reporting airway outcomes after Mohs reconstruction

Author and year	Nasal Subunit	Patients with Nasal Obstruction (%)	Reconstructive Approach	Cartilage Grafting
Reynolds & Gordin,[10] 1998	N = 38 "at risk" site Ala, tip, and sidewall that cross or come within 1 mm of alar groove	N = 8(21.9%)	Local flaps, paramedian forehead flap with and without cartilage grafting	1/8 (12.5%) symptomatic patients
Woodard & Park,[3] 2011	All subsites (n = 213) <1.5 cm • Ala = 84(39.4%) • Sidewall = 15(7%)	N = 3 (1.4% overall) 3% rate among ala and sidewall subunits	Several options depending on site and size: Full thickness skin graft, composite graft, local flaps, or melolabial flap	• 86% of alar sites • 6.7% of sidewall sites
Yong and colleagues,[9] 2014	All subsites (n = 315) 1.5–2.5 cm • Ala = 85(27%) • Sidewall = 17(5.4%)	• 1.3% overall • 3.3% of alar and sidewall subunits	• Ala: Composite grafts, melolabial flaps • Sidewall: Forehead flaps, rotation flaps	• 87.1% of alar sites • 30.8% of sidewall sites
Akdagli et al,[12] 2015	Ala (n = 7) • within 5 mm of margin <1.5 cm	0%	Bilobed Flap	100%
Ezzat & Liu,[11] 2017	Ala and sidewall(N = 38) • Structural support N = 19 • No Structural support N = 19	N= (7.8% overall) • Support group = 0% • Non-support group = 3/19 (16%)	Several options depending on site and size: full thickness skin graft, local flaps, or paramedian forehead flap	50% (graft or suture suspension)

Anatomy of the Nose

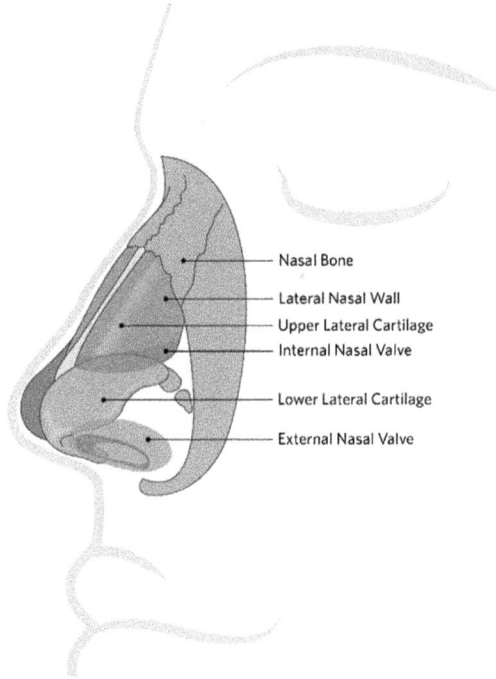

Fig. 2. The internal and external nasal valves. (*Reprinted with permission from* Ishii LE, Toll-efson TT, Basura GJ, Rosenfeld RM, Abramson PJ, Chaiet SR, et al. Clinical Practice Guideline: Improving Nasal Form and Function after Rhinoplasty. Otolaryngol Head Neck Surg. 2017;156(2_suppl):S1-s30.)

wall.[17] LWI is described as occurring at 2 zones—zone 1 at the caudal end of the upper lateral cartilage and zone 2 at the level of the ala.[17] Poiseuille's law describes how resistance to laminar flow of a fluid or gas is inversely proportional to radius of that tube to the fourth power. As relates to the nasal airway, even small changes in the radius of the valve areas can have profound effects on nasal airflow.[7]

Nasal Subunits, Nasal Valves, and Airway Support

The subunits that primarily support the nasal valves include the ala and lateral side-walls.[8] The alar subunit corresponds to the region of the external valve or zone 2 described previously. The alar skin is thick and sebaceous with underlying fibrofatty tissue allowing it to resist collapse. The lateral extent of the alar subunit lacks cartilage as the lateral crus angles toward the pyriform rim (see **Fig. 2**). Challenges in recon-struction of the ala relate to its mobile free edge, which can be superiorly displaced by the forces of secondary movement after flap inset, medially compressed by flap bulk, or pulled medially by factors causing scar contracture at its deep surface. The alar crease is the concave junction between the alar and sidewall subunits. Underlying this crease is the region of the scroll where the cephalic lateral crus and the caudal up-per lateral cartilage overlap (see **Fig. 2**). The alar crease and caudal sidewall regions correspond to the lateral internal valve area (zone 1). Narrowing at this level will decrease the valve angle resulting in a marked rise in airway resistance as defined by Poiseuille's law. The tip, soft tissues facets, and columellar subunits also contribute to the nostril rim and the airway impact of reconstruction of these regions must also be considered. Rates of airway obstruction following Mohs reconstruction of the alar and sidewall subunits vary by case series, ranging from 0% to 21% (see **Table 1**).[3,9–12]

Patient Evaluation

Nasal obstruction after MMS and nasal reconstruction may worsen a pre-existing problem or present as a new complaint. Patient history should document any symptoms of chronic nasal obstruction and any prior nasal procedures.[18] The use of intranasal sprays or other medications for rhinitis must be noted. Smoking history is discussed as current smoking will impact the viability of any local or regional flaps and any substance abuse, especially intranasal, is documented for the same reasons.

The physical examination should note the status of the nasal turbinates, any septal deviation, or pathology and the presence of any abnormal intranasal masses that would result in static narrowing of the nasal airway. Assessment of dynamic collapse is determined by inspection of changes in airway caliber during nasal inspiration looking for evidence of nostril collapse, pinching in the supra-alar region or medial displacement of the lateral nasal wall (zones 1 or 2) seen intranasally.[15] The Cottle maneuver is traditionally performed by laterally displacing the cheek soft tissues adjacent to the nasal sidewall to open the valve area, which will offer subjective relief in symptomatic patients. The modified Cottle maneuver is performed by placing a wax curette against the nasal sidewall to resist collapse that occurs during normal or deep inspiration. The grading of dynamic collapse is performed prior to Mohs excision to establish any baseline airway narrowing. It is also reported during the assessment of patients with post-procedure symptoms of obstruction. Nasal endoscopy will provide a comprehensive evaluation of the nasal airway and is especially important to view areas not well-visualized with anterior rhinoscopy alone. The completion of patient-reported outcomes (PROs) questionnaires will stratify the severity of any pre or post-procedure obstructive symptoms. The Nasal Obstruction Symptom Evaluation (NOSE) scale is a validated 5-item questionnaire that calculates a baseline level of severity of nasal obstruction and is sensitive to change after intervention.[19] More recently, the Nasal Appearance and Function Evaluation Questionnaire was validated to determine patient satisfaction with form and airway function after nasal reconstruction.[20,21] For patients undergoing reconstruction of the subunits that support the nasal valves, a patient-centered assessment of obstruction is important in the reporting of outcomes.

RECONSTRUCTIVE APPROACHES-VALVE PRESERVING

The primary goal of Mohs reconstruction is to replace all resected tissues, which may require reconstitution of nasal lining, cartilaginous/osseous framework, and overlying skin. Preservation of valve support, however, may also require strengthening the valve by placing additional structural support along key areas including the free edge of the ala, which lacks cartilage or regions of the sidewall that support the internal valve. Not only are these maneuvers preventive, they are often necessary to reconstituting contour by adding volume to resected areas that are deep or full thickness.[3,22] We will review specific causes of nasal valve compromise in the reconstructive setting, highlighting concepts of valve preservation with case examples.

Complete Restoration of Resected Lining, Cartilage, and Skin

The size and depth of the resected skin cancer will dictate which grafts or flaps are required for skin cover. Small excisions of 1.5 cm or less are often amenable to skin graft or local flap reconstruction. Interpolated flaps from the cheek or forehead are recruited for intermediate to large size skin defects.[7] Cartilage grafts are harvested from the nasal septum, ear, or rib to replicate the shape of the framework that must be replaced.[23] In a report of outcomes of the reconstruction of intermediate sized (1.5–2.5 cm) nasal defects, alar defects were the most frequent subunit associated full thickness tissue resection.[9] Nasal lining serves as the foundation for nasal reconstruction with scar contraction and airway narrowing resulting from incomplete restoration.[24] Intranasal sources of grafting include the bipedicled vestibular skin flap and mucoperichondrial flaps harvested from the septum. Extranasal sources of lining include the pericranial flap, folded paramedian forehead flap, or facial artery myomucosal flap for larger lining deficits.[24]

Specific Indications for Secondary Intention Healing

Case

MMS of a basal cell carcinoma resulted in a defect of the lateral aspect of the alar crease and caudal sidewall measuring 7 mm x 7 mm (**Fig. 3**A–C). The patient had no pre-existing nasal obstructive symptoms. Of the reconstructive options presented, the patient opted for healing by secondary intention. Significant decrease in the surface area of the defect occurred at 2 weeks and complete closure and epithelialization occured by 6 weeks follow-up with no impact on the position of the alar rim. The patient reported no symptoms of obstruction (see **Fig. 3**).

Secondary intention healing can be applied as a reconstructive option in the nose but in the high-risk zones, several criteria must be met. Healing by secondary intention will result in contraction and ultimate epithelialization of the wound over a period of weeks.[22,25] Advantages are avoidance of scars from local or regional flap elevation, elimination of patient downtime, ease of wound care, minimal pain, and very low rates of infection.[22] Wounds located on concave surfaces such as the alar crease and the sidewalls near the medial canthus are best suited for secondary intention healing as a single modality approach.[22,26] Shallow, small (ideally 1 cm or less) resected areas of the concave alar crease can heal well (see **Fig. 3**) but patients must be informed of the risk of nasal obstruction even when these ideal conditions are met. In their series of 38 patients, Reynolds reported the airway status of 8 patients with small Mohs defects either crossing the alar groove(4 patients, mean defect area = 54 mm^2) or adjacent to it (4 patients, mean defect area = 49.8 mm^2) that were

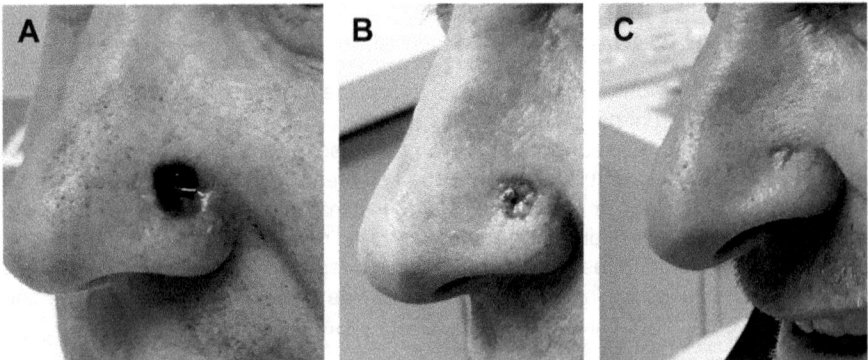

Fig. 3. (A) Secondary intention healing-7x7mm alar crease defect. (B) Two weeks after secondary intention healing (C) Six weeks after healing, the wound is completely healed, with no impact on the alar rim and no obstruction.

allowed to heal by secondary intention.[10] All defects were shallow (none deeper than the muscle layer) and no patient developed nasal valve insufficiency. In addition to its concave contour, the distance of the alar crease from the free edge of the ala minimizes the risk of alar rim retraction (see **Fig. 3**). Larger, more complex defects involving multiple nasal layers and/or subsites are not good candidates for healing by secondary intention nor is the convex alar subunit, which can potentially lead to contracture, landmark distortion, and airway narrowing.[22]

Non-anatomic Cartilage Grafting/Structural Support of The Nasal Valve

Case example

The patient had MMS of a basal cell carcinoma involving greater than 50% of the left alar subunit. The lining and the lateral crus were intact. The remainder of the subunit skin was excised and reconstructed with a melolabial island subcutaneous pedicle flap. A cartilage graft harvested from the conchal bowl was placed along the length of the subunit (**Fig. 4A–C**).

Replacement of resected cartilage is a clear indication for cartilage grafting. The new construct may also require cartilage grafting in areas of the nose placed to provide additional reinforcement and structural support of the external and internal valves. The lateral aspect of the alar subunit does not contain cartilage, but cartilage is often added to this location as a strut when the entirety of the alar subunit is being replaced with an interpolated flap (see **Fig. 4**). Placement of cartilage struts along the alar free margin ("non-anatomic") will prevent valve collapse and alar retraction when reconstructing large or total alar defects.

There is also a role for cartilage grafting in the prevention of alar retraction and valve collapse in smaller alar defects reconstructed with an interpolated flap, local flap, or skin graft.[3,11,12] Akdagli and colleagues reported results of bilobed flap reconstruction of alar skin defects all less than 1.5 cm in diameter and all within 5 mm of the alar rim.[12] All sites had an auricular cartilage graft placed at the rim deep to the bilobed flap. No patients developed rim retraction or had signs or symptoms of external valve collapse. By adding cartilage support, the use of the bilobed flap for an alar defect at high risk for retraction (close to the nostril margin) was made safer. Similarly, Ezzat and Liu, in a series reporting airway outcomes in alar and sidewall defects, found no valve compromise in patients who had cartilage grafting or suture suspension of the nasal ala or sidewall.[11] Of patients who did not have cartilage or suture support placed, 15.7% developed valve collapse. For lesions greater than 1.2 cm, the rate of airway

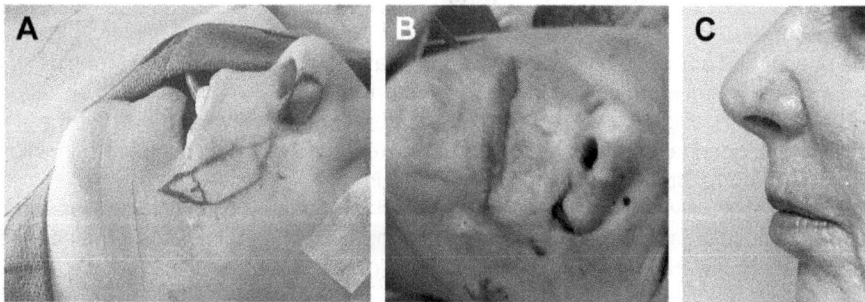

Fig. 4. Graft reconstruction-alar subunit. (*A*) Reconstruction of the entire left alar subunit included placement of an auricular cartilage graft in a "non-anatomic" location along the free-edge, extending along its length. (*B, C*) Melolabial subcutaneous island pedicle flap was placed for skin cover, with good contour and valve patency.

compromise increased to 21% of the group without structural support. In Woodard's report of Mohs defects 1.5 cm or smaller, cartilage grafts were used in 86% of alar defects and 6.7% of sidewall defects with a low, 3% rate of nasal obstruction.[3] (see **Table 1**)

Skin grafts or local flaps alone may restore form and maintain valve function for small or superficial alar lesions.[11,22,27] For small alar defects that do not require replacement of the entire subunit, especially deep lesions near the nostril rim comes the risk of mobility of the nostril margin and compression of the external valve that requires caution when using local flaps as stated previously. For this reason, reconstructive options that do not result in negative vectors of pull are utilized, including the single-staged melolabial flap or the 2-staged melolabial interpolated flap.[9] Another option is the placement of a cartilage graft under a full thickness skin graft (FTSG).[22,28] While skin grafts are associated with some contraction that could distort the ala and narrow the valve, the addition of cartilage can stabilize the ala to prevent these complications. Thin cartilage grafts at the rim are placed and developed to be long enough to secure medially and laterally under intact skin allowing enough exposure of the deep wound bed for contact by the FTSG.[22,27,28] Zopf reported a series of 20 patients using this technique in which all grafts survived with no reports of nasal obstruction.[28] Composite cartilage grafts can also be employed for small alar defects to restore volume, contour, and add rigidity to prevent valve collapse.[3,22]

Suspension suturing techniques to counteract nasal valve collapse have shown benefits in preventing postoperative nasal obstruction. Original concepts of suture suspension of the valves include the technique described by Paniello to suspend the soft tissue of the sidewall to the maxilla at the inferior orbital rim and the upper lateral cartilage flaring suture described by Park.[29,30] Various other suspension suture techniques have since been described. Miladi and colleagues describe a 3-point suturing technique to tent up the deep tissue overlying the internal nasal valve and a modified suspension suture that suspends the fibrofatty tissue of the nasal sidewall to the maxillary periosteum.[31] In their study of 35 patients repaired with either the 3-point suture or Miladi's modified suspension suture, 34 patients did not develop postoperative nasal obstruction. Similarly, Wang and colleagues describe a technique for suspending fibrofatty tissue over the internal nasal valve at the time of resection by anchoring it to the maxillary periosteum at an angle of 15° superiorly and about 2 cm laterally.[32]

RECONSTRUCTIVE APPROACHES-CORRECTING VALVE NARROWING
Alar Retraction/External Valve Narrowing

Case example
The patient had a bilobed flap reconstruction of a right nasal tip (<1.5 cm) Mohs defect close to the nostril margin. Secondary movement of the alar rim resulted in elevation and nasal congestion. To strengthen the rim and external valve and correct the rim retraction, a conchal cartilage graft was harvested and placed through a rim incision (**Fig. 5**A–C) correcting the elevation of the alar rim.

In this case, valve narrowing was corrected secondarily with cartilage grafting. Composite cartilage grafting may need to be employed in certain cases if the needed additional rim lowering results in a gap in lining of the vestibular skin.

Scar Contracture Causing Internal Valve Narrowing

Case example
The patient presented with the chief complaint of right nasal obstruction following Mohs excision several years before at another facility. Examination showed a

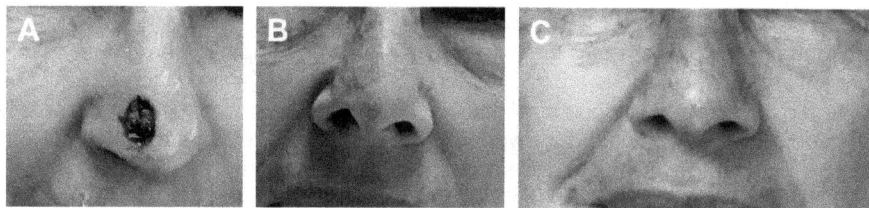

Fig. 5. Alar Retraction (*A*) A bilobed flap was used to reconstruct a caudal nasal tip defect close to the nostril edge. The patient subsequently developed nostril elevation and some nasal congestion. (*B, C*) Auricular cartilage graft was place to correct the secondary nostril retraction.

depressed scar extending from the right nasal tip to the right sidewall in the area of the alar crease (**Fig. 6**A, B). Cottle maneuver was positive on the right. Examination also revealed a deviated septum to the right. The patient opted for septoplasty but declined procedures to revise the scar or reconstruct the internal valve.

Minor notching of the alar rim may be amenable to Z-plasty techniques to lengthen the scar. In cases of external or internal nasal valve collapse, rhinoplasty techniques may be required for placement of spreader grafts (internal nasal valve) or alar batten or lateral crural strut grafts (external nasal valve collapse).[33–35] Composite grafting of depressed/contracted areas of the internal or external valve areas can expand the scarred region while simultaneously adding a cartilage strut to resist the forces of collapse.[22,36] Missing lining must be replaced with local or regional flaps and the overlying skin cover may also need to be expanded if contraction at this level has occurred. Flap bulk may narrow the valve areas due to mass effect. It may be imprudent to thin a flap at initial inset in at risk groups, especially smokers, requiring later flap debulking.[13]

DISCUSSION

Nasal valve obstruction after MMS may be new in onset or worsen pre-existing nasal obstruction. The discussion of this possible complication is important to have with patients as part of the risk/benefit conversation. Appreciation of the impact of reconstruction on the nasal valves has resulted in a growing number of reports focusing on airway

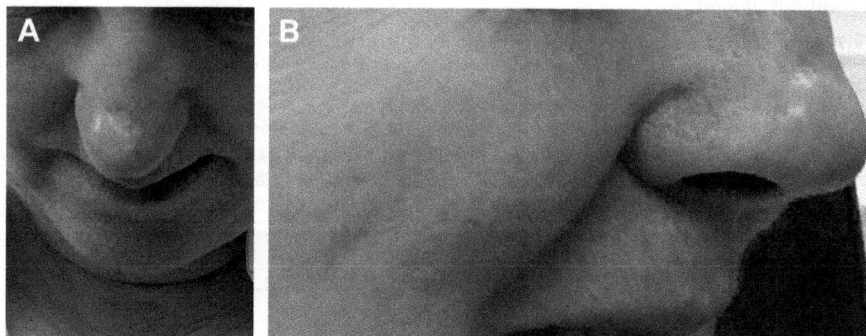

Fig. 6. (*A, B*) Nasal valve narrowing after tip/sidewall scarring-The patient had local flap reconstruction years before and presented with right nasal obstruction. A depressed scar is seen extending along the flap incision to the alar crease.

outcomes and reviews of ways to avoid this complication (see **Table 1**).[3] The elevation and rotation of flaps may result in weakening of nasal valve support. The ligaments that suspend the lateral crus and the upper lateral cartilage to the pyriform aperture may be disrupted during MMS or local flap elevation.[11,37] Nasal dilator muscles may be partially resected during MMS and further weakened during flap development including excision of additional tissue that is performed to prepare the subunit for reconstruction.

Evaluation of the nasal airway that documents possible sites of obstruction, patient symptoms, and utilizes PROs measures should be a part of the patient evaluation before and after treatment.

Based on the current evidence, several valve preserving approaches should be utilized. Outcomes reports show that high rates of cartilage grafting (in addition to replacement of resected cartilage) of alar defects including small and medium sized defects prevents nasal obstruction and valve compromise. Studies with low rates of post-operative nasal obstruction reported grafting of the ala in 86% to 100% of cases.[3,9,11,12] Menick recommended cartilage grafting for any alar defect with at least 30% of the skin surface area resected.[6] Suture suspension techniques have also been utilized in some reports as an alternative to cartilage grafting.

While a low morbidity technique, secondary intention healing can be used for small and shallow alar crease defects. Skin grafting should also be applied for shallow or smaller lesions. When skin grafting is used for larger areas or close to the alar rim, use a composite graft (depending on size of defect), or an FTSG with an alar rim graft.

The prevention of valve compromise is preferable to secondary correction. Valve correction techniques include flap debulking, composite cartilage grafting to expand skin and add cartilage support, nasal lining revision with or without cartilage grafting, and cartilage grafting to correct alar rim retraction. Other rhinoplasty techniques may be required to reconstruct the valves including placement of spreader grafts, correction of septal deviation, or application of batten grafts.

CLINICS CARE POINTS

Several evidence-based recommendations are suggested based on outcomes reports that had low rates of nasal obstruction.

- Sidewall or alar defects greater than 1.2 cm reinforced with cartilage or suture suspension have very low rates of obstruction.[11] No patients who had cartilage or suture suspension in the cohort reported by Ezzat and Liu developed airway obstruction, while 21% of patients without support did.

- Alar defects within 5 mm of the alar margin reconstructed with a bilobed flap should have an alar rim graft placed. Alar retraction, notching, and external valve collapse were avoided with this approach.[12]

- Compared to small (<1.5 cm) defects of the sidewall, medium sized defects (1.5–2.5 cm) require cartilage grafting more frequently to avoid nasal valve compromise. Woodard reported results of sidewall reconstruction (1.5 cm or smaller).[3] Cartilage grafting was placed in 6.7% of cases. For sidewall defects 1.5 cm to 2.5 cm in size, Yong and colleagues used cartilage grafting in 30% of cases[9] suggesting that larger sidewall defects require cartilage grafting more often to prevent valve compromise.

REFERENCES

1. Derebasinlioglu H. Distribution of skin cancers of the head and neck according to anatomical subunit. Eur Arch Oto-Rhino-Laryngol 2022;279(3):1461–6.

2. Kristo B, Krzelj Vidovic I, Krzelj A, et al. Non-melanoma skin carcinomas of the head and neck. Psychiatr Danub 2021;33(Suppl 13):308–13.

3. Woodard CR, Park SS. Reconstruction of nasal defects 1.5 cm or smaller. Arch Facial Plast Surg 2011;13(2):97–102.

4. National Comprehensive Cancer Network. Basal cell skin cancer (version 3.2024). Available at: https://www.nccn.org/professionals/physician_gls/pdf/nmsc.pdf. Accessed August 4, 2024.

5. National Comprehensive Cancer Network. Squamous cell skin cancer (version 1.2024). Available at: https://www.nccn.org/professionals/physician_gls/pdf/squamous.pdf. Accessed August 4, 2024.

6. Burget GC, Menick FJ. The subunit principle in nasal reconstruction. Plast Reconstr Surg 1985;76(2):239–47.

7. Baker SR. Reconstruction of the nose. In: Baker SR, editor. Local flaps in facial reconstruction. 3rd edition. Philadelphia, PA: Elsevier Saunders; 2014. p. 415–80.

8. Robinson JK, Burget GC. Nasal valve malfunction resulting from resection of cancer. Arch Otolaryngol Head Neck Surg 1990;116(12):1419–24.

9. Yong JS, Christophel JJ, Park SS. Repair of intermediate-size nasal defects: a working algorithm. JAMA Otolaryngol Head Neck Surg 2014;140(11):1027–33.

10. Reynolds MB, Gourdin FW. Nasal valve dysfunction after Mohs surgery for skin cancer of the nose. Dermatol Surg 1998;24(9):1011–7.

11. Ezzat WH, Liu SW. Comparative study of functional nasal reconstruction using structural reinforcement. JAMA Facial Plast Surg 2017;19(4):318–22.

12. Akdagli S, Lee MK, Most SP. Bilobe flap with auricular cartilage graft for nasal alar reconstruction. Am J Otolaryngol 2015;36(3):479–83.

13. Rudy SF, Moyer JS. Nasal obstruction after Mohs surgery: prevention and correction. Facial Plast Surg 2020;36(1):84–90.

14. Barbosa NS, Baum CL, Arpey CJ. Nasal valve insufficiency in dermatologic surgery. Dermatol Surg 2020;46(7):904–11.

15. Gassner HG, Sherris DA, Friedman O. Rhinology in rhinoplasty. In: Papel ID, Frodel JL, Holt GR, et al, editors. Facial plastic and reconstructive surgery. 4th edition. New York: Thieme Medical Publishers, Inc.; 2016. p. 385–400.

16. Ishii LE, Tollefson TT, Basura GJ, et al. Clinical practice guideline: improving nasal form and function after rhinoplasty. Otolaryngol Head Neck Surg 2017;156(2_suppl): S1–30.

17. Tsao GJ, Fijalkowski N, Most SP. Validation of a grading system for lateral nasal wall insufficiency. Allergy Rhinol (Providence) 2013;4(2):e66–8.

18. Valero A, Navarro AM, Del Cuvillo A, et al. Position paper on nasal obstruction: evaluation and treatment. J Investig Allergol Clin Immunol 2018;28(2):67–90.

19. Stewart MG, Witsell DL, Smith TL, et al. Development and validation of the nasal obstruction symptom evaluation (NOSE) scale. Otolaryngol Head Neck Surg 2004;130(2):157–63.

20. Veerabagu SA, Perz AM, Lukowiak TM, et al. Patient-reported nasal function and appearance after interpolation flap repair following skin cancer resection: a multicenter prospective cohort study. Facial Plast Surg Aesthet Med 2023;25(2): 113–8.

21. Moolenburgh SE, Mureau MA, Duivenvoorden HJ, et al. Validation of a questionnaire assessing patient's aesthetic and functional outcome after nasal reconstruction: the patient NAFEQ-score. J Plast Reconstr Aesthetic Surg 2009;62(5):656–62.

22. Gruber PJ, Walen S, Massa ST, et al. Using grafts and granulation to improve nasal repair. Facial Plast Surg 2017;33(1):20–6.

23. Constantine FC, Lee MR, Sinno S, et al. Reconstruction of the nasal soft triangle subunit. Plast Reconstr Surg 2013;131(5):1045–50.
24. Graf AE, Kaplowitz L, Butts SC. Nasal lining reconstruction with loco-regional flaps. Facial Plast Surg Clin North Am 2024;32(2):229–37.
25. Fisher E, Frodel JL. Wound healing. In: Papel ID, Frodel JL, Holt GR, et al, editors. Facial plastic and reconstructive surgery. 4th edition. New York: Thieme Medical Publishers, Inc.; 2016. p. 15–25.
26. Zitelli JA. Wound healing by secondary intention. A cosmetic appraisal. J Am Acad Dermatol 1983;9(3):407–15.
27. Tan E, Mortimer N, Salmon P. Full-thickness skin grafts for surgical defects of the nasal ala - a comprehensive review, approach and outcomes of 186 cases over 9 years. Br J Dermatol 2014;170(5):1106–13.
28. Zopf DA, Iams W, Kim JC, et al. Full-thickness skin graft overlying a separately harvested auricular cartilage graft for nasal alar reconstruction. JAMA Facial Plast Surg 2013;15(2):131–4.
29. Paniello RC. Nasal valve suspension. An effective treatment for nasal valve collapse. Arch Otolaryngol Head Neck Surg 1996;122(12):1342–6.
30. Park SS. The flaring suture to augment the repair of the dysfunctional nasal valve. Plast Reconstr Surg 1998;101(4):1120–2.
31. Miladi A, McGowan JW, Donnelly HB. Two suturing techniques for the prevention and treatment of nasal valve collapse after Mohs micrographic surgery. Dermatol Surg 2017;43(3):407–14.
32. Wang JH, Finn D, Cummins DL. Suspension suture technique to prevent nasal valve collapse after Mohs micrographic surgery. Dermatol Surg 2014;40(3):345–7.
33. Gruber RP, Park E, Newman J, et al. The spreader flap in primary rhinoplasty. Plast Reconstr Surg 2007;119(6):1903–10.
34. Gunter JP, Friedman RM. Lateral crural strut graft: technique and clinical applications in rhinoplasty. Plast Reconstr Surg 1997;99(4):943–52, discussion 953-945.
35. Millman B. Alar batten grafting for management of the collapsed nasal valve. Laryngoscope 2002;112(3):574–9.
36. Teltzrow T, Arens A, Schwipper V. One-stage reconstruction of nasal defects: evaluation of the use of modified auricular composite grafts. Facial Plast Surg 2011;27(3):243–8.
37. Craig JR, Bied A, Landas S, et al. Anatomy of the upper lateral cartilage along the lateral pyriform aperture. Plast Reconstr Surg 2015;135(2):406–11.

Moving?

Make sure your subscription moves with you!

To notify us of your new address, find your **Clinics Account Number** (located on your mailing label above your name), and contact customer service at:

Email: journalscustomerservice-usa@elsevier.com

800-654-2452 (subscribers in the U.S. & Canada)
314-447-8871 (subscribers outside of the U.S. & Canada)

Fax number: 314-447-8029

Elsevier Health Sciences Division
Subscription Customer Service
3251 Riverport Lane
Maryland Heights, MO 63043

*To ensure uninterrupted delivery of your subscription, please notify us at least 4 weeks in advance of move.

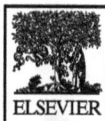

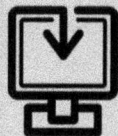

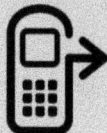

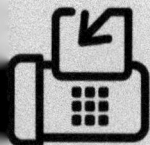

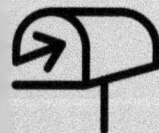

ELSEVIER

www.ingramcontent.com/pod-product-compliance
Lightning Source LLC
Chambersburg PA
CBHW050457190326
41458CB00005B/1327